Atlas of
Human
Anatomy

ISBN 978-3-96298-318-5 (print)
ISBN 978-3-96298-319-2 (ebook pdf)
ISBN 978-3-96298-320-8 (ebook epub)

Printed and bound in India by Replika Press Pvt. Ltd.

10 9 8 7 6 5 4 3 2 1

Illustrations Paul Kim, Irina Münstermann, Liene Znotiņa, Begoña Rodriguez, Samantha Zimmerman, Esther Gollan, Hannah Ely, Mao Miyamoto, Rebecca Betts, and Yousun Koh
Editor Mike Pascoe PhD
Contributors Abdulmalek Albakkar MD, Alexandru Andruşca MD PhD, Claudia Bednarek MD, Declan Tempany BSc (Hons), Dimitrios Mytilinaios MD PhD, Edwin Ocran MBChB MSc, Egle Pirie BSc (Hons), Elisabeth Friesen, Gordana Sendić MD, Jana Vasković MD, Juliana Walek MD, Kevin Kuschel MD, Marcell Laguna, Marta Krzanowski BMedSc, Milena Vujović MD, Muhammed Albakkar DDS, Nicola McLaren MSc, Nila Nikro, Rafael Lourenço do Carmo MD, Rafaela Linhares MD, Roberto Grujičić MD, Sara Ferreira MD, Sophie Stewart MSc

Text design and layout Medlar Publishing Solutions Pvt. Ltd., India

To send correspondence to the authors of this book, contact us directly at **contact@kenhub.com**.

EVOLVING DIVERSITY AND INCLUSION

Diversity is all around us—in nature, culture, art, and in our very being as humans. Society has oftentimes failed to depict the diversity that colors our world, so it's up to everyone as individuals to do their part and contribute towards a diverse and more inclusive culture. We've all seen that this is changing for the better in modern times, since we have come to understand how diversity and inclusion are able to enrich human learning and experience.

Kenhub is a company that greatly values diversity, defined as a broad spectrum of human characteristics and experiences. We foster a culture of inclusion which is reflected in our community of teammates, partners, consumers and customers from all around the world. Our ongoing mission is to create a safe environment for everyone, focusing on cultivating equity, as well as celebrating individual uniqueness and identity.

Representation matters. It is our vision to diversify our content so that everyone feels seen, included, comfortable and respected. We believe that, by representing our differences, we help future healthcare professionals develop and learn new ways of thinking, behaving and caring for their patients. A multicultural exchange of ideas and experiences bolsters new generations, leading to innovation and increased creativity. This is especially pertinent in an educational setting such as Kenhub.

We take pride in making a step towards our vision by diversifying our anatomical models and by shifting away from only featuring the standard white male model of the human body. As many as there are anatomical variations in vessels and nerves of the human body, there can be many different varieties of people, and we're embracing those differences. We understand that we are not exact carbon copies of each other. Thankfully we are all sprinkled with our own unique traits and features and we believe that these individual features should be reflected and celebrated in anatomical education.

In addition, we recognize that the lexicon of anatomy is littered with eponymous terms that primarily represent contributions of white, male scientists. The use of these terms further minimizes the contributions of non-white and non-male scientists and adds cognitive burden required to translate these names into structures. For this reason, we have chosen to use toponyms offered by the *Terminologia Anatomica* (2nd edition, 2019) as primary terms whenever possible.

There are still big steps to be made, both on our platform and in society, but we're moving in the right direction—one step at a time, actively working on changes that we believe will make our audience at Kenhub feel seen and heard.

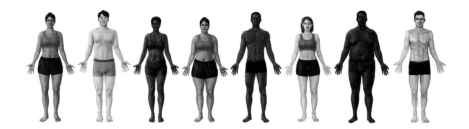

TABLE OF CONTENTS

PREFACE

As of summer 2023, Kenhub.com has helped more than 4 million registered users worldwide to deepen their understanding of the structure and organization of the human body (and pass their exams too). Since launching Kenhub.com in 2012, we've had over 110 million visitors on our website, with this number growing everyday.

Further to this, universities such as Charité—Universitätsmedizin Berlin and the University of Colorado use our learning materials to teach their students, in parallel with textbooks and practical lab teaching.

Kenhub offers you and your university the most accurate and reliable digital anatomy educational tools. Based on regular feedback from our users, it became clear that physical anatomy atlases are still highly valued by students.

That is why we have decided to print a top quality anatomy atlas based on years of experience, constant refinement and user feedback.

OUR QUALITY COMMITMENT

At Kenhub, we are passionate about providing the most accurate and reliable resources for healthcare professionals that are either learning or teaching anatomy and histology. We work hard to ensure that our content rises to the highest academic standards.

We use multiple academic resources as a reference point, with particular emphasis on those which are familiar to the majority of students and instructors alike. Thus for anatomy related content, our main references are two of the most widely respected anatomy textbooks:

- Gray's Anatomy, The Anatomical Basis of Clinical Practice, 42nd Ed. (Editor in chief: Susan Standring)
- Clinically Oriented Anatomy (by Keith L. Moore, Arthur F. Dalley II, and Anne M. R. Agur)

In addition to accuracy, our articles and illustrations on Kenhub.com are continuously updated with the latest findings and discoveries in anatomy and histology. Towards this, our writing and review process involves the appraisal of peer-reviewed scientific literature related to each topic.

Understanding that not everybody enjoys reading dense academic content, we strive to make our articles as light and as easy to read as possible, without scrimping on the details.

Both our atlas of anatomy illustrations and textbook-style articles are available for free upon registration on Kenhub.com. For a faster and more engaging learning experience, we offer hundreds of videos and quizzes as part of our paid Premium product.

REVIEWED BY EXPERTS

In enlisting our content creation team, we follow the highest educational and scientific standards. The authors of our articles are medical students, junior doctors, or postgrads who are passionate about anatomy, histology and medical education. Our talented authors love teaching their younger fellows and have a great ability to simplify complex topics into easy-to-digest articles. The manuscripts are then reviewed by a group of experts in the medical education field. We collaborate with university professors, senior doctors and Ph.D. candidates from around the world who are experts in anatomy, histology and medical education.

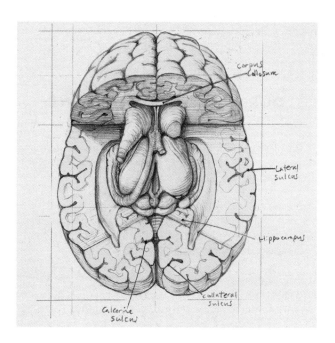

We are also proud to collaborate with some of the world's top medical illustrators, including the Netter award winner Paul Kim, and others like Begoña Rodriguez, Esther Gollan, Hannah Ely, Irina Münstermann, Liene Znotiņa, Mao Miyamoto, Rebecca Betts, Samantha Zimmerman, and Yousun Koh. Referencing Netter's Atlas of Human Anatomy and Sobotta Atlas of Human Anatomy (to name a few), our illustrators create original anatomical or histological illustrations. The original illustrations we create are then subject to a rigorous review process (sometimes it takes more than 6 months for an illustration to be published due to the multiple reviewing steps!).

Atlas content reviewer

For this atlas specifically, we are proud to work together with Dr. Mike Pascoe. Mike is an Associate Professor of Anatomy at the University of Colorado Anschutz Medical Campus.

Dr. Pascoe studied the neurophysiology of movement at the University of Colorado Boulder and defended his doctoral dissertation in 2010. He then joined the faculty at Anschutz in 2011 where he develops and delivers gross anatomy curricula to physical therapy, physician assistant, and medical doctor students.

His primary research interest is the investigation of constructivist approaches in technology-enabled learning environments (e.g., wiki usage, interactive modules, Snapchat, etc) to improve learning outcomes and student satisfaction. Of secondary interest is the determination of "need-to-know" anatomy content for physical therapy students.

Dr. Pascoe's service commitments include mentoring students, organizing anatomy laboratory refresher courses for practicing clinicians, community outreach, and service as a peer-reviewer for many anatomy education journals.

This atlas hasn't been possible without the help of the Kenhub team. It consists of diverse, talented individuals which create Kenhub's unique, interdisciplinary perspective on anatomy education. We are a fully remote company meaning that our team is spread out all around the world.

You can find more information about the team here:

Learn more about the Kenhub Team

Kenhub is grounded on academic literature and research, validated by experts, and trusted by more than 80 million readers worldwide.

HOW TO USE THIS ATLAS

Mike Pascoe PhD

BUILT FOR LEARNERS

This atlas represents a collection of clear, comprehensible and didactically valuable images from Kenhub.com, intuitively organized to aid you in your mastery of the organization of the human body. The features of this modern print atlas were formulated by direct input from students of anatomy and experienced educators. This print atlas was designed by the preferences of anatomy students to assist in the challenges of identifying structures in the anatomy laboratory *and* to assist in studying for written exams.

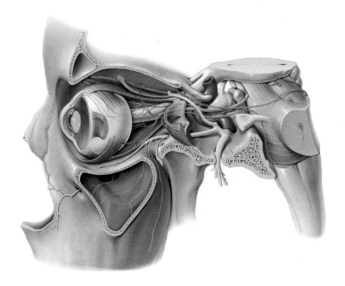

The ease of navigation is the most important feature of an anatomy atlas! Therefore, this atlas has been organized by region (e.g., upper limb), with various body systems presented therein. A color coding system is used throughout the atlas, as this has been recognized as the most efficient way to find a structure quickly in a print atlas. This atlas provides a series of regional overview images that will assist you in identifying structures in and out of the laboratory based on adjacent key anatomical relations. This is how expert anatomists navigate the body, so don't underestimate the power of having a good understanding of neighboring anatomical structures! Additionally, each overview image is accompanied by text captions in order to convey and describe presented structures in a clear and concise manner.

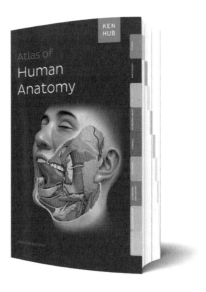

The small size of the atlas enables you to transport it and use it across many different settings beyond your home, such as the anatomy lab and in the lecture hall on campus.

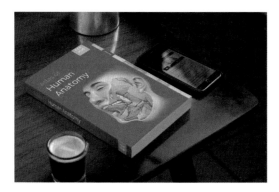

DIGITALLY ENHANCED LEARNING

This atlas can be used in traditional ways, as mentioned above, and in ways you may not have considered before. A big strength of the atlas is the ability to extend its content into the rich resources on the Kenhub website.

The reader can use their smartphone to access any structure on Kenhub through their atlas and view any additional related images, as well as related articles, videos and quizzes. The atlas can also be used as a reference (i.e., "second screen") when reviewing lectures at home or on the go.

This is enabled by the Quick Response (QR) codes, which have been included in the atlas as a quick way to connect you to the extensive online resources on the Kenhub platform. To do this, open the camera app on your smartphone, ensuring the rear-facing camera is selected. Point your camera at the QR code and center the box over the code to scan it. Tap on the URL popup banner at the top of the screen, and you'll be connected directly to the supplemental information on Kenhub.com.

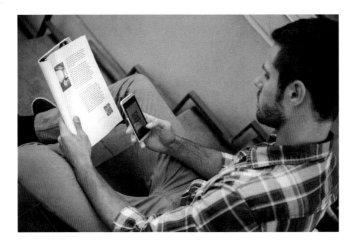

Here we see a learner scanning a QR code in the atlas in order to review further details found on Kenhub. com.

BASICS

1

DIRECTIONAL TERMS AND BODY PLANES

Anatomists use specific terms to help clearly communicate the location of structures within the human body. These are directional terms, regional terms and body planes. To avoid confusion and miscommunication, a standard reference point for these terms is always used, this reference point is the **anatomical position**. The anatomical position is when the body is standing erect, with the face looking forwards, the feet parallel, the arms hanging at the sides, the palms facing forwards and the thumbs pointing away from the body.

Directional terms and body planes allow us to describe the **relationship** between anatomical structures. For example, the wrist is distal to the elbow, the ears are lateral to the eyes, the nose is located in the midsagittal plane.

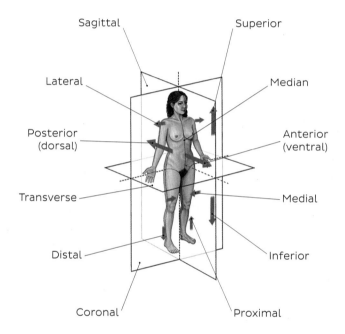

FIGURE 1.1. **Directional terms and body planes.**

Key points about directional terms and body planes	
Body planes	Coronal, sagittal, median, transverse
Directional terms	Superior (cranial), inferior (caudal), anterior (ventral), posterior (dorsal), medial, lateral, proximal, distal, left, right, superficial, deep, central, peripheral, ulnar, radial, rostral, caudal, palmar, plantar

Directional terms and body planes

Basic anatomy and terminology

REGIONS OF THE BODY

The human body can be studied under the umbrella of two primary regions. These are the **axial region**, which encompasses the head, neck and trunk, and the **appendicular region** which describes the upper and lower limbs.

Each of these regions can in turn be broadly divided into a number of smaller sub-regions or parts.

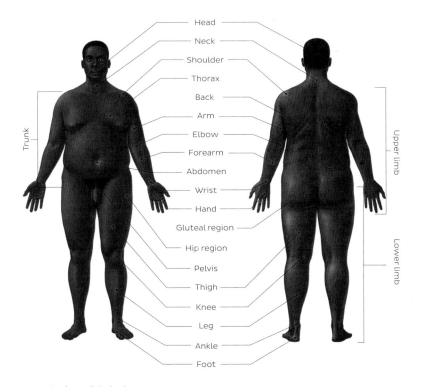

Head
Neck
Shoulder
Thorax
Back
Arm
Elbow
Forearm
Abdomen
Wrist
Hand
Gluteal region
Hip region
Pelvis
Thigh
Knee
Leg
Ankle
Foot

Trunk

Upper limb

Lower limb

FIGURE 1.2. **Regions of the body.**

Key points about the regions of the body	
Axial regions	Head
	Neck
	Trunk (thorax, abdomen, pelvis, back)
Appendicular regions	Upper limb (shoulder, arm, elbow, forearm, wrist, hand)
	Lower limb (hip, gluteal region, thigh, knee, leg, ankle, foot)

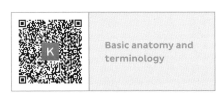

Basic anatomy and terminology

Body regions: Learn with quizzes and labeled diagrams

BODY SURFACE ANATOMY

Surface anatomy teaches about the main anatomical features visible on the surface of the human body. This knowledge helps to identify inner anatomical structures according to their visible features.

A good understanding of surface anatomy is key to interpreting normal and abnormal anatomy in clinical settings, such as medical imaging procedures and physical examination. Many aspects of surface anatomy between the sexes are similar but there are a few differences which mainly relate to sexual differentiation during development.

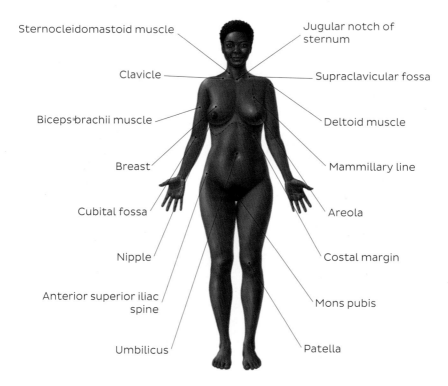

Sternocleidomastoid muscle
Jugular notch of sternum
Clavicle
Supraclavicular fossa
Biceps brachii muscle
Deltoid muscle
Breast
Mammillary line
Cubital fossa
Areola
Nipple
Costal margin
Anterior superior iliac spine
Mons pubis
Umbilicus
Patella

FIGURE 1.3. **Female body surface anatomy (anterior view).**

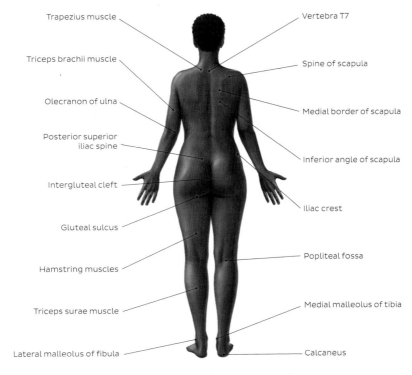

Trapezius muscle

Triceps brachii muscle

Olecranon of ulna

Posterior superior
iliac spine

Intergluteal cleft

Gluteal sulcus

Hamstring muscles

Triceps surae muscle

Lateral malleolus of fibula

Vertebra T7

Spine of scapula

Medial border of scapula

Inferior angle of scapula

Iliac crest

Popliteal fossa

Medial malleolus of tibia

Calcaneus

FIGURE 1.4. **Female body surface anatomy (posterior view).**

Surface landmarks	Anterior surface	Posterior surface
Head, neck and trunk	Larynx, sternocleidomastoid muscle, supraclavicular fossa, clavicle, pectoralis major muscle, jugular notch of sternum, sternum, sternal angle, xiphoid process, breast, areola, nipple, costal margin, rectus abdominis muscle, linea alba, linea semilunaris, umbilicus, mons pubis, anterior superior iliac spine, inguinal ligament, scrotum, penis, glans penis, vulva	External occipital protuberance, vertebra C7 trapezius muscle, spine of scapula, medial border of scapula, inferior angle of scapula, latissimus dorsi muscle, lumbar triangle (of Petit), iliac crest, posterior superior iliac spine, sacral triangle, sacroiliac joint, anal region
Upper limb	Acromion, deltoid muscle, biceps brachii muscle, cubital fossa, radial foveola (anatomical snuffbox), thenar eminence, hypothenar eminence	Triceps brachii muscle, olecranon
Lower limb	Femoral triangle, quadriceps femoris muscle, patella, tibial tuberosity, tibialis anterior muscle, lateral malleolus, medial malleolus	Gluteal region, intergluteal cleft, gluteal sulcus, iliotibial tract, hamstring muscles, popliteal fossa, triceps surae muscle, calcaneal (Achilles) tendon

CAVITIES OF THE BODY

The main body cavities are classified into two groups according to their location: Dorsal cavity and ventral cavity. The **dorsal cavity** consists of the cranial cavity, which houses the brain; and the vertebral canal, which houses the spinal cord. The **ventral cavity** is composed of the thoracic cavity and abdominopelvic cavity. The **thoracic cavity** contains several smaller spaces that house the trachea, lungs, esophagus and heart. The **abdominopelvic cavity** can be subdivided into the abdominal and the pelvic cavities, which contain the abdominal and pelvic organs, respectively.

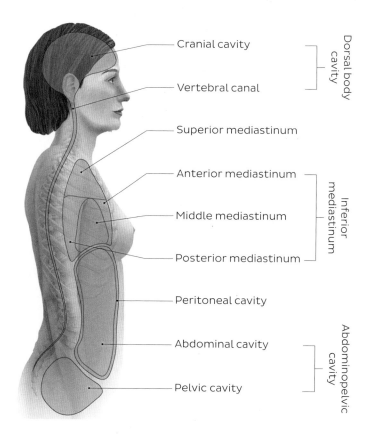

FIGURE 1.5. **Cavities of the body (lateral view).**

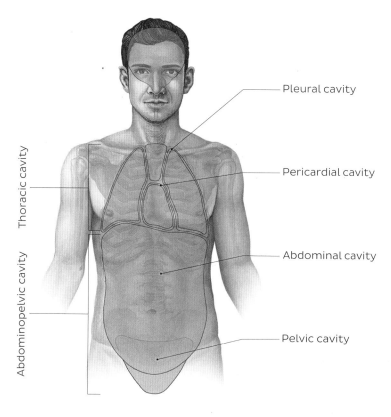

Pleural cavity

Pericardial cavity

Abdominal cavity

Pelvic cavity

Thoracic cavity

Abdominopelvic cavity

FIGURE 1.6. **Cavities of the body (anterior view).**

Key points about the body cavities	
Main cavities of the body	Dorsal cavity: cranial cavity, vertebral canal
	Ventral cavity: thoracic cavity, abdominopelvic cavity
Main contents of body cavities	Cranial cavity: brain
	Vertebral canal: spinal cord
	Thoracic cavity:
	Mediastinum contents: heart, trachea, esophagus
	Mediastinum divisions: superior, inferior (subdivisions: anterior, middle posterior)
	Pleural cavity: lungs
	Abdominopelvic cavity:
	Abdominal cavity: gastrointestinal system
	Pelvic cavity: reproductive organs, urinary bladder, sigmoid colon and rectum

Basic medical
terminology 101:
Learn with quizzes

Basic anatomy and
terminology

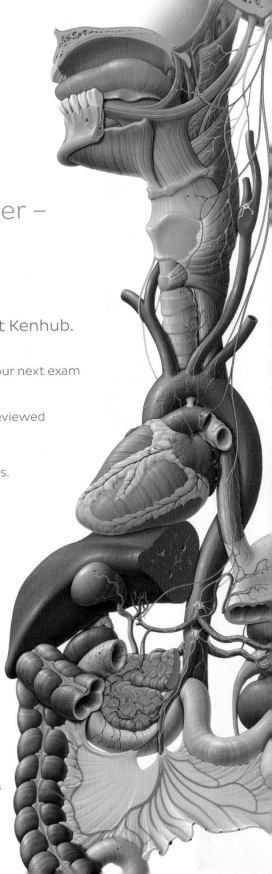

UPPER LIMB

2

REGIONS OF THE UPPER LIMB

Every medical professional needs to know the descriptive terms used for the regions of the whole body in order to localize and diagnose different injuries and diseases, as well as communicate them to other physicians. The same goes for the upper limb, which is divided into several regions on its anterior and posterior aspects. Many of these regions contain various neurovascular structures, which makes them important surgical landmarks.

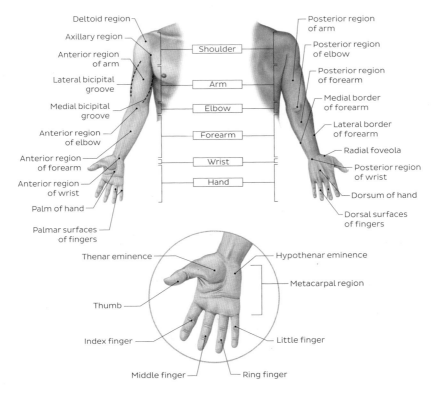

FIGURE 2.1. Regions of the upper limb. The upper limb is divided into 4 main parts—shoulder, arm, forearm and hand. The shoulder contains two important regions: The deltoid region and the axillary (armpit) region. The arm and forearm contain two regions each that correspond to their anterior and posterior surfaces. Found between the arm and forearm are the anterior and posterior cubital regions. Below the forearm is the carpal region, which connects the forearm with the hand. Lastly, the hand consists of the palm anteriorly, and dorsum of hand posteriorly. The hand can be subdivided into the metacarpal region and the digits. The digits are numbered 1–5 from from the thumb to the little finger.

Important terms about the regions of the upper limb	
Shoulder region	Deltoid region (subregion, but in some sources used as synonym)
Axillary region	Axilla, axillary fossa
Arm	Anterior/posterior brachial regions
Elbow region	Cubital region • Anterior cubital region (cubital fossa) • Posterior cubital region (olecranon region)
Forearm	Antebrachial region • Anterior antebrachial region • Posterior antebrachial region • Medial border → ulnar border • Lateral border → radial border
Wrist region	Carpal region • Anterior carpal region • Posterior carpal region
Hand	Radial foveola (anatomical snuffbox) Digits: • Thumb: 1st digit • Index finger: 2nd digit • Middle finger: 3rd digit • Ring finger: 4th digit • Little finger: 5th digit

Regions of the upper limb

CLAVICLE

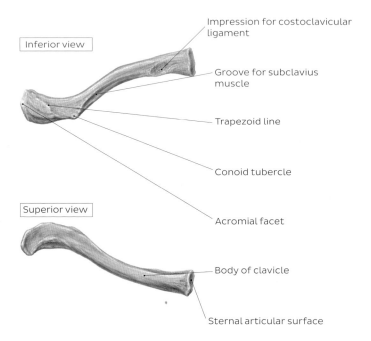

Inferior view

Impression for costoclavicular ligament

Groove for subclavius muscle

Trapezoid line

Conoid tubercle

Superior view

Acromial facet

Body of clavicle

Sternal articular surface

FIGURE 2.2. Clavicle. The clavicle is an S-shaped long bone that connects the upper limb to the trunk resting horizontally between the sternum and the acromion of the scapula. It consists of three main parts: The **shaft**, **sternal end**, and **acromial end**. The sternal end hosts the sternal articular surface (facet) that articulates with the manubrium of sternum, forming the sternoclavicular joint. The acromial end features the acromial articular surface (facet), which forms the acromioclavicular joint together with the acromion of the scapula. The **superior surface** of the clavicle is generally smooth and lies just deep to the skin. In contrast, its **inferior surface** is rough due to several important bony landmarks (namely attachments). From lateral to medial, the following can be observed: Trapezoid line (attachment for the trapezoid ligament), the conoid tubercle (attachment for the conoid ligament), subclavian groove (attachment for the subclavius muscle), and impression for costoclavicular ligament (attachment for the ligament that binds the clavicle to the first rib).

Key points about the clavicle	
Parts	Sternal (medial) end, shaft, acromial (lateral) end
Bony landmarks	Trapezoid line, conoid tubercle, groove for subclavius muscle, impression for costoclavicular ligament
Joints	Sternoclavicular joint – between sternal end of clavicle and manubrium of sternum
	Acromioclavicular joint – between acromial end of clavicle and acromion of scapula
Function	Attachment of upper limb to trunk as part of 'shoulder girdle'
	Protection of underlying neurovascular structures supplying upper limb
	Force transmission from upper limb to axial skeleton

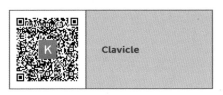

Clavicle

HUMERUS AND SCAPULA

The humerus is a long bone that comprises the bony framework of the arm, while the scapula is a flat bone of the pectoral girdle. The humerus and scapula articulate with each other to form the glenohumeral (shoulder) joint, which is the most mobile joint of the body. Both bones are held together via several ligaments and muscle tendons.

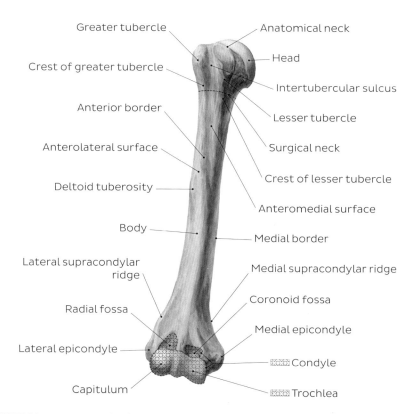

Greater tubercle

Crest of greater tubercle

Anterior border

Anterolateral surface

Deltoid tuberosity

Body

Lateral supracondylar ridge

Radial fossa

Lateral epicondyle

Capitulum

Anatomical neck

Head

Intertubercular sulcus

Lesser tubercle

Surgical neck

Crest of lesser tubercle

Anteromedial surface

Medial border

Medial supracondylar ridge

Coronoid fossa

Medial epicondyle

Condyle

Trochlea

FIGURE 2.3. Humerus (anterior view). The proximal end of the humerus is composed of a large rounded **head**, an **anatomical neck** and a **surgical neck**. Located towards the lateral portion of the proximal humerus is a bony protrusion known as the **greater tubercle**. The greater tubercle has an anterior and posterior surface. The lesser tubercle is much smaller than its greater counterpart and is situated more medially. These prominences act as an important attachment site for the muscles of the shoulder. Both the greater and lesser tubercles extend distally into crests and demarcate a prominent groove called the **intertubercular sulcus**. This sulcus consists of a lateral and medial lip, which function as insertion sites for the latissimus dorsi and pectoralis major muscles. The intertubercular sulcus also acts as a conduit for the tendon of the long head of the biceps brachii muscle and is therefore also known as the bicipital groove.

The anterior shaft of the humerus is marked by the **deltoid tuberosity**, which provides an attachment point for the deltoid muscle. From this anterior perspective, two borders (anterior and medial) and two surfaces (anteromedial and anterolateral) of the humerus can be identified.

The distal end of the humeral shaft widens to form the **medial** and **lateral supracondylar ridges**, which end distally as the **medial** and **epicondyles** of the humerus. The medial and lateral condyles act as important attachment sites for muscles of the forearm.

The distal end of the humerus is marked by a series of fossae and processes. The **condyle** of the humerus is made up of the articulating **trochlea** and **capitulum** and non-articulating **olecranon** (see next image), **coronoid**, and **radial fossae**. The condyle of the humerus plays a key role in the formation of the elbow joint as it articulates with the radius and ulna.

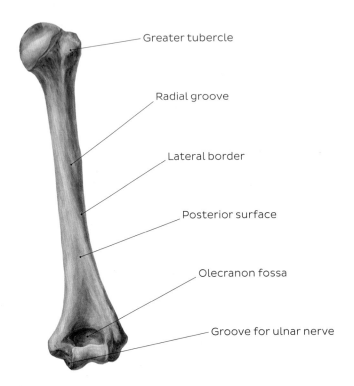

Greater tubercle

Radial groove

Lateral border

Posterior surface

Olecranon fossa

Groove for ulnar nerve

FIGURE 2.4. Humerus (posterior view). Due to its lateral positioning, the greater tubercle of the humerus can also be identified from this posterior view.

Posteriorly, the shaft of the humerus is marked by the oblique **radial groove**, which allows for the passage of the radial nerve and deep brachial artery. In addition, the **lateral border** and **posterior surface** of the humerus can be appreciated from the posterior view.

The distal end of the posterior humerus presents with a large fossa known as the **olecranon fossa**. In elbow extension, the tip of the ulnar olecranon process lodges into this fossa.

The **medial epicondyle** of the humerus contains a shallow ridge on its posterior surface, known as the **groove for ulnar nerve**. As its name suggests, the groove transmits the ulnar nerve.

Key points about the humerus	
Proximal end	Head, anatomical neck, surgical neck, greater tubercle
	Lesser tubercle
	Intertubercular sulcus (crest of greater tubercle, crest of lesser tubercle)
Body	Surfaces: anteromedial, anterolateral, posterior
	Borders: anterior, lateral, posterior
	Landmarks: lateral supracondylar ridge, medial supracondylar ridge, radial groove, supracondylar process
Distal end	Lateral epicondyle
	Medial epicondyle (groove for ulnar nerve)
	Condyle of humerus: capitulum, trochlea, olecranon fossa, coronoid fossa, radial fossa

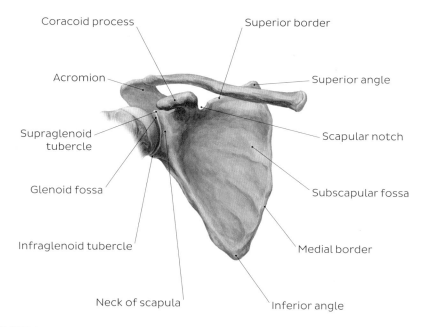

Coracoid process

Superior border

Acromion

Superior angle

Supraglenoid tubercle

Scapular notch

Glenoid fossa

Subscapular fossa

Infraglenoid tubercle

Medial border

Neck of scapula

Inferior angle

FIGURE 2.5. Scapula (anterior view). The scapula is a triangular bone with **three borders** (superior, lateral and medial) and **three angles** (superior, inferior and lateral).

The anterior surface of the scapula leans against the 2nd–7th ribs on the posterolateral aspect of the thorax, and is therefore also known as the **costal surface** of the scapula. The majority of the concave anterior surface of the scapula is occupied by the large **subscapular fossa**, which provides an attachment point for the subscapularis muscle.

The superior border of the scapula is marked by a bony indentation known as the **scapular notch**. The scapular notch allows for the passage of the suprascapular nerve and therefore may also be referred to as the suprascapular notch. Protruding from the superior border of the scapula is the hook-like projection known as the **coracoid process**. This structure allows for the attachment of various muscles and ligaments.

The lateral surface of the scapula contains the **neck** of scapula, which extends to form the glenoid fossa. The shallow glenoid fossa articulates with the humeral head to form the highly dynamic but resultantly unstable glenohumeral joint. Superior and inferior to the glenoid fossa are the **supra-** and **infraglenoid tubercles**, respectively. These act as important attachment points for the long head of the biceps and triceps brachii muscles.

Key points about the scapula	
Surfaces	Costal surface: subscapular fossa
	Posterior surface: spine of scapula, deltoid tubercle, spinoglenoid notch, supraspinous fossa, infraspinous fossa, acromion
Borders	Medial border
	Lateral border
	Superior border: scapular notch, coracoid process
Angles	Superior angle
	Inferior angle
	Lateral angle: glenoid fossa, supraglenoid tubercle, infraglenoid tubercle, neck of scapula

UPPER LIMB

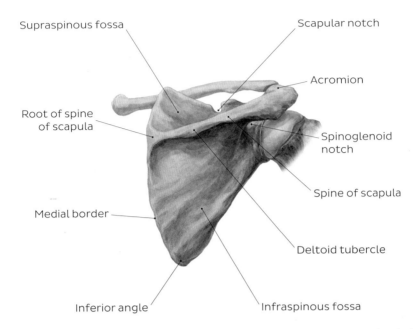

Supraspinous fossa

Scapular notch

Acromion

Root of spine of scapula

Spinoglenoid notch

Spine of scapula

Medial border

Deltoid tubercle

Inferior angle

Infraspinous fossa

FIGURE 2.6. Scapula (posterior view). The posterior surface of the scapula is convex and marked by a protruding ridge of bone known as the **spine of scapula**. This ridge unevenly separates the posterior surface of the scapula into two divisions: The **supraspinous fossa** and the much bigger, **infraspinous fossa**. The supraspinatus muscle sits within the supraspinous fossa, while the infraspinous fossa is occupied by the infraspinatus and teres minor muscles of the rotator cuff complex.

The spine of the scapula begins at the **root** of the spine and extends and widens to form the **acromion** process of the scapula. The acromion articulates with the clavicle to form the acromioclavicular joint. The spine and acromion of the scapula serve as important attachment points for muscles of the back and shoulder and function as levers for these muscles, particularly the trapezius muscle.

Connecting the supraspinous and infraspinous fossa together is the **spinoglenoid notch**. The suprascapular artery and nerve travel through this notch to supply structures of the scapular region.

Humerus

Scapula

GLENOHUMERAL (SHOULDER) JOINT

The glenohumeral joint, also known as the shoulder joint, is a **ball-and-socket** type of synovial joint, in which the head of the humerus (ball) articulates with the glenoid fossa of the scapula (socket). The surface of the humeral head is much larger than the surface of glenoid fossa, which allows for the **greatest range of motion** seen in any joint. This mobility comes at the cost of joint stability, with the shoulder joint being one of the most frequently dislocated joints of the body.

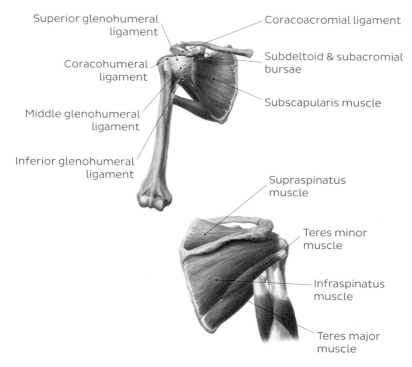

Superior glenohumeral ligament

Coracoacromial ligament

Coracohumeral ligament

Subdeltoid & subacromial bursae

Middle glenohumeral ligament

Subscapularis muscle

Inferior glenohumeral ligament

Supraspinatus muscle

Teres minor muscle

Infraspinatus muscle

Teres major muscle

FIGURE 2.7. Shoulder joint (anterior/posterior views). Three **glenohumeral ligaments** (superior, middle, inferior) form as a thickening of the articular capsule and connect the humeral head to the glenoid fossa of the scapula. The **coracohumeral ligament** connects the coracoid process of the scapula with the greater tubercle of the humerus and reinforces the superior portion of the glenohumeral articular capsule. The **transverse humeral ligament** extends between the lesser and greater tubercles and stabilizes the tendon of the long head of the biceps brachii muscle. Lastly, the joint is also stabilized by four muscles (supraspinatus, infraspinatus, teres minor and subscapularis muscles [faded]) collectively known as the **rotator cuff** which form a musculotendinous sleeve around the joint.

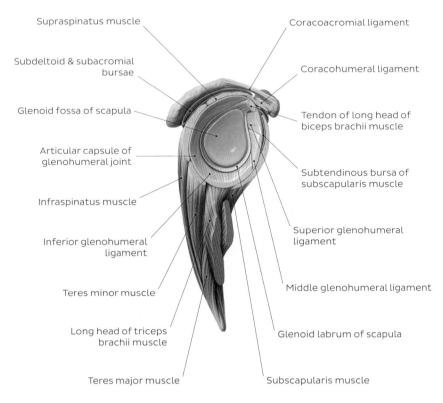

Supraspinatus muscle

Subdeltoid & subacromial bursae

Glenoid fossa of scapula

Articular capsule of glenohumeral joint

Infraspinatus muscle

Inferior glenohumeral ligament

Teres minor muscle

Long head of triceps brachii muscle

Teres major muscle

Coracoacromial ligament

Coracohumeral ligament

Tendon of long head of biceps brachii muscle

Subtendinous bursa of subscapularis muscle

Superior glenohumeral ligament

Middle glenohumeral ligament

Glenoid labrum of scapula

Subscapularis muscle

UPPER LIMB

FIGURE 2.8. Shoulder joint (lateral view).

Key points about shoulder joint	
Joint type	Synovial ball–and–socket joint
Articular surfaces	Glenoid fossa of scapula, head of humerus
Ligaments	Superior glenohumeral, middle glenohumeral, inferior glenohumeral, coracohumeral, transverse humeral
Important muscles	**Rotator cuff muscles**: supraspinatus, infraspinatus, teres minor, subscapularis
Functions	Flexion, extension, abduction, adduction, external rotation, internal rotation and circumduction

Glenohumeral joint

MUSCLES OF THE ARM AND SHOULDER

The muscles of the arm and shoulder act on the shoulder and elbow joints, ensuring the mobility of the upper limb relative to the trunk. They are divided into the following groups:

- The **muscles of the shoulder**, specifically the scapulohumeral muscles, consist of the deltoid, teres major, and muscles of the rotator cuff (supraspinatus, infraspinatus, teres minor, and subscapularis). All these muscles support movement and stabilization of the shoulder joint.
- The **muscles of the arm** are divided into anterior and posterior compartments. Depending on their bony attachments and line of pull, the muscles will serve either as flexors (anterior group) or extensors (posterior group) of the arm and/or forearm.

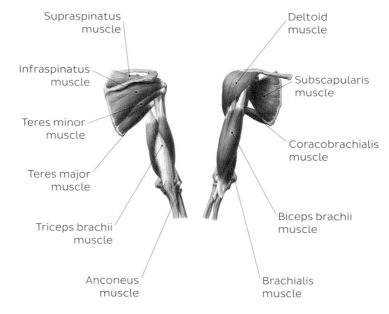

Supraspinatus muscle

Deltoid muscle

Infraspinatus muscle

Subscapularis muscle

Teres minor muscle

Coracobrachialis muscle

Teres major muscle

Triceps brachii muscle

Biceps brachii muscle

Anconeus muscle

Brachialis muscle

FIGURE 2.9. Muscles of the arm and shoulder.

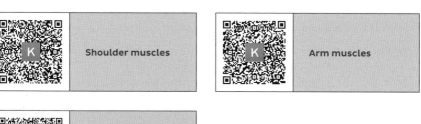

Shoulder muscles

Arm muscles

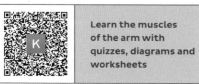

Learn the muscles of the arm with quizzes, diagrams and worksheets

UPPER LIMB

Arm muscles	Origin	Insertion	Innervation	Function
Deltoid	**Clavicular part**: lateral third of clavicle **Acromial part**: acromion of scapula **Spinal part**: spine of scapula	Deltoid tuberosity of humerus	Axillary nerve (C5–C6)	**Shoulder joint**: arm flexion, arm internal rotation (clavicular part), arm abduction (acromial part), arm extension, arm lateral rotation (spinal part)
Teres major	Inferior angle and lower part of lateral border of scapula	Crest of lesser tubercle of humerus (a.k.a. Medial lip of intertubercular sulcus)	Lower subscapular or thoracodorsal nerves (C5–C7)	**Shoulder joint**: arm internal rotation, arm extension, arm adduction
Coracobrachialis	Coracoid process of scapula	Anteromedial surface of humeral shaft		**Shoulder joint**: arm flexion, arm adduction
Biceps brachii	**Long head**: supraglenoid tubercle of scapula **Short head**: coracoid process of scapula	Radial tuberosity of radius	Musculocutaneous nerve (C5–C6)	**Elbow joint**: forearm flexion and supination; **Shoulder joint**: weak arm flexion
Brachialis	Distal half of anterior surface of humerus	Ulnar tuberosity, Coronoid process of ulna	Musculocutaneous nerve, Radial nerve (C5–C7)	**Elbow joint**: forearm flexion (in all positions)
Triceps brachii	**Long head**: infraglenoid tubercle of scapula **Lateral head**: posterior surface of humerus (superior to radial groove) **Medial head**: posterior surface of humerus (inferior to radial groove)	Olecranon of ulna and fascia of forearm	Radial nerve (C6–C8)	**Shoulder joint**: arm extension and adduction (long head); **Elbow joint**: forearm extension
Anconeus	Lateral epicondyle of humerus	Lateral surface of olecranon	Radial nerve (C7, C8)	**Elbow joint**: assists in forearm extension; stabilization of elbow joint

Rotator cuff muscles	Origin	Insertion	Innervation	Function
Subscapularis	Subscapular fossa of scapula	Lesser tubercle of humerus	Upper and lower subscapular nerves (C5–C6)	**Shoulder joint**: arm internal rotation; stabilizes humeral head in glenoid cavity
Teres minor	Lateral border of scapula	Greater tubercle of humerus	Axillary nerve (C5, C6)	**Shoulder joint**: arm external rotation, arm adduction; stabilizes humeral head in glenoid cavity
Supraspinatus	Supraspinous fossa of scapula		Suprascapular nerve (C5, C6)	**Shoulder joint**: arm abduction; stabilizes humeral head in glenoid cavity
Infraspinatus	Infraspinous fossa of scapula			**Shoulder joint**: arm external rotation; stabilizes humeral head in glenoid cavity

UPPER LIMB

RADIUS AND ULNA

The radius and ulna are the two bones of the forearm. They articulate proximally with the humerus at the **elbow**, and distally with the carpal bones at the **wrist**. In the anatomical position, the radius is positioned on the lateral aspect of the forearm, while the ulna is found medially.

The radius and ulna articulate with each other at the proximal and distal **radioulnar joints**, while their bodies are connected by an **interosseous membrane**. These two joints allow the radius to move around the ulna, allowing for a palm facing up (supinated) or palm facing down (pronated) positioning of the forearm.

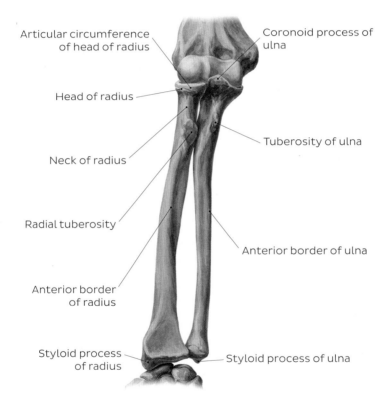

Articular circumference of head of radius

Coronoid process of ulna

Head of radius

Tuberosity of ulna

Neck of radius

Radial tuberosity

Anterior border of ulna

Anterior border of radius

Styloid process of radius

Styloid process of ulna

FIGURE 2.10. Radius and ulna (anterior view). The **radius** is the shorter of the two bones of the forearm and consists of a proximal extremity, shaft and a distal extremity. The **proximal end** of radius consists of a head and neck. The discoid **head** of the radius articulates superiorly with the capitulum of the humerus, contributing to the formation of the elbow joint. At the same time, the head of the radius also articulates with the ulna forming the proximal radioulnar joint. In this joint, the circumference of the head of the radius is situated on the radial notch of ulna. The **neck** of radius is a narrowing of the radius that lies just distal to the head. Distal to the medial aspect of the neck is an oval bony protrusion known as the **radial tuberosity**, onto which the biceps brachii inserts. The **shaft** of the radius acts as an important attachment point for muscles of the forearm, some of which include the supinator and pronator teres muscles. From this anterior view, the anterior border of the shaft of the radius can be appreciated.

The **distal extremity** of the radius widens to form three smooth, concave surfaces. The medial aspect of the distal radius forms a concavity known as the **ulnar notch**, which articulates with the distal ulna. The lateral aspect of the distal radius forms a ridge and terminates distally as the radial **styloid process**.

The **ulna** is similarly composed of a proximal end, shaft and distal end. The **proximal end** of the ulna is particularly wide to accommodate the trochlea of humerus. Projecting anteriorly from the proximal portion of the ulna is the **coronoid process**. The coronoid process aids in stabilizing the elbow joint and preventing hyperflexion of the forearm. Inferior to the coronoid process is the **tuberosity of ulna**, which functions as an attachment point for the brachialis muscle. The **distal end** of the ulna tapers to form the disc-like head of the ulna. The **head** of the ulna does not articulate with the carpal bones and is therefore not a component of the wrist joint. Projecting from the head of the ulna is a small bony protrusion known as the **styloid process** of ulna.

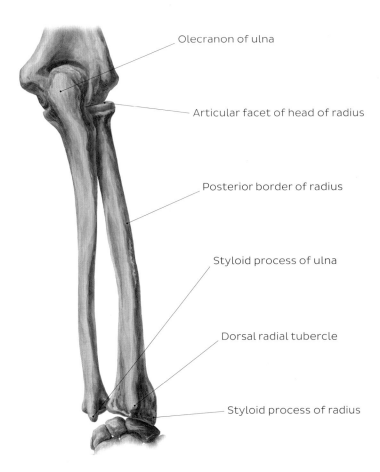

Olecranon of ulna

Articular facet of head of radius

Posterior border of radius

Styloid process of ulna

Dorsal radial tubercle

Styloid process of radius

FIGURE 2.11. Radius and ulna (posterior view). Posteriorly, the **posterior** and **interosseous borders of radius** can be identified. The interosseous border of the radius forms the radial attachment point for the interosseous membrane of the forearm, that spans the space between the radius and ulna. The **dorsal tubercle** protrudes on the posterior aspect of the head of the radius and is seated between the grooves for the tendons of the extensor carpi radialis longus and brevis, as well as the tendon of the extensor pollicis longus. The **styloid process** of radius can also be identified from this posterior view.

From a posterior aspect, the ulna is rounded and smooth and can be palpated subcutaneously along the entire length of the medial antebrachial region. The proximal end of the posterior ulna presents a hook-shaped process known as the **olecranon**. This bony protrusion serves as a short lever for extension of the elbow. The **posterior** and **interosseous borders of ulna** can also be appreciated from this view.

UPPER LIMB

Key points about the radius	
Proximal end	**Head**: articular facet of head of radius (for capitulum of humerus), articular circumference of head of radius (for radial notch of ulna) **Neck**
Body	**Surfaces**: anterior, lateral, superior **Borders**: anterior, interosseous, posterior **Landmarks**: radial tuberosity, pronator tuberosity, suprastyloid crest
Distal end	Radial styloid process, dorsal radial tubercle, ulnar notch, carpal articular surface

Key points about the ulna	
Proximal end	Olecranon, coronoid process (tuberosity of ulna, radial notch), trochlear notch, sublime tubercle
Body	**Surfaces**: anterior, posterior, medial **Borders**: anterior, interosseous, posterior **Landmarks**: supinator crest
Distal end	**Head of ulna** (articular circumference for ulnar notch of radius, ulnar styloid process)

Ligaments between the radius and ulna	
Ligaments	Interosseous membrane of forearm Oblique cord Anular ligament of radius Radial collateral ligament of elbow joint Ulnar collateral ligament of elbow joint Dorsal radioulnar ligament Palmar radioulnar ligament

Radius and ulna

ELBOW JOINT

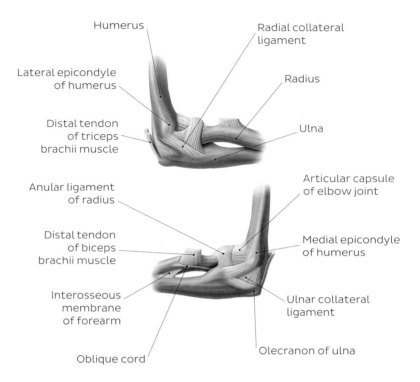

Humerus

Radial collateral ligament

Lateral epicondyle of humerus

Radius

Distal tendon of triceps brachii muscle

Ulna

Anular ligament of radius

Articular capsule of elbow joint

Distal tendon of biceps brachii muscle

Medial epicondyle of humerus

Interosseous membrane of forearm

Ulnar collateral ligament

Oblique cord

Olecranon of ulna

UPPER LIMB

FIGURE 2.12. Elbow joint (medial/lateral views). The elbow joint is made up of three joints including the humeroulnar, humeroradial and proximal radioulnar joints. The **humeroulnar joint** is between the trochlea on the medial aspect of the distal end of the humerus and the trochlear notch on the proximal ulna. The **humeroradial joint** is formed between the capitulum on the lateral aspect of the distal end of the humerus with the head of the radius. The proximal ends of the radius and ulna articulate with each other at the **proximal radioulnar joint**. There are three main ligaments that support the elbow joint: The ulnar collateral ligament, radial collateral ligament and anular ligament. The ulnar and radial collateral ligaments are each made up of three component parts:

- **Ulnar collateral ligament**: Anterior bundle, posterior bundle, and transverse bundle (Cooper's ligament).

- **Radial collateral ligament**: Annular ligament, radial collateral ligament (proper), and lateral ulnar collateral ligament.

UPPER LIMB

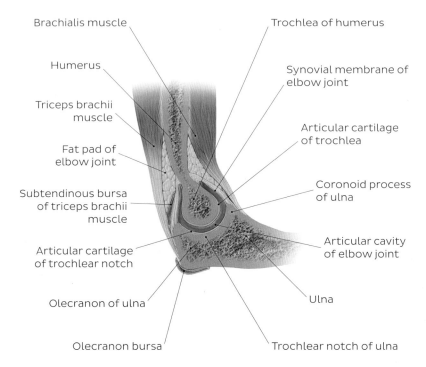

Brachialis muscle

Humerus

Triceps brachii muscle

Fat pad of elbow joint

Subtendinous bursa of triceps brachii muscle

Articular cartilage of trochlear notch

Olecranon of ulna

Olecranon bursa

Trochlea of humerus

Synovial membrane of elbow joint

Articular cartilage of trochlea

Coronoid process of ulna

Articular cavity of elbow joint

Ulna

Trochlear notch of ulna

FIGURE 2.13. Elbow joint (sagittal section through trochlea). The elbow joint is enveloped in an **articular capsule** composed of an outer fibrous layer and lined internally by a synovial membrane. During movement (flexion and extension), the fat pads are pulled away by the tendinous attachments of the brachialis and triceps brachii muscles to allow space for bony processes. Extension of the elbow is facilitated by the **olecranon bursa** which serves as a lubricating component between the olecranon of the ulna and the overlying skin.

Key points about the elbow joint	
Bones	Humerus, radius, ulna
Joints	Humeroulnar joint, humeroradial joint, proximal radioulnar joint
Ligaments	Ulnar collateral ligament, radial collateral ligament, anular ligament
Movements	Flexion, extension, supination, pronation

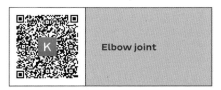

Elbow joint

FOREARM MUSCLES: ANTERIOR COMPARTMENT

The forearm is divided into anterior and posterior compartments. The muscles of the anterior compartment, also known as the *flexor-pronator* muscles, are divided into two groups:

- **Superficial group:** Pronator teres, flexor carpi radialis, flexor carpi ulnaris, palmaris longus and flexor digitorum superficialis muscles.
- **Deep group:** Flexor digitorum profundus, flexor pollicis longus and pronator quadratus muscles.

These muscles act on different joints of the upper limb, enabling movements of the forearm, hand and fingers. Most of the anterior muscles are innervated by the branches of the **median nerve**. The exceptions are the flexor carpi ulnaris, which is supplied by the ulnar nerve, and the flexor digitorum profundus, which is innervated by branches of both the median and the ulnar nerves.

Although the brachioradialis muscle is present in the following image, it does not belong to the anterior forearm muscles. Functionally it is a flexor of the elbow joint, however, based on its location, it belongs to the superficial group of posterior compartment muscles.

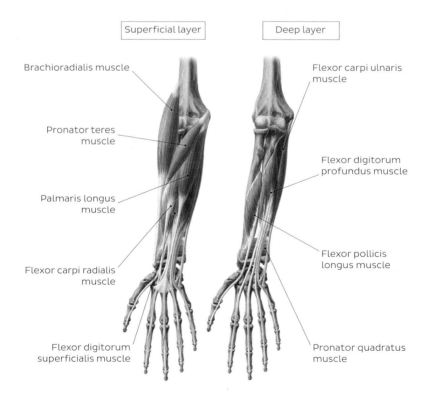

Superficial layer | Deep layer

Brachioradialis muscle

Flexor carpi ulnaris muscle

Pronator teres muscle

Flexor digitorum profundus muscle

Palmaris longus muscle

Flexor pollicis longus muscle

Flexor carpi radialis muscle

Flexor digitorum superficialis muscle

Pronator quadratus muscle

FIGURE 2.14.

UPPER LIMB

UPPER LIMB

Muscles of the anterior compartment of the forearm		Origin	Insertion	Innervation	Function
Superficial group	Pronator teres	**Humeral head**: medial supracondylar ridge of humerus **Ulnar head**: coronoid process of ulna	Lateral surface of radius (distal to supinator)	Median nerve (C6, C7)	**Elbow joint**: forearm flexion; **Proximal radioulnar joint**: forearm pronation
	Flexor carpi radialis	Medial epicondyle of humerus	Bases of metacarpal bones 2–3		**Wrist joint**: wrist flexion, wrist abduction
	Flexor carpi ulnaris	Medial epicondyle of humerus, Olecranon and posterior border of ulna	Pisiform bone, Hamate bone, Base of metacarpal bone 5	Ulnar nerve (C7–T1)	**Wrist joint**: wrist flexion, wrist adduction
	Palmaris longus	Medial epicondyle of humerus	Flexor retinaculum, Palmar aponeurosis	Median nerve (C7, C8)	**Wrist joint**: wrist flexion; tenses palmar aponeurosis
	Flexor digitorum superficialis	**Humeroulnar head**: medial epicondyle of humerus, Coronoid process of ulna **Radial head**: proximal half of anterior border of radius	Sides of middle phalanges of digits 2–5	Median nerve (C8, T1)	**Metacarpophalangeal and proximal interphalangeal joints 2–5**: finger flexion
Deep group	Flexor digitorum profundus	Proximal half of anterior surface of ulna, Interosseous membrane	Palmar surfaces of distal phalanges of digits 2–5	Digits 2–3: median nerve (anterior interosseous nerve); Digits 4–5: ulnar nerve (C8, T1)	**Metacarpophalangeal and interphalangeal joints 2–5**: finger flexion
	Flexor pollicis longus	Anterior surface of radius and interosseous membrane	Palmar surface of distal phalanx of thumb	Median nerve (anterior interosseous nerve) (C7, C8)	**Metacarpophalangeal and interphalangeal joint 1**: thumb flexion
	Pronator quadratus	Distal anterior surface of ulna	Distal anterior surface of radius		**Radioulnar joints**: forearm pronation

Superficial anterior forearm muscles

Deep anterior forearm muscles

FOREARM MUSCLES: POSTERIOR COMPARTMENT

The muscles of the posterior compartment, also known as the *extensor-supinator* muscles, are divided into two groups:

- **Superficial group:** Brachioradialis, extensor carpi radialis longus, extensor carpi radialis brevis, extensor digitorum, extensor digiti minimi and extensor carpi ulnaris muscles.
- **Deep group:** Supinator, abductor pollicis longus, extensor pollicis brevis, extensor pollicis longus and extensor indicis muscles.

Most of the muscles in the superficial layer have a common origin on the lateral epicondyle of the humerus, while the muscles of the deep layer typically originate from the distal part of the ulna. All are innervated by branches of the radial nerve.

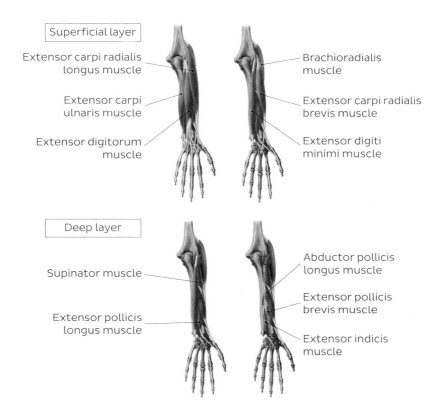

Superficial layer

Extensor carpi radialis longus muscle

Brachioradialis muscle

Extensor carpi ulnaris muscle

Extensor carpi radialis brevis muscle

Extensor digitorum muscle

Extensor digiti minimi muscle

Deep layer

Supinator muscle

Abductor pollicis longus muscle

Extensor pollicis brevis muscle

Extensor pollicis longus muscle

Extensor indicis muscle

FIGURE 2.15.

Superficial posterior forearm muscles

Deep posterior forearm muscles

Posterior compartment muscles		Origin	Insertion	Innervation	Function
Superficial group	Brachioradialis	Lateral supracondylar ridge of humerus, Lateral intermuscular septum of arm	(Proximal to) Styloid process of radius	Radial Nerve (C5–C8)	Elbow joint: forearm flexion (when semi pronated)
	Extensor carpi radialis longus		Posterior aspect of base of metacarpal bone 2		Wrist joints: hand extension, Hand abduction (radial deviation)
	Extensor carpi radialis brevis		Posterior aspect of base of metacarpal bone 3		
	Extensor digitorum	Lateral epicondyle of humerus (common extensor tendon)	Extensor expansions of digits 2–5		Metacarpophalangeal/interphalangeal joints 2–5: finger extension
	Extensor digiti minimi		Extensor expansion of digit 5		Metacarpophalangeal joint 5: finger extension
	Extensor carpi ulnaris	Lateral epicondyle of humerus, Posterior border of the ulna	Base of metacarpal bone 5		Wrist joint: hand extension and adduction
Deep group	Supinator	Lateral epicondyle of humerus, Radial collateral ligament, Anular ligament, Supinator crest of ulna	Lateral, posterior, and anterior surfaces of proximal third of radius	Posterior interosseous nerve (C7, C8)	Proximal radioulnar joint: forearm supination
	Abductor pollicis longus	Posterior surface of proximal half of radius, ulna and interosseous membrane	Base of metacarpal bone 1, (Trapezium Bone)		Radiocarpal joint: hand abduction (radial deviation); Carpometacarpal joint of thumb: thumb abduction and extension
	Extensor pollicis longus	Posterior surface of middle third of ulna and interosseous membrane	Posterior aspect of base of distal phalanx of thumb		Wrist joint: weak hand extension; Metacarpophalangeal and interphalangeal joint of thumb: thumb extension
	Extensor pollicis brevis	Posterior surface of distal third of radius and interosseous membrane	Posterior aspect of base of proximal phalanx of thumb		Carpometacarpal and Metacarpophalangeal joint 1: thumb extension
	Extensor indicis	Posterior surface of distal third of ulna and interosseous membrane	Extensor expansion of index finger		Wrist joint: weak hand extension; Metacarpophalangeal and interphalangeal joints of index finger: finger extension

BONES OF THE WRIST AND HAND

The wrist and hand are the most distal parts of the upper limb. They consist of several groups of bones connected via numerous articulations that facilitate fine movements of the hand, such as writing or drawing. From proximal to distal, these bones are divided into three groups:

- **Carpal bones:** Eight short bones arranged into proximal and distal rows (4 each). **Metacarpal bones:** Five long bones, each form the root of the corresponding digit. **Phalanges:** Fourteen long bones subdivided into three sets: Proximal, middle and distal. (Note that the thumb is devoid of a middle phalanx)

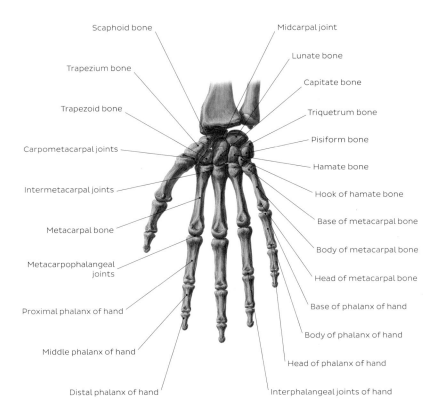

Scaphoid bone
Midcarpal joint
Trapezium bone
Lunate bone
Capitate bone
Trapezoid bone
Triquetrum bone
Carpometacarpal joints
Pisiform bone
Hamate bone
Intermetacarpal joints
Hook of hamate bone
Metacarpal bone
Base of metacarpal bone
Metacarpophalangeal joints
Body of metacarpal bone
Head of metacarpal bone
Proximal phalanx of hand
Base of phalanx of hand
Middle phalanx of hand
Body of phalanx of hand
Distal phalanx of hand
Head of phalanx of hand
Interphalangeal joints of hand

FIGURE 2.16.

UPPER LIMB

Key points about the bones of the wrist and hand	
Carpal bones	8 short bones that comprise the root of the hand
	Proximal row: scaphoid, lunate, triquetrum, pisiform
	Distal row: trapezium, trapezoid, capitate, hamate
	Joints: radiocarpal, intercarpal, midcarpal, carpometacarpal
Metacarpal bones	5 long bones of the hand
	Parts: metacarpal base, body, head
	Joints: carpometacarpal, intermetacarpal, metacarpophalangeal
Phalanges	14 long bones of the fingers (5 proximal, 4 middle, 5 distal)
	Parts: base, body, head
	Joints: metacarpophalangeal, interphalangeal

 Carpal bones

 Metacarpal bones

 Phalanges of the hand

LIGAMENTS OF THE WRIST AND HAND

The ligaments participate in the stabilization of joints, but can also limit certain movements based on their position around the joint. The wrist and hand feature several joints. Proximal to distal, the first one is the radiocarpal (wrist) joint which connects the forearm and the hand. The rest of the joints are in the hand, connecting groups of bones to each other (e.g. carpal and metacarpal), as well as individual bones amongst themselves (e.g. scaphoid and lunate). Namely, these joints are: Intercarpal, carpometacarpal, intermetacarpal, metacarpophalangeal and interphalangeal joints.

The proper function of the ligaments is crucial for the normal mobility and function of the wrist and hand.

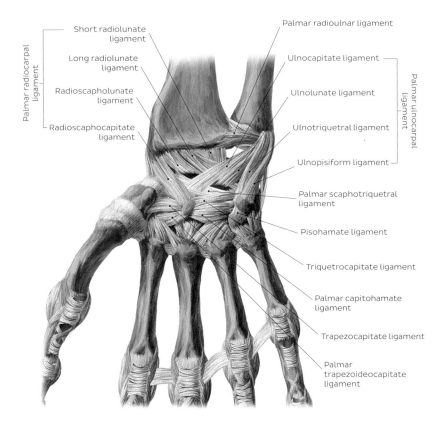

FIGURE 2.17. Ligaments of the wrist and hand (palmar view). The **radiocarpal joint (wrist joint)** is stabilized by a number of ligaments, namely the palmar and dorsal radiocarpal ligaments, the palmar ulnocarpal ligament and the radial and ulnar collateral ligaments. These ligaments extend from the distal portion of either the radius or ulna, respectively, to insert onto the carpal bones of the hand.

The **intercarpal joints** formed between the carpal bones are stabilized by numerous sets of ligaments. The palmar intercarpal ligaments stretch between adjacent carpal bones and are made up of the radiate carpal ligament, the palmar scaphotriquetral and pisohamate ligaments as well as a few others which are not visible from this view. The radiate carpal ligament is formed by a set of five ligaments: The scaphocapitate (not seen), triquetrocapitate, palmar capitohamate, palmar trapezoideocapitate and trapezocapitate ligaments.

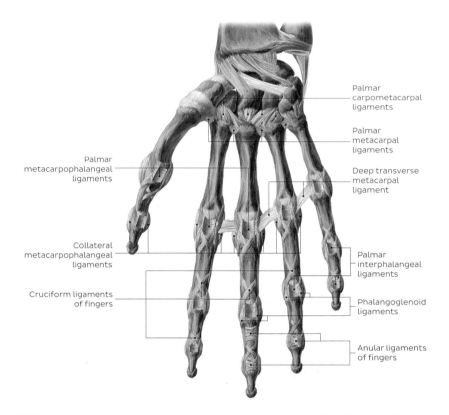

Palmar
carpometacarpal
ligaments

Palmar
metacarpal
ligaments

Deep transverse
metacarpal
ligament

Palmar
metacarpophalangeal
ligaments

Collateral
metacarpophalangeal
ligaments

Cruciform ligaments
of fingers

Palmar
interphalangeal
ligaments

Phalangoglenoid
ligaments

Anular ligaments
of fingers

FIGURE 2.18. Ligaments of the metacarpals and phalanges (palmar view). The distal row of the palmar surface of carpal bones and metacarpal bones are bridged by the **palmar carpometacarpal ligaments**. The palmar carpometacarpal ligaments are comprised of a series of ligamentous bands. There are 2 bands associated with the 2nd metacarpal, one of which is connected to the trapezoid and one to the trapezium bone. The 4th metacarpal is connected to the capitate and the hamate, while the 5th metacarpal only has one band anchoring it to the hamate bone. In contrast, the 3rd metacarpal has three associated ligaments which anchor it to the trapezoid, capitate and hamate bones on the palmar surface of the hand.

The four **palmar metacarpal ligaments** attach to the palmar surfaces of the bases of adjacent metacarpal bones, connecting the 5 metacarpal bones to each other.

Located on the palmar aspect of the metacarpophalangeal (MCP) joints are the **palmar metacarpophalangeal ligaments**, which are dense fibrocartilaginous thickenings of the metacarpophalangeal joint capsule.

The **anular ligaments** of the phalanges form small hoops on the palmar surface of the digits, through which the tendons of flexor digitorum muscle pass. There are 2-3 annular ligaments associated with the phalanges of the thumb and 5 annular ligaments in each of the four fingers.

The **cruciform ligaments** consist of two obliquely crossed bands and there are 3 sets associated with each digit. The annular and cruciform ligaments of the phalanges work together to prevent bowstringing of the flexor tendons.

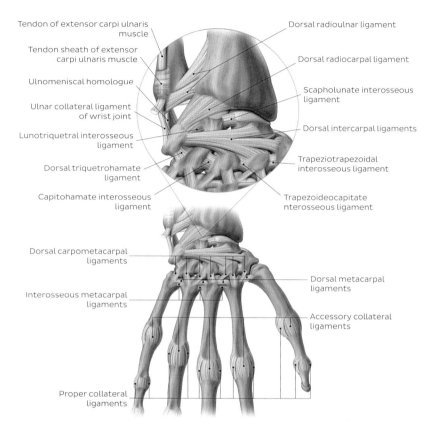

Tendon of extensor carpi ulnaris muscle

Tendon sheath of extensor carpi ulnaris muscle

Ulnomeniscal homologue

Ulnar collateral ligament of wrist joint

Lunotriquetral interosseous ligament

Dorsal triquetrohamate ligament

Capitohamate interosseous ligament

Dorsal carpometacarpal ligaments

Interosseous metacarpal ligaments

Proper collateral ligaments

Dorsal radioulnar ligament

Dorsal radiocarpal ligament

Scapholunate interosseous ligament

Dorsal intercarpal ligaments

Trapeziotrapezoidal interosseous ligament

Trapezoideocapitate nterosseous ligament

Dorsal metacarpal ligaments

Accessory collateral ligaments

FIGURE 2.19. Ligaments of the wrist and hand (dorsal view). The **interosseous intercarpal ligaments** are visible. These ligaments lie within the joint capsule and provide stability to the intercarpal joints. The interosseous intercarpal ligaments include the scapholunate, lunotriquetral, trapeziotrapezoidal, trapezoideocapitate and the capitohamate interosseous ligaments.

Located between the dorsal and palmar metacarpal ligaments are the **interosseous metacarpal ligaments**. These ligaments stretch between adjacent metacarpal bones aiding in stabilizing movement.

The **dorsal carpometacarpal ligaments** of metacarpals 2-4 are composed of two ligaments each of which attach to the base of the metacarpals. Similar to its palmar counterpart, the 5th metacarpal has only one dorsal carpometacarpal ligament.

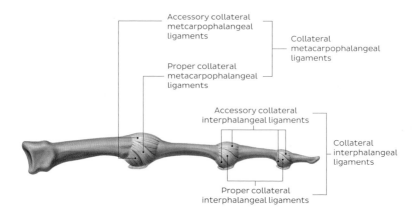

Accessory collateral metcarpophalangeal ligaments

Collateral metacarpophalangeal ligaments

Proper collateral metacarpophalangeal ligaments

Accessory collateral interphalangeal ligaments

Collateral interphalangeal ligaments

Proper collateral interphalangeal ligaments

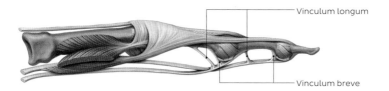

Vinculum longum

Vinculum breve

FIGURE 2.20. Ligaments of the metacarpals and phalanges (lateral view). Contributing to the stabilization of the metacarpophalangeal (MCP) and interphalangeal (IP) joints are the **proper and accessory collateral ligaments of the MCP and IP joints**. These ligaments are located on the radial and ulnar aspects of each joint and help to prevent excessive adduction–abduction movements of associated joints.

Key points about the ligaments and supporting structures of the wrist and hand	
Distal radioulnar joint	Palmar radioulnar ligament
	Dorsal radioulnar ligament
Radiocarpal (wrist) joint	**Palmar radiocarpal ligament** (radioscaphocapitate ligament, short and long radiolunate ligaments, radioscapholunate ligament)
	Palmar ulnocarpal ligament (ulnocapitate, ulnolunate, ulnotriquetral, ulnopisiform ligaments)
	Dorsal radiocarpal ligament
	Triangular fibrocartilage complex (palmar ulnocarpal ligaments, palmar radioulnar ligament, articular disc, ulnomeniscal homologue, tendon sheath of extensor carpi ulnaris muscle)
	Collateral ligaments of wrist (radial/ulnar collateral ligaments of wrist joint)
Intercarpal joints	**Fascial bands**:
	Flexor retinaculum of wrist
	Extensor retinaculum of wrist
	Palmar ligaments:
	Palmar intercarpal ligaments: radiate carpal ligament (scaphocapitate, triquetrocapitate, palmar capitohamate, palmar trapezoideocapitate, trapezocapitate ligaments), palmar scaphotriquetral, palmar lunotriquetral, palmar triquetrohamate, pisotriquetral and pisohamate ligaments
	Dorsal ligaments:
	Dorsal intercarpal ligaments
	Interosseous ligaments:
	Intercarpal interosseous ligaments: scapholunate interosseous ligament, lunotriquetral interosseous ligament, trapeziotrapezoidal interosseous ligament, trapezoideocapitate interosseous ligament, capitohamate interosseous ligament
Carpometacarpal joints	Dorsal carpometacarpal ligaments
	Palmar carpometacarpal ligaments
Intermetacarpal joints	Palmar metacarpal ligaments
	Dorsal metacarpal ligaments
	Interosseous metacarpal ligaments
Metacarpophalangeal joints	Proper collateral metacarpophalangeal ligaments
	Accessory collateral metacarpophalangeal ligaments
	Phalangoglenoid ligaments
	Palmar metacarpophalangeal ligaments
	Deep transverse ligament
Interphalangeal joints	Palmar interphalangeal ligaments
	Proper collateral interphalangeal ligaments
	Accessory collateral interphalangeal ligaments
	Annular ligaments
	Cruciform ligaments

Joints and ligaments
of the upper limb

MRI of the wrist
normal anatomy

MUSCLES OF THE HAND

The muscles of the hand are organized into five compartments: The thenar, adductor, hypothenar, central, and interosseous compartments.

Thenar compartment
- Adductor pollicis brevis
- Flexor pollicis brevis
- Opponens pollicis

Adductor compartment
- Adductor pollicis

Hypothenar compartment
- Abductor digiti minimi
- Flexor digiti minimi
- Opponens digiti minimi

Central compartment
- Lumbricals (4)

Interosseous compartments
- Dorsal interossei (4)
- Palmar interossei (3)

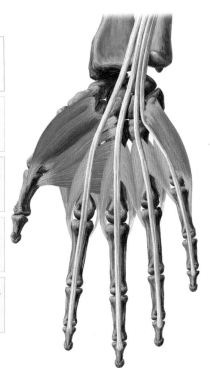

FIGURE 2.21. **Muscular compartments of the hand.** The **thenar compartment** contains the short muscles of the thumb and includes the abductor pollicis brevis, flexor pollicis brevis, and opponens pollicis muscles. The **adductor compartment** contains the adductor pollicis muscle. The **hypothenar muscles** move the little finger and include the abductor digiti minimi, flexor digiti minimi and opponens digiti minimi muscles. The palmaris brevis is sometimes considered with the hypothenar muscles, however is functionally not related to movement of the little finger. The **central compartment** contains the lumbrical muscles (4), which are found between the metacarpals and attach proximally to the tendons of flexor digitorum profundus muscle. The **interosseous compartments** contain either the dorsal interossei (4), which are small muscles found between the metacarpal bones on the dorsal surface of the hand, or the palmar interossei (3), which represent their palmar counterparts.

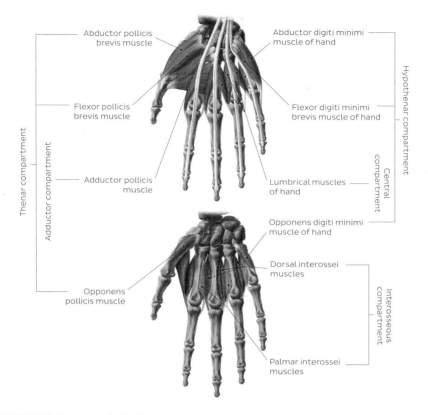

FIGURE 2.22. Muscles of the hand. The majority of the muscles of the hand lie superficially in the palm and are depicted on the upper image. The lower image shows four muscles that lie deep within the hand: The opponens pollicis (of the thenar compartment), palmar and dorsal interossei (of the interosseous compartment) and opponens digiti minimi (of the hypothenar group). The attachments, innervation and functions of each muscle are in the tables following.

Thenar muscles	Origin	Insertion	Innervation	Function
Opponens pollicis	Tubercle of trapezium bone, Flexor retinaculum	Radial border of metacarpal bone 1	Recurrent branch of median nerve (C8, T1)	**Carpometacarpal joint 1**: thumb opposition
Abductor pollicis brevis	Tubercles of scaphoid and trapezium bones, Flexor retinaculum	Lateral aspect of base of proximal phalanx 1 (via radial sesamoid bone)		**Carpometacarpal joint 1**: thumb abduction
Flexor pollicis brevis	**Superficial head**: flexor retinaculum, Tubercle of trapezium bone **Deep head**: trapezoid and capitate bones		**Superficial head**: recurrent branch of median nerve **Deep head**: deep branch of ulnar nerve (C8, T1)	**Carpometacarpal and metacarpophalangeal joint 1**: thumb flexion

Hypothenar muscles	Origin	Insertion	Innervation	Function
Abductor digiti minimi	Pisiform bone (Pisohamate ligament, Tendon of flexor carpi ulnaris)	Ulnar side of base of proximal phalanx of digit 5, Extensor expansion of digit 5	Deep branch of ulnar nerve (C8, T1)	**Metacarpophalangeal joint 5**: finger abduction and flexion; **Interphalangeal joints**: finger extension
Flexor digiti minimi	Hook of hamate, Flexor retinaculum	Base of proximal phalanx of digit 5		**Metacarpophalangeal joint 5**: finger flexion (+ Finger lateral rotation/opposition)
Opponens digiti minimi		Ulnar aspect of metacarpal bone 5		**Carpometacarpal joint 5**: finger flexion, finger lateral rotation/opposition
(Palmaris brevis)	Palmar aponeurosis, Flexor retinaculum	Dermis of skin of hypothenar region	Superficial branch of ulnar nerve (C8, T1)	Tightens palmar aponeurosis, Tightens grip

Central, interosseous and adductor muscles	Origin	Insertion	Innervation	Function
Lumbricals (4)	**1 & 2**: radial aspects of tendons 1 & 2 of flexor digitorum profundus; **3 & 4**: opposing aspects of tendons 2–4 of flexor digitorum profundus	Radial aspect of extensor expansion of digits 2–5	**1 & 2**: median nerve (C8, T1) **3 & 4**: deep branch of ulnar nerve (C8–T1)	**Metacarpophalangeal joints 2-5**: finger flexion; **Interphalangeal joints 2-5**: finger extension
Dorsal interossei (4)	Adjacent sides of metacarpal bones 1-5	**1 & 2**: radial bases of proximal phalanges/ extensor expansions of digits 2 & 3 **3 & 4**: ulnar bases of proximal phalanges/ extensor expansions of digits 3 and 4	Deep branch of ulnar nerve (C8–T1)	**Metacarpophalangeal joints 2-4**: finger abduction, finger flexion; **Interphalangeal joints 2-4**: finger extension
Palmar interossei (3)	Ulnar side of metacarpal bone 2, Radial side of metacarpal bones 4 and 5	**1**: ulnar base of proximal phalanx/extensor expansion of digit 2 **2 & 3**: radial base of proximal phalanges/ extensor expansions of digits 4 and 5		**Metacarpophalangeal joints 2, 4 & 5**: finger adduction, finger flexion; **Interphalangeal joints 2, 4 & 5**: finger extension
Adductor pollicis	**Transverse head**: palmar base of metacarpal bone 3 **Oblique head**: capitate bone, Palmar bases of metacarpal bones 2 & 3	Medial base of proximal phalanx 1 (via ulnar sesamoid bone)	Deep branch of ulnar nerve (C8, T1)	**Carpometacarpal joint 1**: thumb adduction

 Thenar muscles

 Hypothenar muscles

BRACHIAL PLEXUS

The brachial plexus is a network of nerves originating in the neck region, passing between the anterior and middle scalene muscles. It passes through the axilla where many peripheral nerves arise that course through the upper limb to innervate the muscles, joints and skin. It can be divided into two main parts: Supraclavicular and infraclavicular. The **supraclavicular part** (roots and trunks with their branches) of the brachial plexus is located in the posterior triangle of the neck, while its **infraclavicular part** (cords and their branches) is in the axilla. The brachial plexus gives off lateral branches (anterior and posterior) and five major terminal branches.

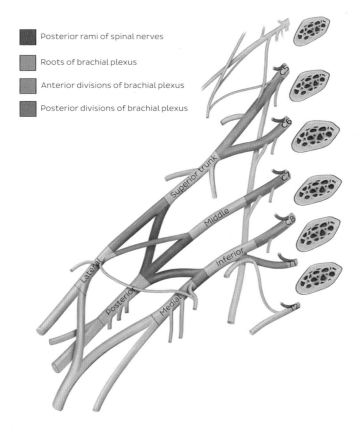

Posterior rami of spinal nerves

Roots of brachial plexus

Anterior divisions of brachial plexus

Posterior divisions of brachial plexus

FIGURE 2.23. Brachial plexus: Overview. The brachial plexus is formed by five anterior rami that originate from the spinal nerves C5-T1 (roots of the brachial plexus). These **roots** merge to form three trunks: Superior (C5-6), middle (C7) and inferior (C8-T1). Each trunk then divides into an anterior and posterior **division**, therefore forming six divisions altogether. The six divisions then reform, resulting in three **cords**: Posterior, lateral and medial.

Brachial plexus

Clinical case: Brachial plexus injury

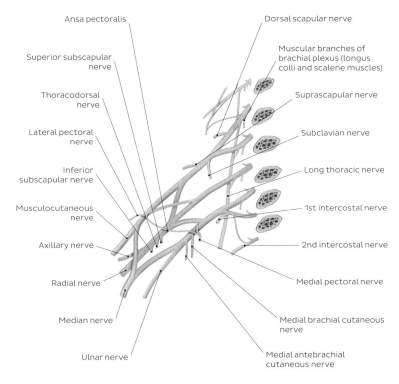

Ansa pectoralis

Superior subscapular nerve

Thoracodorsal nerve

Lateral pectoral nerve

Inferior subscapular nerve

Musculocutaneous nerve

Axillary nerve

Radial nerve

Median nerve

Ulnar nerve

Dorsal scapular nerve

Muscular branches of brachial plexus (longus colli and scalene muscles)

Suprascapular nerve

Subclavian nerve

Long thoracic nerve

1st intercostal nerve

2nd intercostal nerve

Medial pectoral nerve

Medial brachial cutaneous nerve

Medial antebrachial cutaneous nerve

FIGURE 2.24. Brachial plexus: Branches. With respect to their position relative to the clavicle, the branches of the brachial plexus can be divided into supraclavicular and infraclavicular groups. The **supraclavicular** branches include the dorsal scapular nerve, suprascapular nerve, long thoracic nerve and subclavian nerve. The **infrascapular** branches can be further divided into preterminal and terminal branches. The **preterminal** infraclavicular branches emerge from the lateral, medial and posterior cords of the brachial plexus. The lateral cord gives rise to the lateral pectoral nerve while the medial cord gives rise to the medial pectoral nerve and medial brachial/antebrachial cutaneous nerves forearm. The posterior cord of the brachial plexus gives off the upper subscapular nerve, thoracodorsal nerve and lower subscapular nerve. Finally, the five main **terminal** branches include the musculocutaneous, axillary, radial, median and ulnar nerves.

Key points about the brachial plexus	
Roots	C5, C6, C7, C8, T1
Structural organization	**Trunks**: superior, middle, inferior **Divisions**: three anterior and three posterior **Cords**: posterior, lateral and medial
Supraclavicular preterminal branches	Dorsal scapular nerve, suprascapular nerve, long thoracic nerve and subclavian nerve
Infraclavicular preterminal branches	Lateral pectoral nerve, medial pectoral nerve, medial cutaneous nerve of arm, medial cutaneous nerve of forearm, upper subscapular nerve, thoracodorsal nerve, lower subscapular nerve.
Terminal branches	Musculocutaneous nerve, axillary nerve, median nerve, radial nerve, ulnar nerve
Function	Complete sensory and motor innervation of the upper limb

NEUROVASCULATURE OF THE ARM AND SHOULDER

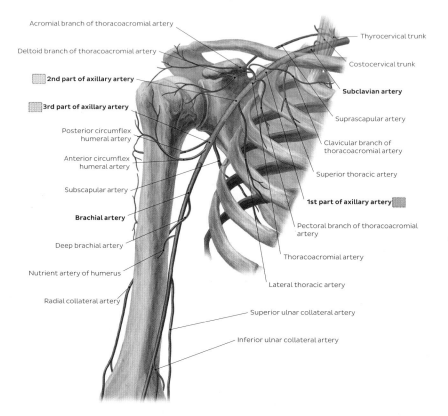

Acromial branch of thoracoacromial artery

Deltoid branch of thoracoacromial artery

2nd part of axillary artery

3rd part of axillary artery

Posterior circumflex humeral artery

Anterior circumflex humeral artery

Subscapular artery

Brachial artery

Deep brachial artery

Nutrient artery of humerus

Radial collateral artery

Thyrocervical trunk

Costocervical trunk

Subclavian artery

Suprascapular artery

Clavicular branch of thoracoacromial artery

Superior thoracic artery

1st part of axillary artery

Pectoral branch of thoracoacromial artery

Thoracoacromial artery

Lateral thoracic artery

Superior ulnar collateral artery

Inferior ulnar collateral artery

FIGURE 2.25. Arteries of the arm and shoulder (anterior view). The subclavian artery conveys oxygenated blood to the upper limb, axilla and lateral aspect of the thorax. It exits the thorax at the lateral border of the first rib where it becomes the axillary artery which can be divided into three parts relative to the pectoralis minor muscle. The first part is proximal to the pectoralis minor and has one branch: The superior thoracic artery, which supplies the pectoralis minor and major muscles. The second part lies posterior to the pectoralis minor and has two main branches: The thoracoacromial artery, which further divides into four terminal branches (acromial, clavicular, deltoid and pectoral) and the lateral thoracic artery supplying the pectoralis and serratus anterior muscles. The third part has three branches: The subscapular artery, the anterior circumflex humeral artery and posterior circumflex humeral artery. The axillary artery terminates at the inferior border of the teres major muscle where it becomes the brachial artery. Branches of the brachial artery in the arm include the deep brachial artery, the nutrient artery of humerus as well as the superior and inferior ulnar collateral arteries.

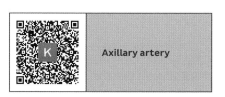

Axillary artery

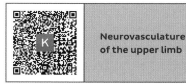

Neurovasculature of the upper limb

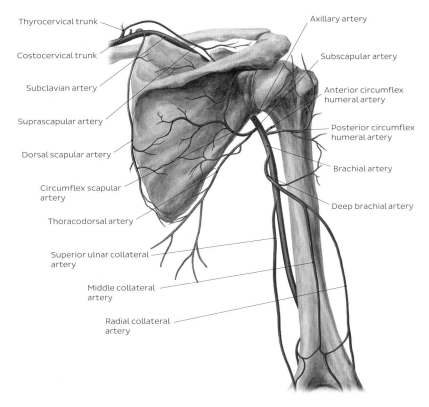

Thyrocervical trunk

Costocervical trunk

Subclavian artery

Suprascapular artery

Dorsal scapular artery

Circumflex scapular
artery

Thoracodorsal artery

Superior ulnar collateral
artery

Middle collateral
artery

Radial collateral
artery

Axillary artery

Subscapular artery

Anterior circumflex
humeral artery

Posterior circumflex
humeral artery

Brachial artery

Deep brachial artery

UPPER LIMB

FIGURE 2.26. Arteries of the arm and shoulder (posterior view). Oxygenated blood is supplied to the proximal upper limb (pectoral girdle region) by arterial branches originating from the **subclavian artery**. The **thyrocervical trunk**, a short and wide vessel arising from the first segment of the subclavian artery, vascularizes the deep cervical and shoulder muscles as well as the skin of the neck and shoulders. A branch of the thyrocervical trunk, the **suprascapular artery**, courses inferolaterally towards the superior border of the scapula to supply muscles in the shoulder and scapular region, including skin of the upper thoracic cage and shoulder. The **dorsal scapular artery**, an independent branch of the subclavian artery, supplies two superficial muscles of the back, the **levator scapulae** and **rhomboid** muscles. It anastomoses with the suprascapular artery in the posterior scapular region. Together with the subscapular artery and its branch, the **circumflex scapular artery**, they form the scapular anastomosis. The **thoracodorsal artery**, a branch of the subscapular artery, descends with the thoracodorsal nerve to supply muscles of the back and skin in the axillary region. The largest branch of the brachial artery is the **deep brachial artery** which supplies the posterior arm muscles. It divides into two branches, the **middle collateral** and the **radial collateral arteries** which contribute to the arterial anastomosis of the elbow. Specifically, the **radial collateral artery** supplies the **radial nerve**, the **brachioradialis** and **brachialis** muscles.

Key points about the arteries of the arm and shoulder	
Axillary artery	Superior thoracic artery
	Thoracoacromial artery
	Lateral thoracic artery
	Subscapular artery
	Anterior/posterior circumflex humeral arteries
	Brachial artery
Brachial artery	Deep brachial artery
	Superior ulnar collateral artery
	Inferior ulnar collateral artery
	Radial artery
	Ulnar artery

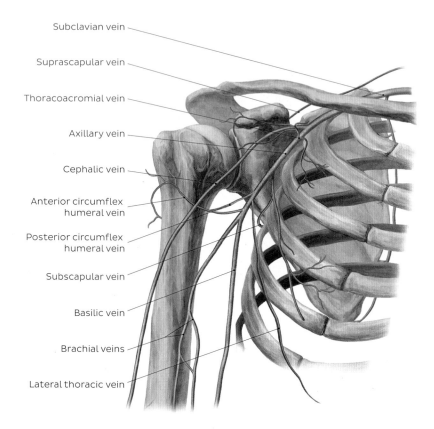

Subclavian vein

Suprascapular vein

Thoracoacromial vein

Axillary vein

Cephalic vein

Anterior circumflex
humeral vein

Posterior circumflex
humeral vein

Subscapular vein

Basilic vein

Brachial veins

Lateral thoracic vein

FIGURE 2.27. Veins of the arm and shoulder (anterior view). Deoxygenated blood from the hand, forearm and arm is drained via the superficial and deep veins of the arm. The main superficial veins of the upper limb are the cephalic and basilic veins which are continuations of the same veins in the forearm. Deep veins of the upper limb, such as the brachial, axillary and subclavian veins, and their tributaries accompanying their arterial counterparts (i.e. venae comitantes). At the inferior border of the teres major muscle, the basilic vein unites with the brachial vein(s) to form the axillary vein. At the lateral border of the first rib, it continues as the subclavian vein transporting deoxygenated blood to the brachiocephalic vein. Venous blood is returned to the heart via the superior vena cava.

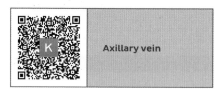

K   **Axillary vein**

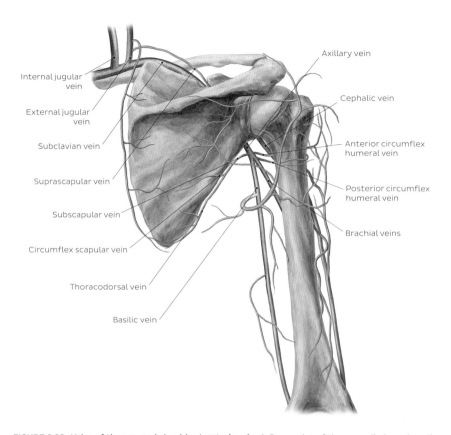

Internal jugular vein

External jugular vein

Subclavian vein

Suprascapular vein

Subscapular vein

Circumflex scapular vein

Thoracodorsal vein

Basilic vein

Axillary vein

Cephalic vein

Anterior circumflex humeral vein

Posterior circumflex humeral vein

Brachial veins

FIGURE 2.28. Veins of the arm and shoulder (posterior view). Deep veins of the upper limb, such as the **brachial, axillary** and **subclavian** veins, transport deoxygenated blood to the **superior vena cava**. The paired **brachial veins** along with their tributaries, the veins of the forearm, empty into the **axillary vein** which in turn conveys the majority of blood from the arm and shoulder. The **anterior** and **posterior circumflex humeral veins** accompany their arterial counterparts, passing anterior to the surgical neck of the humerus to enter the **axillary vein**. In the scapular region, accompanying veins of the arteries contributing to the scapular anastomosis equally form a rich venous plexus to drain the scapular and shoulder region.

Key points about the veins of the arm and shoulder	
Axillary vein	Formed by: basilic vein, brachial veins
	Tributaries: thoracoacromial, subscapular, anterior circumflex humeral and posterior circumflex humeral veins, cephalic vein
	Drains into: subclavian vein

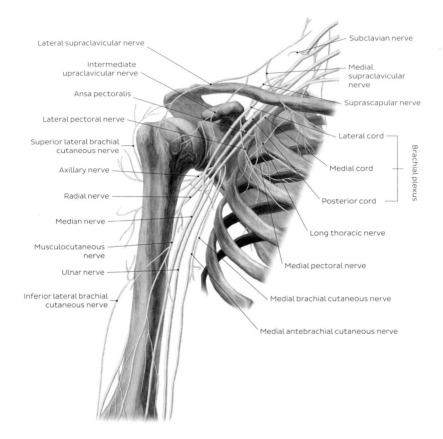

Lateral supraclavicular nerve

Intermediate supraclavicular nerve

Ansa pectoralis

Lateral pectoral nerve

Superior lateral brachial cutaneous nerve

Axillary nerve

Radial nerve

Median nerve

Musculocutaneous nerve

Ulnar nerve

Inferior lateral brachial cutaneous nerve

Subclavian nerve

Medial supraclavicular nerve

Suprascapular nerve

Lateral cord

Medial cord

Posterior cord

Brachial plexus

Long thoracic nerve

Medial pectoral nerve

Medial brachial cutaneous nerve

Medial antebrachial cutaneous nerve

UPPER LIMB

FIGURE 2.29. Nerves of the arm and shoulder (anterior view). A major component of the axilla are the cords and branches of the brachial plexus, a major network of nerves supplying the upper limb. The lateral pectoral nerve arises from the lateral cord of brachial plexus and primarily innervates the pectoralis major muscle (fibers may also pass to the medial pectoral nerve via the ansa pectoralis, when present). The musculocutaneous nerve is a terminal branch of the lateral cord which provides motor innervation to the muscles of the anterior arm (namely the biceps brachii, coracobrachialis and brachialis muscles) as well as sensory innervation of the lateral forearm. The median nerve arises from medial and lateral roots; it is branchless within the arm. Branches of the medial cord of the brachial plexus include the medial pectoral nerve (which provides motor innervation to the pectoralis minor and sternocostal head of the pectoralis major muscle), medial brachial cutaneous nerve (provides sensory innervation to the skin of the medial aspect of the arm) and medial antebrachial cutaneous nerve providing sensory innervation to the skin of the arm overlying the biceps brachii and medial forearm.

Axillary nerve

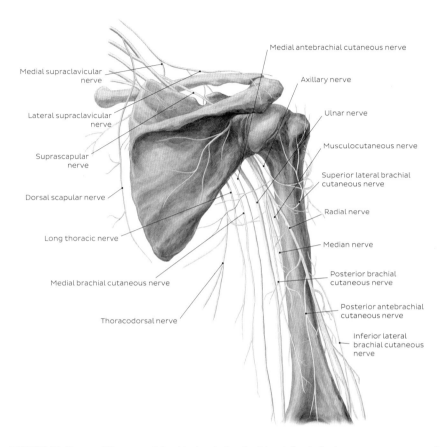

Medial antebrachial cutaneous nerve

Medial supraclavicular nerve

Axillary nerve

Lateral supraclavicular nerve

Ulnar nerve

Musculocutaneous nerve

Suprascapular nerve

Superior lateral brachial cutaneous nerve

Dorsal scapular nerve

Radial nerve

Long thoracic nerve

Median nerve

Medial brachial cutaneous nerve

Posterior brachial cutaneous nerve

Thoracodorsal nerve

Posterior antebrachial cutaneous nerve

Inferior lateral brachial cutaneous nerve

FIGURE 2.30. Nerves of the arm and shoulder (posterior view). In relation to the humerus, many nerves of the brachial plexus arise and course posterior to it. The **ulnar nerve** is a terminal branch of the medial cord of the brachial plexus; it is branchless within the arm. The posterior cord of the brachial plexus gives rise to the **subscapular** (not depicted here), **thoracodorsal** and **axillary nerves** innervating the **subscapularis** and **teres major** muscles, the **latissimus dorsi** and **deltoid muscles**, respectively. The **radial nerve**, a larger terminal branch of the posterior cord, supplies all muscles of the posterior compartment of the arm and forearm. It equally provides sensory innervation to the skin of the posterior and inferolateral arm and forearm (posterior/inferior lateral brachial cutaneous nerves). In the clavicular and shoulder region, the **supraclavicular nerves** arising from the cervical plexus provide sensation over the clavicle, anteromedial shoulder and medial chest. The **suprascapular nerve** arises from the superior trunk of the brachial plexus and passes through the scapular notch to innervate the **supraspinatus** and **infraspinatus** muscles, as well as the glenohumeral joint along its course. The **long thoracic nerve** originates from the posterior aspect of anterior rami of spinal nerves C5, C6 and C7 and supplies the **serratus anterior** muscle. Arising from the anterior ramus of spinal nerve C5, the **dorsal scapular nerve** descends deep to the **levator scapulae** and **rhomboid** muscles to supply them.

Key points about the nerves of the arm and shoulder	
Cervical plexus	Supraclavicular nerves
Supraclavicular/ preterminal branches of brachial plexus	Dorsal scapular nerve
	Long thoracic nerve
	Suprascapular nerve
	Subclavian nerve
Lateral cord of brachial plexus	Lateral pectoral nerve
	Musculocutaneous nerve
	(Lateral root of) Median nerve

Key points about the nerves of the arm and shoulder	
Posterior cord of brachial plexus	Subscapular nerves
	Thoracodorsal nerve
	Radial nerve
	• Posterior brachial cutaneous nerve
	• Inferior lateral cutaneous brachial nerve
	Axillary nerve
	• Superior lateral brachial cutaneous nerve
Medial cord of brachial plexus	Medial pectoral nerve
	Medial brachial cutaneous nerve (anastomoses with intercostobrachial nerve)
	Medial antebrachial cutaneous nerve
	Ulnar nerve
	(Medial root of) Median nerve

NEUROVASCULATURE OF THE ELBOW AND FOREARM

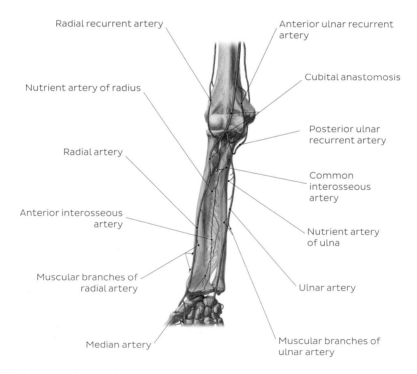

FIGURE 2.31. Arteries of the forearm (anterior view). Oxygenated blood reaches the elbow and forearm via the **brachial artery**, and its largest branch, the **deep brachial artery**. Upon entering the cubital fossa the brachial artery immediately divides into the two major arteries of the forearm: The ulnar and radial arteries. Branches from the brachial, ulnar and radial arteries anastomose to form the cubital anastomosis. Shortly after its origin, the ulnar artery gives off the common interosseous artery which further bifurcates into anterior and posterior interosseous arteries. The anterior interosseous artery extends along the interosseous membrane of the forearm. The ulnar and radial arteries then descend through the forearm, giving off several muscular branches along their lengths, before terminating in the arterial arches of the hand.

UPPER LIMB

Radial artery

Ulnar artery

UPPER LIMB

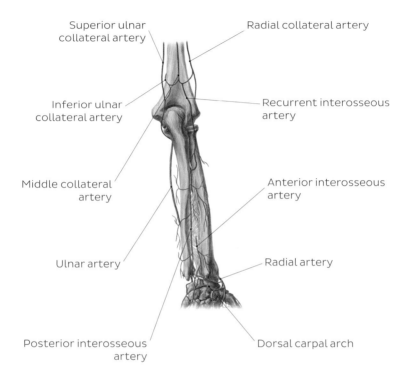

Superior ulnar
collateral artery

Radial collateral artery

Inferior ulnar
collateral artery

Recurrent interosseous
artery

Middle collateral
artery

Anterior interosseous
artery

Ulnar artery

Radial artery

Posterior interosseous
artery

Dorsal carpal arch

FIGURE 2.32. Arteries of the forearm (posterior view). The **anastomotic network** encompassing the elbow joint is formed by branches of the brachial, radial and ulnar arteries. Component vessels of the cubital anastomosis include: The radial, middle, superior ulnar and inferior ulnar collateral arteries of the arm which anastomose with the radial, interosseous, anterior ulnar and posterior ulnar recurrent arteries of the forearm, respectively. These arteries provide arterial supply to structures of the elbow joint. The posterior interosseous artery arises from the common interosseous artery and passes dorsally across the proximal border of the interosseous membrane to reach the posterior compartment of the forearm. It continues distally between the deep and superficial muscles of the posterior forearm and gives off several muscular and cutaneous branches. Near the wrist it anastomoses with the anterior interosseous artery and contributes to the formation of the dorsal carpal arch of the hand.

Key points about the arteries of the elbow and forearm	
Radial artery	Radial recurrent artery
	Muscular branches of radial artery
Ulnar artery	Anterior ulnar recurrent artery
	Posterior ulnar recurrent artery
	Muscular branches of ulnar artery
	Nutrient artery of ulna
	Common interosseous artery
	Anterior interosseous artery (→ nutrient artery of radius, median artery)
	Posterior interosseous artery (→ recurrent interosseous artery)

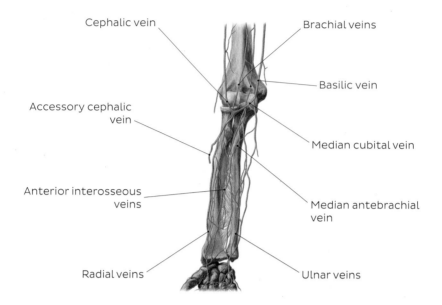

Cephalic vein

Brachial veins

Accessory cephalic vein

Basilic vein

Median cubital vein

Anterior interosseous veins

Median antebrachial vein

Radial veins

Ulnar veins

FIGURE 2.33. Veins of the forearm (anterior view). The upper limb is drained by both deep and superficial venous systems. The main **superficial veins** include the cephalic and basilic veins, both of which arise from the dorsal venous network of the hand. The cephalic vein communicates with the basilic vein via the median cubital vein and drains superficial regions of the hand, wrist and forearm. The median antebrachial vein drains the anterior forearm, usually emptying into the median cubital/basilic vein in the region of the cubital fossa. The **deep venous system** arises from the venous palmar arches and comprises the paired radial, ulnar and anterior interosseous veins which empty into the brachial veins of the arm. The deep veins of the forearm communicate with the superficial veins via perforating veins.

Key points about the veins of the elbow and forearm	
Cephalic vein	Tributaries: dorsal venous network, Accessory cephalic vein
	Drains into: axillary vein
Basilic vein	Tributaries: median cubital vein (median antebrachial vein)
	Drains into: axillary vein
Brachial veins	Tributaries: anterior interosseous veins, posterior interosseous veins, ulnar veins, radial veins, deep brachial veins
	Drains into: axillary vein

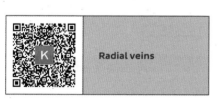

Radial veins

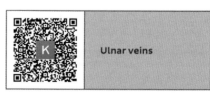

Ulnar veins

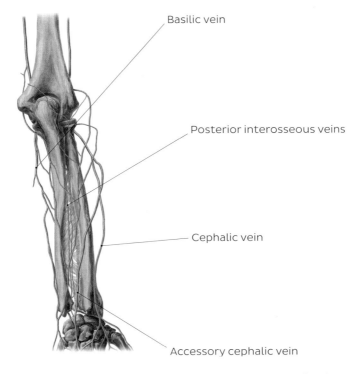

Basilic vein

Posterior interosseous veins

Cephalic vein

Accessory cephalic vein

FIGURE 2.34. Veins of the forearm (posterior view). The cephalic and basilic veins of the forearm originate from the **dorsal venous network** of the hand. Also arising from the medial aspect of the dorsal venous network is the accessory cephalic vein. It courses in a superolateral direction to unite with the cephalic vein variably around the level of the elbow joint, when present. The deep veins of the forearm seen from this posterior view include the posterior interosseous veins, which arise from the dorsal venous network and drain to a collateral vein at the elbow joint.

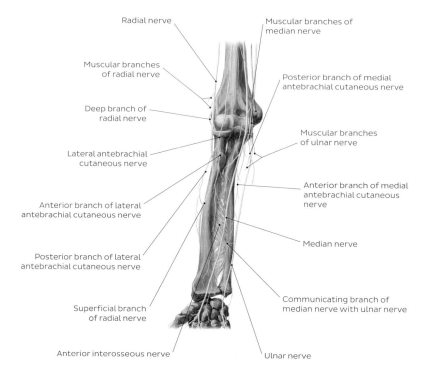

Radial nerve

Muscular branches of median nerve

Muscular branches of radial nerve

Posterior branch of medial antebrachial cutaneous nerve

Deep branch of radial nerve

Muscular branches of ulnar nerve

Lateral antebrachial cutaneous nerve

Anterior branch of medial antebrachial cutaneous nerve

Anterior branch of lateral antebrachial cutaneous nerve

Median nerve

Posterior branch of lateral antebrachial cutaneous nerve

Superficial branch of radial nerve

Communicating branch of median nerve with ulnar nerve

Anterior interosseous nerve

Ulnar nerve

FIGURE 2.35. **Nerves of the forearm (anterior view).** The **median nerve** is the principal nerve of the anterior compartment of the forearm. It gives rise to the anterior interosseous nerve as well as several muscular branches. The **ulnar nerve** travels through the forearm, supplying only the flexor carpi ulnaris and part of flexor digitorum profundus muscles as it travels to supply structures of the hand. The **radial nerve** divides into its superficial and deep branches just before it enters the forearm. **Cutaneous innervation** of the anterior forearm is supplied by the medial and lateral antebrachial cutaneous nerves and their associated branches. The medial antebrachial cutaneous nerve arises from the medial cord of the brachial plexus while the lateral antebrachial cutaneous nerve is a continuation of the musculocutaneous nerve.

Key points about the nerves of the elbow and forearm	
Radial nerve	Posterior antebrachial cutaneous nerve
	Muscular branches of radial nerve
	Deep branch of radial nerve (Posterior interosseous nerve)
	Superficial branch of radial nerve
Lateral antebrachial cutaneous nerve	Anterior branch of lateral antebrachial cutaneous nerve
	Posterior branch of lateral antebrachial cutaneous nerve
Median nerve	Muscular branches of median nerve
	Anterior interosseous nerve
	Communicating branch of median nerve and ulnar nerve
Ulnar nerve	Muscular branches of ulnar nerve
Medial antebrachial cutaneous nerve	Anterior branch of medial antebrachial cutaneous nerve
	Posterior branch of medial antebrachial cutaneous nerve

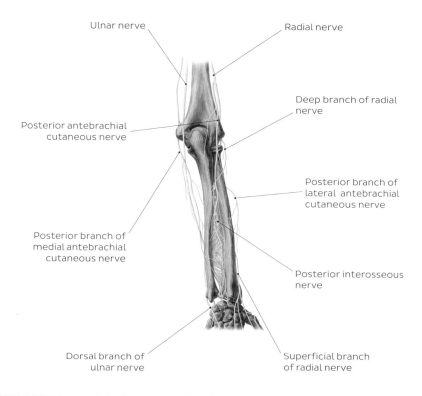

Ulnar nerve

Radial nerve

Deep branch of radial nerve

Posterior antebrachial cutaneous nerve

Posterior branch of lateral antebrachial cutaneous nerve

Posterior branch of medial antebrachial cutaneous nerve

Posterior interosseous nerve

Dorsal branch of ulnar nerve

Superficial branch of radial nerve

FIGURE 2.36. Nerves of the forearm (posterior view). The **radial nerve** divides into superficial and deep branches just anterior to the lateral epicondyle of the humerus. The **superficial branch** descends along the anterior forearm curving around the radius between the brachioradialis and pronator teres muscles to enter the posterior distal third of the forearm. The **deep branch** of the radial nerve enters the posterior forearm by passing between the humeral and ulnar heads of the supinator muscle, at which point it becomes known as the posterior interosseous nerve. This nerve provides motor innervation to muscles of the posterior forearm. The posterior antebrachial cutaneous nerve arises from radial nerve in the posterior compartment of the arm and descends distally to provide cutaneous innervation to the skin of the posterolateral forearm. Posterior branches of the medial and lateral antebrachial nerves also contribute to the cutaneous innervation of the posterior forearm. The ulnar nerve can be seen passing posterior to the medial epicondyle of the distal humerus where it is prone to compression.

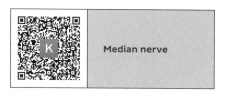

Median nerve

Ulnar nerve

NEUROVASCULATURE OF THE HAND

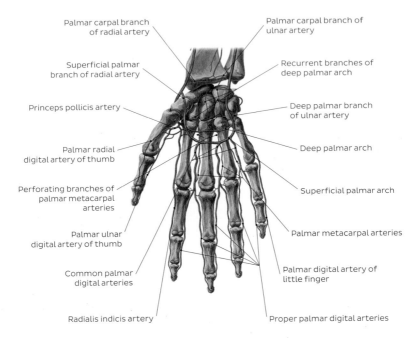

Palmar carpal branch of radial artery

Palmar carpal branch of ulnar artery

Superficial palmar branch of radial artery

Recurrent branches of deep palmar arch

Princeps pollicis artery

Deep palmar branch of ulnar artery

Palmar radial digital artery of thumb

Deep palmar arch

Perforating branches of palmar metacarpal arteries

Superficial palmar arch

Palmar ulnar digital artery of thumb

Palmar metacarpal arteries

Common palmar digital arteries

Palmar digital artery of little finger

Radialis indicis artery

Proper palmar digital arteries

FIGURE 2.37. Arteries of the hand (palmar view). The arterial supply of the hand is provided by the **ulnar** and **radial arteries**, whose terminal branches contribute to the formation of superficial and deep palmar arches. The **superficial palmar arch** is formed by the terminal branch of the ulnar artery and the superficial branch of the radial artery. The superficial palmar arch gives rise to the common palmar digital arteries which travel distally between fingers 2-4. It also gives rise to the palmar digital artery of little finger. At the level of the metacarpophalangeal joints, the common palmar digital arteries bifurcate to form proper palmar digital arteries. The **deep palmar arch** is formed by the terminal branch of the radial artery and the deep branch of the ulnar artery. The deep palmar arch gives off three palmar arteries which join with the common palmar digital arteries to supply the fingers. At the base of the palmar metacarpal arteries are the perforating branches of the palmar metacarpal arteries which anastomose with the dorsal metacarpal arteries. The palmar aspect of the thumb receives its arterial supply from a branch of the radial artery known as the princeps pollicis artery.

UPPER LIMB

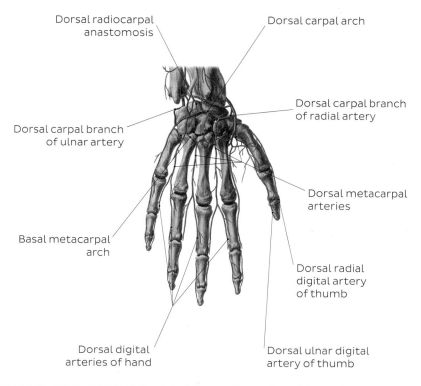

Dorsal radiocarpal anastomosis

Dorsal carpal arch

Dorsal carpal branch of radial artery

Dorsal carpal branch of ulnar artery

Dorsal metacarpal arteries

Basal metacarpal arch

Dorsal radial digital artery of thumb

Dorsal digital arteries of hand

Dorsal ulnar digital artery of thumb

FIGURE 2.38. Arteries of the hand (dorsal view). There are three main arterial networks on the dorsum of the hand: The dorsal radiocarpal anastomosis, the dorsal carpal arch and the basal metacarpal arch. The **dorsal radiocarpal anastomosis** is formed by contributions from the radial, ulnar and anterior/posterior interosseous arteries. The **dorsal carpal arch** is formed by the dorsal carpal branches of the radial and ulnar arteries as well as contributions from the dorsal radiocarpal anastomosis. Arising from the dorsal carpal arch are the 2nd-4th dorsal metacarpal arteries, which are often linked via anastomosing vessels at the bases of the metacarpal bones, forming a **basal metacarpal arch**. The dorsal metacarpal arteries extend distally along the metacarpal bones and bifurcate to form the dorsal digital arteries of the hand. The dorsal surface of the thumb receives its arterial supply from the dorsal radial and ulnar digital arteries, which arise from the radial artery and 1st dorsal metacarpal artery, respectively.

Hand: arteries	Palmar branches	Dorsal branches
Radial artery	Palmar carpal branch of radial artery	Dorsal carpal branch of radial artery
	Superficial palmar branch of radial artery	1st dorsal metacarpal artery (Dorsal ulnar digital artery of thumb)
	Princeps pollicis artery (→ radialis indicis artery, palmar ulnar digital artery of thumb, palmar radial digital artery of thumb)	Dorsal radial digital artery of thumb
Ulnar artery	Palmar carpal branch of ulnar artery	Dorsal carpal branch of ulnar artery (→ dorsal digital artery of little finger)
	Deep palmar branch of ulnar artery	
Arterial arches	Palmar arches	Dorsal radiocarpal anastomosis
	Superficial palmar arch (→ common palmar digital arteries, proper palmar digital arteries, palmar digital artery of little finger)	Dorsal carpal arch (→ dorsal metacarpal arteries, dorsal digital arteries)
	Deep palmar arch (→ palmar metacarpal arteries, perforating branches of palmar metacarpal arteries)	Basal metacarpal arch

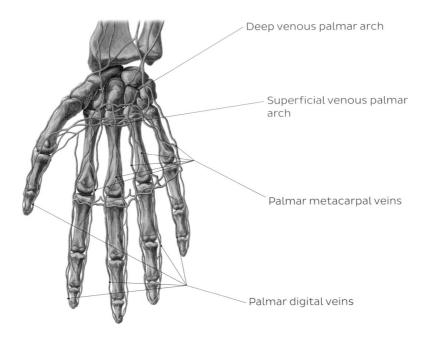

FIGURE 2.39. Veins of the hand (palmar view). Palmar digital veins drain the palmar aspect of the fingers and empty into either the superficial venous palmar arch or the dorsal venous network via communicating intercapitular veins. **Palmar metacarpal veins** drain into the deep venous palmar arch. The superficial and deep venous **palmar networks** follow their arterial counterparts draining blood into the ulnar and radial veins.

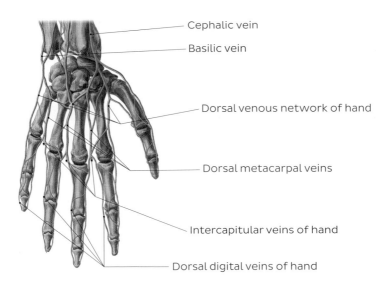

FIGURE 2.40. Veins of the hand (dorsal view). The **dorsal digital veins** travel along the sides of the fingers and are joined by the oblique intercapitular veins which collect blood from the palmar digital veins. The dorsal digital veins empty into the dorsal metacarpal veins which ultimately drain to the **dorsal venous network** of the hand. The dorsal venous network gives rise to the **superficial veins of the forearm** which include the cephalic and basilic veins.

Hand: veins	
Cephalic vein	Dorsal venous network, lateral dorsal metacarpal veins, dorsal digital veins
Basilic vein	Dorsal venous network, medial dorsal metacarpal veins, dorsal digital veins
Radial veins	Deep venous palmar arch, palmar metacarpal veins
Ulnar veins	Superficial venous palmar arch, palmar digital veins

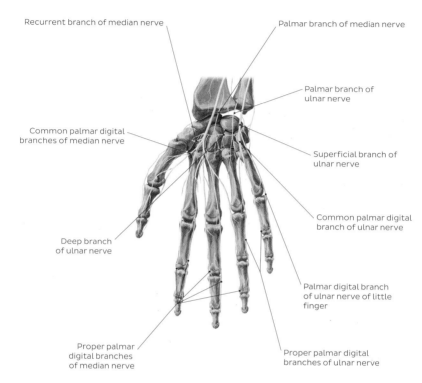

Recurrent branch of median nerve

Palmar branch of median nerve

Palmar branch of ulnar nerve

Common palmar digital branches of median nerve

Superficial branch of ulnar nerve

Common palmar digital branch of ulnar nerve

Deep branch of ulnar nerve

Palmar digital branch of ulnar nerve of little finger

Proper palmar digital branches of median nerve

Proper palmar digital branches of ulnar nerve

FIGURE 2.41. Nerves of the hand (palmar view). Motor innervation to the hand is supplied by the median and ulnar nerves. The radial nerve only contributes to its cutaneous innervation. The **ulnar nerve** gives off a palmar branch in the distal forearm before bifurcating into superficial and deep branches when it reaches the hand. The superficial branch of the ulnar nerve gives off a common palmar digital branch and a palmar digital branch to the [ulnar side of the] little finger. The common palmar digital branch further bifurcates to form two proper palmar digital branches of the ulnar nerve which supply the adjoining sides of the ring and little fingers. Therefore, the ulnar nerve provides sensory innervation to the medial one third of the palm of the hand and palmar surfaces of medial one and a half digits. As the **median nerve** enters the hand it divides into palmar, recurrent and common palmar digital branches. The common palmar digital branches divide into proper palmar digital branches to supply the thumb through middle fingers as well as the radial aspect of the ring finger. The median nerve provides sensory innervation to the lateral two thirds of the palm of the hand and the palmar surface and dorsal distal one third of the lateral three and a half digits.

Hand: main nerves	Branches	Innervation field
Median nerve	Palmar branch, recurrent branch, common palmar digital branches (→ proper palmar digital branches)	**Motor**: thenar muscles and lumbrical muscles (1st & 2nd) **Sensory**: lateral ⅔ of palm; palmar surface and dorsal distal ⅓ of lateral 3 ½ digits
Ulnar nerve	Dorsal branch, dorsal digital branches, palmar branch, superficial branch (→ common palmar digital nerves → proper palmar digital nerves), deep branch	**Motor**: hypothenar, interossei muscles and lumbricals (3rd & 4th) **Sensory**: medial ⅓ of palm; palmar surfaces of medial 1 ½ digits, Medial ⅓ of dorsum of hand; dorsal surfaces of medial 2 ½ digits
Radial nerve	Superficial branch (→ dorsal digital branches)	**Motor**: none **Sensory**: lateral ⅔ of dorsum of hand; dorsal proximal ⅔ of lateral 3 ½ digits

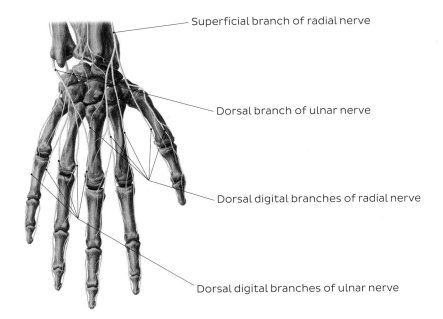

Superficial branch of radial nerve

Dorsal branch of ulnar nerve

Dorsal digital branches of radial nerve

Dorsal digital branches of ulnar nerve

FIGURE 2.42. Nerves of the hand (dorsal view). Cutaneous innervation on the dorsum of the hand is mainly supplied by the ulnar and radial nerves. The dorsal branch of the **ulnar nerve** arises from the ulnar nerve approximately 5cm proximal to the wrist joint. It extends dorsally and divides into several dorsal digital branches. The dorsal digital branches of the ulnar nerve provide cutaneous innervation to the skin of the medial half of the dorsum of the hand and the skin on the dorsal aspect of the medial two and a half fingers. The superficial branch of the **radial nerve** extends dorsally and gives off several dorsal digital branches. The dorsal digital branches of the radial nerve provide cutaneous innervation to the lateral two thirds of the dorsum of the hand and dorsal proximal two thirds of the lateral two and a half digits The 5th dorsal digital branch of radial nerve usually communicates with adjacent ulnar r. digitalis dorsalis which supplies the adjoining sides of the middle and ring fingers. The terminal parts of the dorsal aspect of the lateral three and a half digits are supplied by branches of the median nerve.

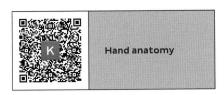

Hand anatomy

LOWER LIMB 3

REGIONS OF THE LOWER LIMB

Like the rest of the body, the **lower limb** is divided into many smaller regions that help clinicians describe, diagnose and treat pathologic conditions of the lower limb. The lower limb has an anterior and a posterior surface. Each surface consists of different regions that have their own **boundaries** and clinically important **contents**, such as muscles, bones and neurovascular structures.

LOWER LIMB

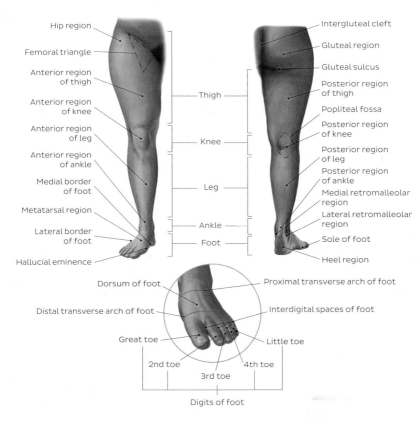

FIGURE 3.1. Regions of the lower limb. The lower limb is divided into 7 main **regions**: The gluteal, hip, femoral (thigh), knee, leg, talocrural (ankle) and foot regions. Some of these regions are divided in accordance to their anterior and posterior surfaces, while others have specific subregions through which clinically significant neurovascular structures pass. e.g., femoral triangle, which contains the femoral nerve, artery and vein.

Regions of the lower limb

Human anatomy terminology

HIP BONE

The hip bone is the large flat bone forming the left and right aspects of the pelvis. It is made from three primary bones: The **ilium**, **ischium** and **pubis**. These primary bones fuse into a single hip bone during the adolescent stage of development. Sometimes called the pelvic bone, each hip bone articulates anteriorly with its contralateral counterpart at the pubic symphysis and posteriorly with the sacrum. On its inferolateral surface is the acetabulum, a concave socket that articulates with the femur to form the hip joint. The hip bone has a number of important bony landmarks and provides attachment for many muscles, including muscles of the abdomen, back, buttocks, hip and thigh. It transfers body weight between the lower limbs and axial skeleton and thus has an important role to play in locomotion.

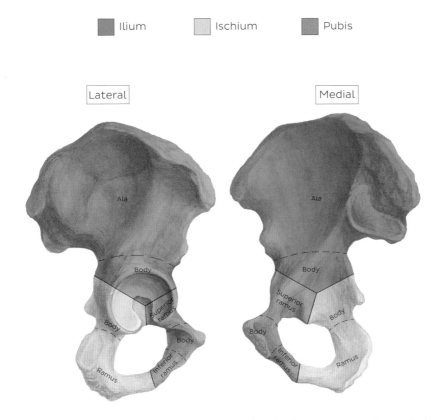

FIGURE 3.2. Hip bone. Three primary bones fuse together to form the hip bone, the ilium, ischium and pubis. All three bones meet at the acetabulum. The **ilium** is the largest of the three hip bone components and is located superior to both the ischium and pubis. The body of the ilium forms its inferior portion, fusing with the ischium and pubis at the acetabulum. Its upper part forms the wing, or ala, of the ilium. The pubis is the smallest of the three bones. It is positioned on the anterior aspect of the pelvic girdle and articulates with its fellow at the pubic symphysis. The **pubis** consists of a body from which two projections extend: The superior and inferior pubic rami. The **ischium**, sometimes called the "sitting bone", is the inferoposterior component of the hip bone. Superiorly, the body of the ischium meets the body of the ilium and superior ramus of the pubis, while inferiorly the ramus arches anteriorly to meet the inferior pubic ramus forming the ischiopubic ramus. This arch forms the inferior boundary of the obturator foramen.

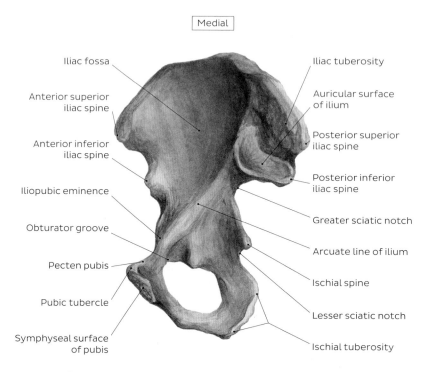

Medial

Iliac fossa

Anterior superior
iliac spine

Anterior inferior
iliac spine

Iliopubic eminence

Obturator groove

Pecten pubis

Pubic tubercle

Symphyseal surface
of pubis

Iliac tuberosity

Auricular surface
of ilium

Posterior superior
iliac spine

Posterior inferior
iliac spine

Greater sciatic notch

Arcuate line of ilium

Ischial spine

Lesser sciatic notch

Ischial tuberosity

FIGURE 3.3. Medial surface. The internal surface of the iliac ala/wing features the large, concave **iliac fossa** which provides attachment for the iliacus muscle. It is limited inferiorly by the arcuate line, which contributes to the pelvic inlet/superior pelvic aperture. Also visible is the medially facing **sacropelvic surface** of ilium, which bears the iliac tuberosity as well as an ear-shaped auricular surface for articulation with the sacrum at the sacroiliac joint. The **greater sciatic notch** is found along the posterior border of the ilium and ischium. Moving inferiorly, the **lesser sciatic notch** can be identified between the ischial spine and tuberosity. The pubis is located anteriorly; its superior ramus extends laterally to meet the ilium at the iliopubic eminence. The medial, oval-shaped **symphyseal surface** of the pubis is separated from its contralateral fellow by an interpubic disc, forming the pubic symphysis.

Key points about the hip bone	
Bones	Ilium, Ischium, Pubis
	(Shared landmarks: acetabulum, greater sciatic notch, obturator foramen)
Ilium	**Body**: supraacetabular groove
	Ala: iliac fossa, iliac crest, anterior superior iliac spine, anterior inferior iliac spine, posterior superior iliac spine, posterior inferior iliac spine
	Sacropelvic surface: iliac tubercle, auricular surface of ilium
	Gluteal surface: anterior gluteal line, posterior gluteal line, inferior gluteal line
Ischium	**Body**: ischial spine, lesser sciatic notch
	Ramus: ischial tuberosity
Pubis	**Body**: pubic tubercle, pubic crest, symphyseal surface
	Superior ramus: iliopubic eminence, pecten pubis, obturator crest, obturator groove, anterior/posterior obturator tubercles
	Inferior ramus: contributes to ischiopubic ramus

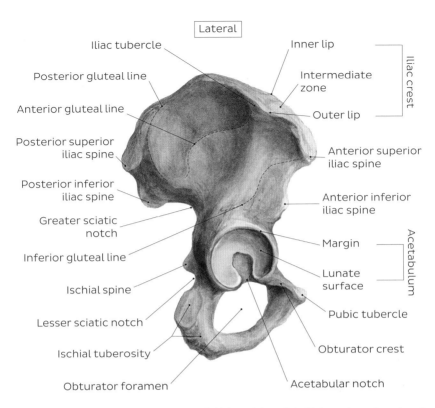

Lateral

Iliac tubercle

Posterior gluteal line

Anterior gluteal line

Posterior superior iliac spine

Posterior inferior iliac spine

Greater sciatic notch

Inferior gluteal line

Ischial spine

Lesser sciatic notch

Ischial tuberosity

Obturator foramen

Inner lip

Intermediate zone

Outer lip

Iliac crest

Anterior superior iliac spine

Anterior inferior iliac spine

Margin

Lunate surface

Acetabulum

Pubic tubercle

Obturator crest

Acetabular notch

LOWER LIMB

FIGURE 3.4. Lateral surface. The superior part of this lateral view of the hip bone shows the external or gluteal surface of the ilium. It is marked by three elevations (the anterior, posterior and inferior gluteal lines) which mark the boundaries between attachment sites for the gluteal muscles. The most superior aspect of the ilium forms a well defined rim called the **iliac crest**, which extends between the anterior and posterior superior iliac spines (ASIS/PSIS). The anterior superior iliac spine provides the lateral attachment for the inguinal ligament. Just inferior to these spines we can find their inferior counterparts, the anterior and posterior inferior iliac spines. The lateral view also presents a cup-shaped cavity known as the **acetabulum**, in which the hip bone articulates with the femur at the hip joint. Four main elements of the acetabulum can be identified: The margin, fossa, lunate surface and acetabular notch. Also seen is a large bony aperture known as the **obturator foramen**; this is closed by the obturator membrane, except for a small opening (canal) giving passage to the obturator artery, veins and nerve from the pelvis into the medial compartment of the thigh.

Hip bone

FEMUR

The femur is the longest and **strongest bone** of the human body. It forms the skeletal framework of the thigh and contributes to two major body joints: The hip and knee. The majority of the muscles of the hip and thigh attach to the femur in order to produce the movements on these joints.

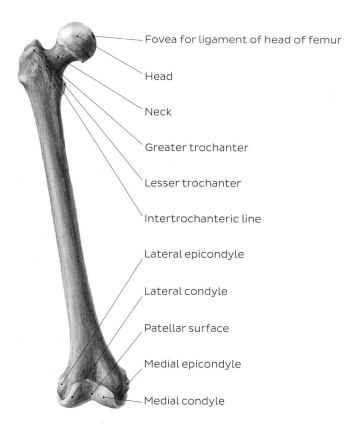

Fovea for ligament of head of femur

Head

Neck

Greater trochanter

Lesser trochanter

Intertrochanteric line

Lateral epicondyle

Lateral condyle

Patellar surface

Medial epicondyle

Medial condyle

FIGURE 3.5. Femur (anterior view). The anterior view of the femur features several important landmarks. The most proximal portion of the head of the femur features a small dimple, known as the **fovea** for the ligament of head of femur. Below the neck of the femur are the **greater** and **lesser trochanters**, with the **intertrochanteric line** spanning between them. These bony prominences act as important attachment sites for the muscles of the hip and thigh. The distal end of the femur contains the **medial** and **lateral condyles** that articulate with the tibia, as well as the **medial** and **lateral epicondyles** above them. Between the medial and lateral condyle is the **patellar surface** of the femur, which as its name suggests, articulates with the patella, contributing to the formation of the knee joint. Notice how some of these landmarks are better seen on the posterior view (2nd image), such as the lesser trochanter, and the medial and lateral condyles.

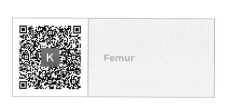

Femur

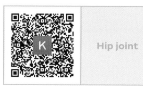

Hip joint

LOWER LIMB

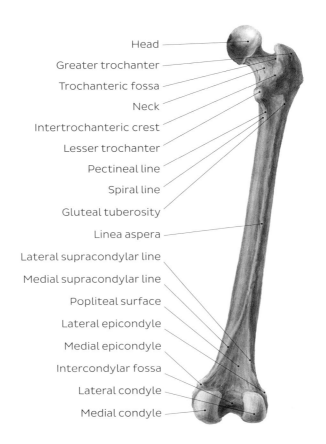

Head
Greater trochanter
Trochanteric fossa
Neck
Intertrochanteric crest
Lesser trochanter
Pectineal line
Spiral line
Gluteal tuberosity
Linea aspera
Lateral supracondylar line
Medial supracondylar line
Popliteal surface
Lateral epicondyle
Medial epicondyle
Intercondylar fossa
Lateral condyle
Medial condyle

LOWER LIMB

FIGURE 3.6. **Femur (posterior view).** The **lesser trochanter** is clearly seen on the posterior view, separated from the greater trochanter by the **intertrochanteric crest**. The intertrochanteric crest and intertrochanteric line (anterior view) mark the transition between the neck of the femur and the shaft of the femur. Found on the medial surface of the greater trochanter is the crescent-shaped depression known as the **trochanteric fossa**. Seen below the lesser trochanter are the 3 small bony ridges called **pectineal line**, **spiral line** and **gluteal tuberosity**. These 3 ridges converge inferiorly to form the **linea aspera** that runs along the entire shaft of the femur. Near the distal end of the femur, the linea aspera diverges into 2 ridges: The medial and lateral **supracondylar lines**. The posterior surface of the distal end of the femur provides a better visual of the medial and lateral condyles, which in this view are separated by the **intercondylar fossa**.

Key points about the femur	
Proximal end	Head of femur, fovea for ligament of head of femur, neck of femur, greater trochanter, trochanteric fossa, lesser trochanter, intertrochanteric line, intertrochanteric crest
Shaft	Spiral line, pectineal line, gluteal tuberosity, linea aspera (with medial and lateral lips, medial supracondylar line, lateral supracondylar line, popliteal surface
Distal end	**Medial condyle**: medial epicondyle, adductor tubercle
	Lateral condyle: lateral epicondyle, groove for popliteus muscle
	Intercondylar fossa
	Intercondylar line
	Patellar surface
Joints	Hip joint, knee joint

HIP JOINT

The hip joint is a large articulation between the head of the **femur** and acetabulum of the **hip bone**. It is the most proximal joint of the free lower limb and is classified as a ball-and-socket type of synovial joint capable of a wide range of movements. Compared to the shoulder joint, the hip joint sacrifices a part of its mobility for stability, since it needs to bear the entire weight of the upper body while standing. Hence, the hip joint is the **most stable joint** in the body.

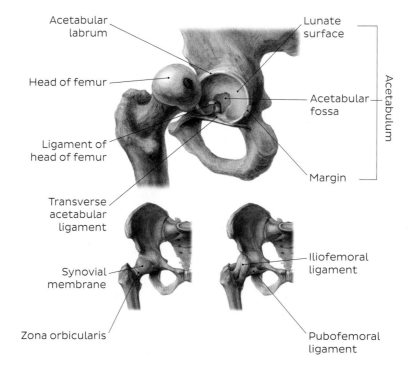

FIGURE 3.7. Overview of the hip joint. The hip joint has several ligaments that play an important role in stabilizing the joint during various movements. The ligaments of the hip joint are divided into two groups: Capsular and intracapsular. The capsular ligaments reinforce the joint capsule and include the **iliofemoral**, **pubofemoral** and **ischiofemoral** ligaments. The intracapsular ligaments are situated inside of the joint capsule and include the **transverse ligament of the acetabulum** and **ligament of the head of the femur**.

Key points about the hip joint	
Joint type	Synovial ball-and-socket joint
Articulating surfaces	Head of femur, lunate surface of acetabulum
Ligaments	**Capsular**: iliofemoral, pubofemoral, ischiofemoral ligaments **Intracapsular**: transverse ligament of acetabulum, ligament of head of femur
Movements	Flexion, extension, abduction, adduction, external rotation, internal rotation and circumduction

MUSCLES OF THE HIP AND THIGH

The muscles of the hip and thigh are divided into three major groups:

- **Iliopsoas muscle**
- **Gluteal muscles**, comprised of superficial and deep groups
- **Thigh muscles**, subdivided into the anterior, medial and posterior groups.

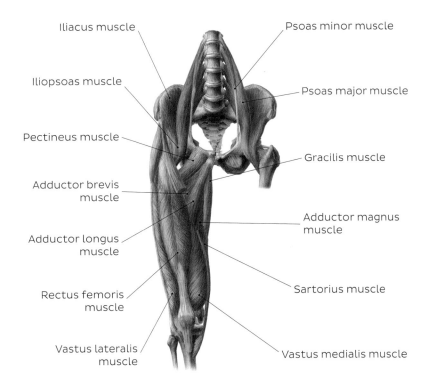

Iliacus muscle

Iliopsoas muscle

Pectineus muscle

Adductor brevis muscle

Adductor longus muscle

Rectus femoris muscle

Vastus lateralis muscle

Psoas minor muscle

Psoas major muscle

Gracilis muscle

Adductor magnus muscle

Sartorius muscle

Vastus medialis muscle

FIGURE 3.8. Anterior view. From this anterior perspective the **iliopsoas muscle** as well as the muscles of the anterior and medial compartments can be identified. The iliopsoas muscle group consists of the iliacus, psoas major, and psoas minor muscles which function to flex the trunk and thigh at the hip joint. The **quadriceps femoris muscle** forms the great anterior muscle of the thigh. It consists of four parts: The vastus lateralis, vastus intermedius, vastus medialis, and rectus femoris muscles. The quadriceps femoris muscle is a powerful extensor of the knee. The rectus femoris muscle of this group also works together with the sartorius muscle of the anterior thigh to produce flexion of the thigh at the hip joint. The **medial thigh muscles** mainly function to adduct the thigh at the hip joint. Muscles of this region include the gracilis, pectineus, adductor longus, adductor brevis, and adductor magnus. This group of muscles may also be known as the adductor muscle group. The obturator externus muscle is also classified as a member of the medial compartment of the thigh due to its innervation by the obturator nerve, however, is often grouped with the other lateral rotators of the hip joint (deep gluteal muscles) due to its shared function with these muscles.

LOWER LIMB

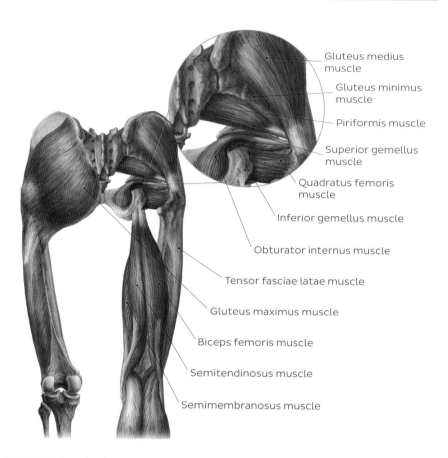

Gluteus medius muscle

Gluteus minimus muscle

Piriformis muscle

Superior gemellus muscle

Quadratus femoris muscle

Inferior gemellus muscle

Obturator internus muscle

Tensor fasciae latae muscle

Gluteus maximus muscle

Biceps femoris muscle

Semitendinosus muscle

Semimembranosus muscle

FIGURE 3.9. Posterior view. The muscles of the gluteal region are divided into superficial and deep groups. The **superficial gluteal muscles** include the large gluteus maximus muscle as well as the gluteus medius and minimus muscles; the tensor fascia latae muscle which is positioned laterally. The superficial gluteal muscles collectively contribute to extension, internal and external rotation and abduction and adduction of the thigh at the hip joint. The **deep gluteal muscles** are located beneath the superficial gluteal muscles and include the piriformis, gemellus superior, obturator internus, gemellus inferior, obturator externus, and quadratus femoris muscles. The deep gluteal muscles function to externally rotate and abduct the thigh at the hip joint whilst also contributing to stabilization of the head of the femur with the acetabulum.

The posterior muscles of the thigh are also known as the **ischiocrural**, or more commonly, the hamstring muscles. They include: The biceps femoris, semimembranosus and semitendinosus muscles. The ischiocrural muscles work together to extend the thigh, flex the knee joint and stabilize the hip joint.

Iliopsoas muscles	Origin	Insertion	Innervation	Function
Iliacus	Iliac fossa		Femoral nerve (L2–L4)	**Hip joint**: thigh/ trunk flexion, thigh external rotation; trunk lateral flexion
Psoas major	Vertebral bodies of T12–L4, Intervertebral discs between T12–L4, Costal processes of L1–L5 vertebrae	Lesser trochanter of femur	Anterior rami of spinal nerves L1–L3 (Psoas minor: L1 only)	
Psoas minor	Vertebral bodies of T12 & L1 vertebrae	Iliopubic eminence, Pecten pubis		Weak trunk flexion

LOWER LIMB

Gluteal muscles		Origin	Insertion	Innervation	Function
Superficial group	**Gluteus maximus**	Lateroposterior surface of sacrum and coccyx, Gluteal surface of ilium (behind posterior gluteal line), Thoracolumbar fascia, Sacrotuberous ligament	Iliotibial tract, Gluteal tuberosity of femur	Inferior gluteal nerve (L5–S2)	**Hip joint**: thigh extension, thigh external rotation, thigh abduction (superior part), thigh adduction (inferior part)
	Gluteus medius	Gluteal surface of ilium (between anterior and posterior gluteal lines)	Lateral aspect of greater trochanter of femur		**Hip joint**: thigh abduction, thigh internal rotation (anterior part); pelvis stabilization
	Gluteus minimus	Gluteal surface of ilium (between anterior and inferior gluteal lines)	Anterior aspect of greater trochanter of femur	Superior gluteal nerve (L4–S1)	
	Tensor fasciae latae	Anterior superior iliac spine (ASIS), Outer lip of iliac crest	Iliotibial tract		**Hip joint**: thigh internal rotation, (weak abduction); **Knee joint**: leg external rotation, (weak leg flexion/extension); stabilizes hip & knee joints
Deep group	**Piriformis**	Anterior surface of sacrum (between the S2 and S4), Gluteal surface of ilium (near posterior inferior iliac spine), (Sacrotuberous ligament)	Apex of greater trochanter of femur	Nerve to piriformis (S1–S2)	
	Superior gemellus	Ischial spine	Medial surface of greater trochanter of femur, (via tendon of obturator internus)	Nerve to obturator internus (L5, S1)	**Hip joint**: thigh external rotation, thigh abduction (from flexed hip); stabilizes head of femur in acetabulum
	Inferior gemellus	Ischial tuberosity		Nerve to quadratus femoris (L4–S1)	
	Obturator internus	Ischiopubic ramus, Posterior surface of obturator membrane	Medial surface of greater trochanter of femur	Nerve to obturator internus (L5, S1)	
	Obturator externus	Anterior surface of obturator membrane, Bony boundaries of obturator foramen	Trochanteric fossa of femur	Obturator nerve (L3, L4)	
	Quadratus femoris	Ischial tuberosity	Intertrochanteric crest of femur	Nerve to quadratus femoris (L4–S1)	**Hip joint**: thigh external rotation; stabilizes head of femur in acetabulum

LOWER LIMB

LOWER LIMB

Anterior thigh muscles	Origin	Insertion	Innervation	Function
Sartorius	Anterior superior iliac spine (ASIS)	Proximal end of tibia below medial condyle (via pes anserinus)	Femoral nerve (L2-L4) (Sartorius L2-L3 only)	**Hip joint**: thigh flexion, thigh abduction, thigh external rotation; **Knee joint**: leg flexion, leg internal rotation
Rectus femoris	Anterior inferior iliac spine, Supracetabluar groove	Tibial tuberosity (via patellar ligament), Patella (Lateral condyle of tibia)		**Hip joint**: thigh flexion; **Knee joint**: leg extension
Vastus intermedius	Anterior surface of femoral shaft			
Vastus lateralis	Intertrochanteric line, Gluteal tuberosity, Greater trochanter, Linea aspera of femur	Tibial tuberosity (via patellar ligament), Patella, (Lateral condyle of tibia)		**Knee joint**: leg extension
Vastus medialis	Intertrochanteric line, spiral line and linea aspera, medial supracondylar line of femur	Tibial tuberosity (via patellar ligament), Patella, (Medial condyle of tibia)		

Medial thigh muscles	Origin	Insertion	Innervation	Function
Pectineus	Superior pubic ramus (Pectineal line of pubis)	Pectineal line of femur, Linea aspera of femur	Femoral nerve (L2, L3) (Obturator nerve (L2, L3)	**Hip joint**: thigh flexion, thigh adduction, thigh external rotation, thigh internal rotation; pelvis stabilization
Adductor magnus	Adductor part: inferior pubic ramus, Ischial ramus Ischiocondylar part: ischial tuberosity	Adductor part: gluteal tuberosity, Linea aspera (medial lip), Medial supracondylar line; Ischiocondylar part: adductor tubercle of femur	Adductor part: obturator nerve (L2-L4); Ischiocondylar part: tibial division of sciatic nerve (L4)	**Hip joint**: thigh flexion, thigh adduction, thigh external rotation (adductor part), thigh extension, thigh internal rotation (ischiocondylar part); pelvis stabilization

Medial thigh muscles	Origin	Insertion	Innervation	Function
Adductor minimus	Inferior public ramus	Gluteal tuberosity of femur		**Hip joint**: thigh adduction, thigh external rotation
Adductor longus	Anterior body of pubis		Obturator nerve (L2-L4)	**Hip joint**: thigh flexion, thigh adduction, thigh external rotation; pelvis stabilization
Adductor brevis	Anterior body of pubis, Inferior pubic ramus	Linea aspera of femur (medial lip)		**Hip joint**: thigh flexion, thigh adduction, thigh external rotation; pelvis stabilization
Gracilis	Anterior body of pubis, Inferior pubic ramus, Ischial ramus	Medial surface of proximal tibia (via pes anserinus)	Obturator nerve (L2-L3)	**Hip joint**: thigh flexion, thigh adduction; **Knee joint**: leg flexion, leg internal rotation

Posterior thigh muscles	Origin	Insertion	Innervation	Function
Semimembranosus	(Superolateral impression of) Ischial tuberosity	Medial condyle of tibia	Tibial division of sciatic nerve (L5-S2)	**Hip joint**: thigh extension, thigh internal rotation; **Knee joint**: leg flexion, leg internal rotation; stabilizes pelvis
Semitendinosus	(Posteromedial impression of) Ischial tuberosity	Proximal end of tibia below medial condyle (via pes anserinus)		
Biceps femoris	Long head: (Inferomedial impression of) Ischial tuberosity, Sacrotuberous ligament; Short head: linea aspera of femur (lateral lip), Lateral supracondylar line of femur	(Lateral aspect of) Head of fibula	Long head: tibial division of sciatic nerve (L5-S2); Short head: common fibular division of sciatic nerve (L5-S2)	**Hip joint**: thigh extension, thigh external rotation; **Knee joint**: leg flexion, leg external rotation; stabilizes pelvis

Hip and thigh muscles

The quadriceps femoris muscle

TIBIA AND FIBULA

The tibia and fibula are the two long bones of the leg, positioned parallel to each other. The **tibia** is the second largest bone in the body (after the femur) and the primary weight-bearing bone of the leg. The **fibula** is the more slender of the two bones, located lateral to the tibia. These two bones articulate with each other, making the three following joints:

1. **Superior tibiofibular joint:** Plane synovial joint
2. **Middle tibiofibular joint:** Fibrous joint, attached by the interosseous membrane
3. **Inferior tibiofibular joint:** Syndesmosis

The tibia and fibula articulate with the talus to form the **ankle joint**, while only the tibia articulates with the femur and participates in the formation of the **knee joint**.

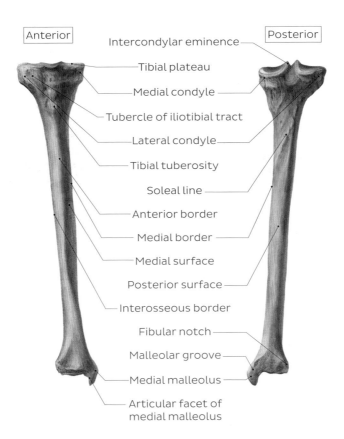

Anterior · Posterior

- Intercondylar eminence
- Tibial plateau
- Medial condyle
- Tubercle of iliotibial tract
- Lateral condyle
- Tibial tuberosity
- Soleal line
- Anterior border
- Medial border
- Medial surface
- Posterior surface
- Interosseous border
- Fibular notch
- Malleolar groove
- Medial malleolus
- Articular facet of medial malleolus

FIGURE 3.10. Tibia. The tibia articulates proximally at the knee joint with the distal end of the femur which rests upon the **tibial plateau**, formed by the medial and lateral tibial condyles. The **tibial tuberosity** is a large roughened prominence on the anterior proximal tibia which serves as the attachment point for the patellar ligament (and indirectly for the tendon of the quadriceps femoris muscle). The **body**, or shaft, of the tibia has three surfaces (medial, lateral and posterior), which are separated by three borders (anterior, interosseous and medial). The posterior surface of the tibia bears a ridge known as the **soleal line** which gives attachment to the soleus muscle. The distal end of the tibia bears a projection known as the **medial malleolus** which articulates with the body of the talus; its medial surface can be palpated as the medial 'knob' of the ankle.

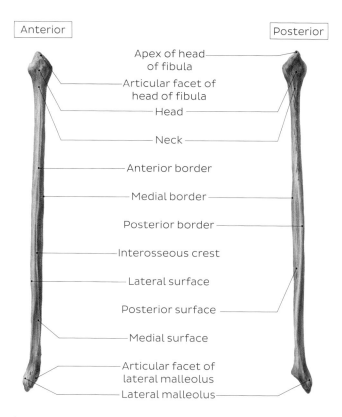

Anterior | Posterior

Apex of head of fibula
Articular facet of head of fibula
Head
Neck
Anterior border
Medial border
Posterior border
Interosseous crest
Lateral surface
Posterior surface
Medial surface
Articular facet of lateral malleolus
Lateral malleolus

FIGURE 3.11. **Fibula.** The **head** forms the enlarged proximal end of the fibula. It bears two main landmarks: An apex (a.k.a., styloid process) which projects proximally from its posterior surface, and a small, medially oriented articular surface for the lateral condyle of the tibia, which contributes to the superior tibiofibular joint. The **body** of the fibula forms a long thin shaft, with three surfaces (medial, lateral and posterior) separated by three ill-defined borders (anterior, posterior and medial). The medial surface of the fibula is marked by an **interosseous crest**, which is connected to the interosseous border of the tibia via the interosseous membrane of the leg to form the middle tibiofibular joint. The distal end of the fibula articulates once again with the tibia to form the inferior tibiofibular joint, before expanding to form the **lateral malleolus** which constitutes the lateral 'knob' of the ankle. Like its medial counterpart, the lateral malleolus articulates with the body of the talus to collectively form the talocrural joint.

Key points about the tibia	
Proximal end	Lateral condyle, medial condyle, tibial plateau, anterior and posterior intercondylar areas, tubercle of iliotibial tract, tibial tuberosity
Shaft	**Three borders** (anterior, medial, interosseous); **three surfaces** (posterior, medial, lateral), **soleal line** (posterior surface)
Distal end	Medial malleolus, fibular notch

Key points about the fibula	
Proximal end	Apex (styloid process), head of fibula, (with articular facet for lateral condyle of tibia), neck
Shaft	**Three borders** (anterior, medial, posterior); **three surfaces** (medial, lateral, posterior)
Distal end	Lateral malleolus

Intracrural joints	
Superior/proximal tibiofibular joint	Proximal tibia ↔ proximal fibula
Middle tibiofibular joint	Shaft of tibia ↔ shaft of fibula (via interosseous membrane)
Inferior/distal tibiofibular joint	Distal tibia ↔ distal fibula

Tibia

Fibula

LOWER LIMB

KNEE JOINT

The knee joint is a complex synovial joint that connects three bones (the femur, tibia and patella) which together form a pair of articulations:

1. The **tibiofemoral** joint, formed between the tibia and the femur.
2. The **patellofemoral** joint, formed between the patella and the femur.

The knee joint is the largest joint of the body, responsible for bearing a considerable amount of biomechanical stress every time we stand or walk. Its integrity is supported by many extracapsular and intracapsular ligaments, menisci, as well as surrounding muscles that provide the knee joint with the stability needed to bear the weight of the whole body.

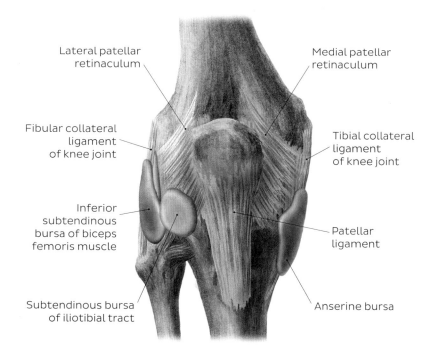

Lateral patellar retinaculum

Medial patellar retinaculum

Fibular collateral ligament of knee joint

Tibial collateral ligament of knee joint

Inferior subtendinous bursa of biceps femoris muscle

Patellar ligament

Subtendinous bursa of iliotibial tract

Anserine bursa

FIGURE 3.12. **Bursae and extracapsular ligaments (anterior view).** Knee bursae are small fluid-filled sacs whose function is to reduce friction and accommodate gliding of muscles or tendons as they cross over bony prominences of the knee joint. Two groups of bursae are associated with the knee joint: Bursae around the patella (anterior/patellar ligaments) and bursae located elsewhere. The nonpatellar group consists of a group of superficial bursae, most notable being the **inferior subtendinous bursa of biceps femoris muscle** and **anserine bursa**. The former is located on the lateral side of the joint, between the tendon of biceps femoris and fibular collateral ligament. The anserine bursa is found on the medial side, cushioning the space between the tibial collateral ligament and combined tendinous expansions of the sartorius, gracilis and semitendinosus muscles (pes anserinus).

As many as fourteen bursae may be present, including the **subtendinous bursa of iliotibial tract** found between tibia and the distal part of iliotibial tract.

The **extracapsular ligaments** of the knee are located outside the joint capsule. They are the patellar ligament, fibular and tibial collateral ligaments, and oblique and arcuate popliteal ligaments (depicted on the posterior view).

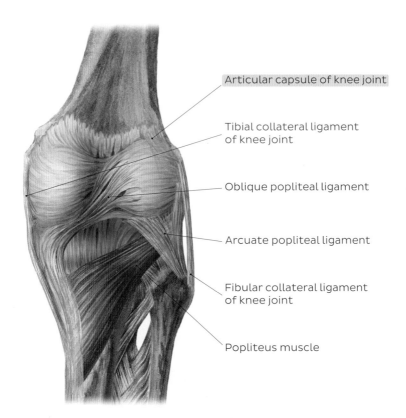

Articular capsule of knee joint

Tibial collateral ligament
of knee joint

Oblique popliteal ligament

Arcuate popliteal ligament

Fibular collateral ligament
of knee joint

Popliteus muscle

FIGURE 3.13. **Extracapsular ligaments and popliteus muscle (posterior view).** Right knee, capsule in situ. The articular capsule extends posteriorly between the intercondylar line of the femur to the posterior border of the tibial plateau. It strengthened posteriorly by the **arcuate** and **oblique popliteal ligaments**, medially by the tibial collateral ligament and laterally by the fibular collateral ligament. The popliteus muscle provides additional stabilization to the knee joint as it ascends superolaterally across its posterior aspect. Its tendon enters the lateral part of the articular capsule, deep to the arcuate popliteal ligament, therefore making it an intracapsular structure.

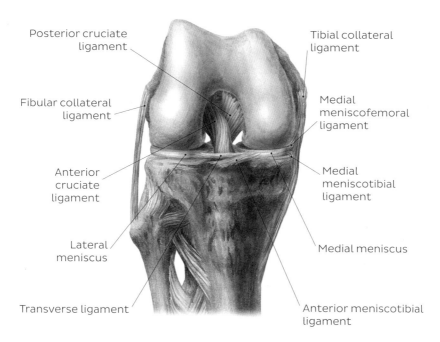

Posterior cruciate ligament

Tibial collateral ligament

Fibular collateral ligament

Medial meniscofemoral ligament

Anterior cruciate ligament

Medial meniscotibial ligament

Lateral meniscus

Medial meniscus

Transverse ligament

Anterior meniscotibial ligament

FIGURE 3.14. Intracapsular ligaments and menisci (anterior view). Right knee, flexed position with capsule removed. The **intracapsular ligaments** of the knee joint are located within the joint capsule, with the most notable being the anterior and posterior cruciate ligaments (discussed in next image). The **menisci** are paired, crescent-shaped fibrocartilaginous structures located between the articular surfaces of tibia and femur. They are supported by several accessory ligaments which include anterior and medial meniscotibial ligaments, medial meniscofemoral and posterior meniscofemoral (depicted on posterior view) and transverse ligament of knee.

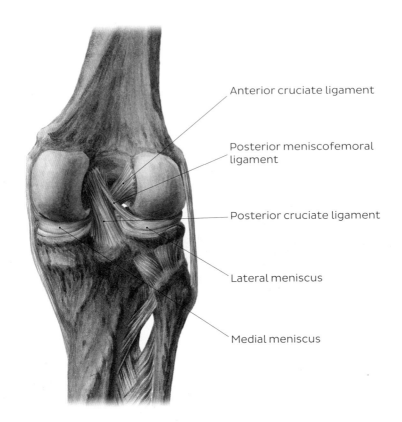

Anterior cruciate ligament

Posterior meniscofemoral ligament

Posterior cruciate ligament

Lateral meniscus

Medial meniscus

FIGURE 3.15. **Intracapsular ligaments and menisci (posterior view).** Right knee, capsule removed. The cruciate ligaments of the knee extend between the intercondylar fossa of the femur and intercondylar areas of the tibia, crossing each other to form an 'X' shape (cross: Latin = crux). The posterior cruciate ligament is the shorter, thicker and stronger of the pair. They function to stabilize the knee joint by resisting translation of the femur on the tibia and preventing hyperflexion/hyperextension.

Key points about the knee joint	
Type	**Tibiofemoral joint**: synovial hinge joint
	Patellofemoral joint: plane joint
Articular surfaces	**Tibiofemoral joint**: lateral and medial condyles of femur, tibial plateau
	Patellofemoral joint: patellar surface of femur, articular surface of patella
Ligaments and menisci	**Extracapsular ligaments**: patellar ligament, medial and lateral patellar retinacula, tibial (medial) collateral ligament, medial meniscofemoral ligament, medial meniscotibial ligament, fibular (lateral) collateral ligament, oblique popliteal ligament, arcuate popliteal ligament, anterolateral ligament
	Intracapsular ligaments/menisci: anterior cruciate ligament (ACL), posterior cruciate ligament (PCL), medial meniscus, lateral meniscus, transverse ligament of the knee, anterior meniscotibial ligament, posterior meniscofemoral ligament
Movements	Extension, flexion, internal/external rotation

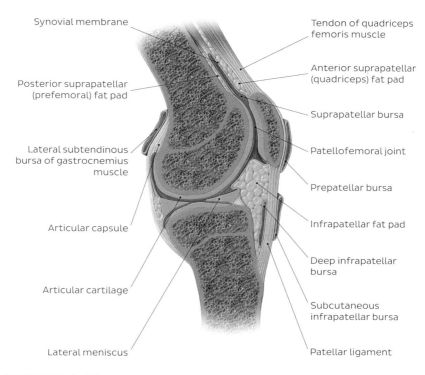

Synovial membrane

Tendon of quadriceps femoris muscle

Anterior suprapatellar (quadriceps) fat pad

Posterior suprapatellar (prefemoral) fat pad

Suprapatellar bursa

Lateral subtendinous bursa of gastrocnemius muscle

Patellofemoral joint

Prepatellar bursa

Articular capsule

Infrapatellar fat pad

Articular cartilage

Deep infrapatellar bursa

Subcutaneous infrapatellar bursa

Lateral meniscus

Patellar ligament

FIGURE 3.16. **Sagittal view of the knee joint (mid patella).** Sagittal view of the knee joint, with articulating surfaces clearly visible. The lateral and medial **condyles of the femur** articulate with the tibial plateau inferiorly forming the tibiofemoral joint. Anteriorly, the patellar surface of the femur articulates with the articular surface of patella forming the **patellofemoral joint**. This view of the knee joint is best for examining the structure of the articular capsule and its two parts, the outer fibrous layer and inner synovial membrane which encloses the articular cavity.

The **articular capsule** forms several pouches called **bursae**, that cushion and reduce friction between muscle tendons and bones of the knee. Additional important structures are the menisci situated between the lateral and medial condyles of the femur and tibial plateau, increasing congruency between these articulating surfaces. A large, intracapsular **infrapatellar fat pad** can be identified between the patellar ligament and synovial membrane. It works to reduce friction between surrounding adjacent structures i.e. patella bone, patellar ligament and underlying bones.

Knee joint

Patella

MUSCLES OF THE LEG

The muscles of the leg are divided into three compartments based on their location and primary functions.

- The **anterior (dorsiflexor) compartment**, which consists of the tibialis anterior, extensor digitorum longus, fibularis tertius and extensor hallucis longus muscles. Crossing the ankle from the anterior aspect, these muscles primarily cause **dorsiflexion** of the foot.
- The **lateral (fibular) compartment**, which houses the fibularis longus and fibularis brevis muscles. The major function of this compartment is to **evert** the foot.
- The **posterior (plantar flexor) compartment**, which is divided into the superficial and deep parts. The former contains the triceps surae (gastrocnemius and soleus) and plantaris muscles, while the latter consists of the popliteus, tibialis posterior, flexor digitorum longus and flexor hallucis longus muscles. The main function of this compartment is **plantar flexion** of the foot at the ankle joint.

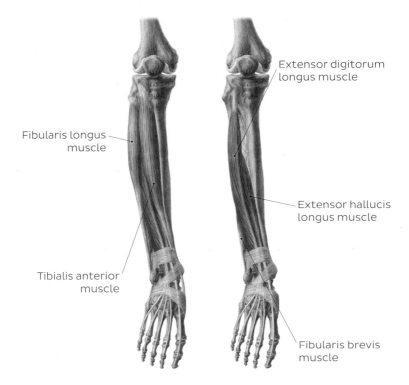

Fibularis longus muscle

Extensor digitorum longus muscle

Extensor hallucis longus muscle

Tibialis anterior muscle

Fibularis brevis muscle

FIGURE 3.17. **Muscles of the leg (anterior view).** The four muscles of the **anterior compartment** of the leg include the tibialis anterior, extensor digitorum longus, extensor hallucis longus, and fibularis tertius (not shown/illustrated) muscles. These muscles pass anterior to the ankle joint to insert at the foot, therefore eliciting dorsiflexion at the ankle joint on contraction. The extensor digitorum longus and extensor hallucis longus extend distally to insert onto the dorsal surface of the phalanges and therefore also function in extension of the digits at the metatarsophalangeal and interphalangeal joints.

The fibularis longus and brevis muscles form the **lateral compartment of the leg**. The fibularis longus muscle travels along the lateral portion of the leg, crossing onto the plantar aspect of the foot, before inserting onto the first metatarsal and medial cuneiform bones. The fibularis brevis muscle inserts onto the tuberosity of the fifth metatarsal bone. The fibularis longus and brevis muscles are both evertors of the foot (occurring at the subtalar joint), therefore functioning to elevate the lateral border of the foot on contraction.

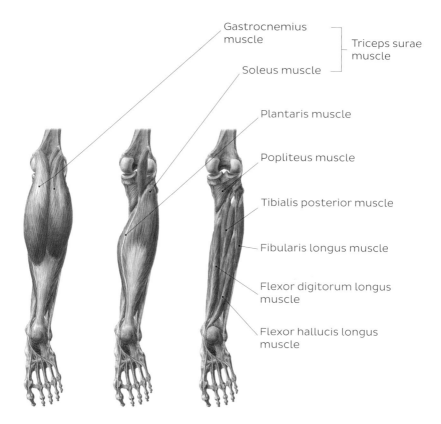

Gastrocnemius muscle

Triceps surae muscle

Soleus muscle

Plantaris muscle

Popliteus muscle

Tibialis posterior muscle

Fibularis longus muscle

Flexor digitorum longus muscle

Flexor hallucis longus muscle

FIGURE 3.18. Muscles of the leg (posterior view). The posterior compartment of the leg can be divided into superficial and deep parts by the transverse intermuscular septum. The **superficial muscles** of the posterior leg include the gastrocnemius, soleus and plantaris. The large gastrocnemius and soleus collectively form the **triceps surae muscle** which is a powerful plantar flexor of the foot at the ankle joint. A large shared common tendon, the calcaneal tendon (a.k.a. **Achilles tendon**), extends from the muscle bellies of the triceps surae muscle to insert onto the posterior aspect of the calcaneus. The plantaris muscle has a short belly and a long tendon which extends along the posterior leg to also insert onto the posterior calcaneus. This muscle contributes to proprioception during plantarflexion of the ankle joint.

The **deep muscles** of the posterior leg comprise four muscles: The popliteus, flexor digitorum longus, flexor hallucis longus, and tibialis posterior. The short popliteus muscle acts on the knee joint, while the rest of the deep muscles of the posterior leg contribute to plantarflexion of the foot at the ankle joint, in addition to other individual functions. The flexor digitorum longus and flexor hallucis longus muscles also contribute to flexion of the toes at the metatarsophalangeal and interphalangeal joints.

Anterior leg muscles	Origin	Insertion	Innervation	Function
Tibialis anterior	Lateral tibial condyle, proximal half of lateral surface of tibia, Interosseous membrane	Medial cuneiform bone, Base of metatarsal bone 1	Deep fibular nerve (L4, L5)	**Talocrural Joint**: foot dorsiflexion; **Subtalar joint**: foot inversion; supports medial longitudinal arch of foot
Extensor hallucis longus	(Middle third of) Medial surface of fibula, Interosseous membrane	Base of distal phalanx of great toe		**Metatarsophalangeal and interphalangeal joint 1**: toe extension; **Talocrural joint**: foot dorsiflexion
Extensor digitorum longus	(Proximal half of) Medial surface of fibula, Lateral tibial condyle, Interosseous membrane	Distal and middle phalanges of digits 2-5	Deep fibular nerve (L5, S1)	**Metatarsophalangeal and interphalangeal joints 2-5**: toe extension; **Talocrural joint**: foot dorsiflexion; **Subtalar joint**: foot eversion
Fibularis tertius	(Distal third of) Medial surface of fibula, Anterior intermuscular septum	Dorsal surface of base of metatarsal bone 5		**Talocrural joint**: foot dorsiflexion; **Subtalar joint**: foot eversion

Lateral leg muscles	Origin	Insertion	Innervation	Function
Fibularis longus	Head of fibula, Proximal 2/3 of lateral surface of fibula, Anterior and posterior intermuscular septa	Medial cuneiform bone, Metatarsal bone 1	Superficial fibular nerve (L5, S1)	**Talocrural joint**: foot plantar flexion; **Subtalar joint**: foot eversion; supports longitudinal and transverse arches of foot
Fibularis brevis	Distal 2/3 of lateral surface of fibula, Anterior intermuscular septum	Tuberosity of metatarsal bone 5		**Talocrural joint**: foot plantar flexion; **Subtalar joint**: foot eversion

LOWER LIMB

Posterior leg muscles	Origin	Insertion	Innervation	Function
Gastrocnemius	**Lateral head**: posterolateral surface of lateral femoral condyle; **Medial head**: posterior surface of medial femoral condyle, Popliteal surface of femoral shaft	Posterior surface of calcaneus (via calcaneal tendon)	Tibial nerve (S1, S2)	**Talocrural joint**: foot plantar flexion; **Knee joint**: leg flexion
Soleus	Soleal line, Medial border of tibia, Head of fibula, Posterior border of fibula			**Talocrural joint**: foot plantar flexion; **Subtalar joint**: foot eversion
Plantaris	Lateral supracondylar line of femur, Oblique popliteal ligament of knee			**Talocrural joint**: foot plantar flexion; **Knee joint**: knee flexion
Popliteus	Lateral condyle of femur, Posterior horn of lateral meniscus of knee joint	Posterior surface of proximal tibia	Tibial nerve (L4–S1)	Unlocks knee joint; Knee joint stabilization
Tibialis posterior	Posterior surface of tibia, Posterior surface of fibula, Interosseous membrane	Tuberosity of navicular bone, All cuneiform bones, bases of metatarsal bones 2-4 (Cuboid bone)	Tibial nerve (L4, L5)	**Talocrural joint**: foot plantar flexion; **Subtalar joint**: foot inversion; supports medial longitudinal arch of foot
Flexor digitorum longus	Posterior surface of tibia, (inferior to soleal line)	Bases of distal phalanges of digits 2-5	Tibial nerve (L5–S2)	**Metatarsophalangeal and interphalangeal joints 2–5**: toe flexion; **Talocrural joint**: foot plantar flexion; **Subtalar joint**: foot inversion
Flexor hallucis longus	(Distal 2/3 of) Posterior surface of fibula, Interosseous membrane, Posterior intermuscular septum, Fascia of tibialis posterior muscle	Base of distal phalanx of great toe	Tibial nerve (S2, S3)	**Metatarsophalangeal and interphalangeal joint 1**: toe flexion; **Talocrural joint**: foot plantar flexion; **Subtalar joint**: foot inversion

Leg muscles

Learn the muscles of the leg fast with these quizzes diagrams and labeling exercises

3d muscle anatomy videos

LOWER LIMB

BONES OF THE FOOT

The human foot contains 26 bones that are divided into 3 groups. The most proximal are the tarsal bones, which consist of seven irregularly shaped short bones, homologous to the carpal bones of the hand. Next are the five long metatarsal bones which are equivalent to the metacarpals of the hand. Finally, the phalanges of the foot form the toes in an identical manner to which the phalanges of the hand form the fingers. The lateral four toes are made up of three phalanges (proximal, middle and distal), while the great toe consists of only two phalanges (proximal and distal).

The foot can also be divided into 3 regions; the hindfoot, midfoot and forefoot. The tarsal bones are contained in the hindfoot and midfoot, while the metatarsals and phalanges lie in the forefoot.

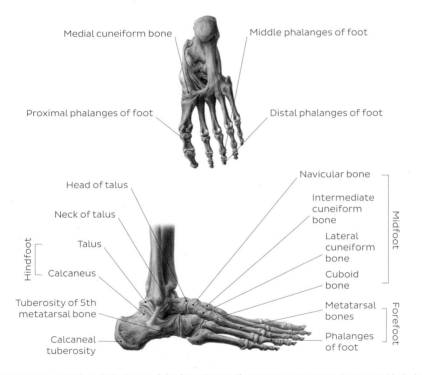

FIGURE 3.19. **Overview of the bones of the foot.** The hindfoot is the most proximal group and includes only two bones: The **talus** and **calcaneus**. The talus forms the ankle joint superiorly with the tibia and fibula, while the calcaneus forms the heel. Anterior to the talus and calcaneus are the next set of tarsal bones, which belong to the midfoot: The **navicular**, **cuboid** and three **cuneiform bones** (lateral, intermediate and medial). The last group of bones make up the forefoot and include the **metatarsal bones** and **phalanges**. There are three consecutive sets of phalanges for each toe (proximal, middle and distal), except for the great toe that contains two phalanges (proximal and distal).

Key points about the bones of the foot

Bones	**Tarsal bones**: talus, calcaneus, navicular, medial cuneiform, intermediate cuneiform, lateral cuneiform, cuboid
	Metatarsal bones 1-5
	Phalanges of foot: proximal, middle and distal phalanx (toes 2-5); proximal and distal phalanx (great toe)
Joints	**Talocrural joint**: talus ↔ tibia/fibula (a.k.a. ankle joint)
	Subtalar joint: talus ↔ calcaneus
	Calcaneocuboid joint: calcaneus ↔ cuboid
	Talonavicular joint: talus ↔ navicular bone
	Tarsometatarsal joints: medial, intermediate and lateral cuneiform, cuboid bones ↔ metatarsal bones
	Metatarsophalangeal joints: metatarsal bones ↔ proximal phalanges
	Proximal interphalangeal joints: proximal phalanges ↔ middle phalanges
	Distal interphalangeal joints: middle phalanges ↔ distal phalanges

Ankle and foot anatomy

Talus

Calcaneus

Navicular bone

Cuboid

LOWER LIMB

TALUS

The **talus** is the most proximal bone of the foot that belongs to the group of bones collectively known as the **tarsus**. It articulates with four bones: The tibia, fibula, calcaneus and navicular. In articulating with the tibia and fibula superiorly, the talus forms the **ankle/talocrural joint** and thereby establishes a link between the leg and the foot. Inferiorly, the talus articulates with the calcaneus forming the **subtalar/talocalcaneal joint**, while anteriorly it articulates with the navicular bone where it forms the talonavicular joint. In these articulations, the talus represents the cornerstone of the longitudinal arch formed by the tarsal and metatarsal bones, that transmits the entire weight of the body evenly to the heel and forefoot when standing.

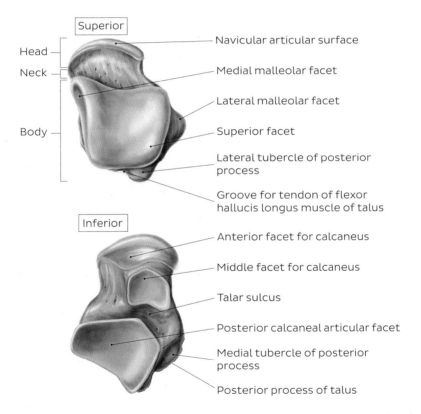

Superior

Head
Neck
Body

Navicular articular surface

Medial malleolar facet

Lateral malleolar facet

Superior facet

Lateral tubercle of posterior process

Groove for tendon of flexor hallucis longus muscle of talus

Inferior

Anterior facet for calcaneus

Middle facet for calcaneus

Talar sulcus

Posterior calcaneal articular facet

Medial tubercle of posterior process

Posterior process of talus

FIGURE 3.20. Talus (superior and inferior views). The talus consists of three main parts: **Head, neck** and **body**. The head of the talus is the most distal part and presents the **navicular articular surface**. The inferior aspect of the head of the talus features the **anterior and middle facets**, which articulate with corresponding facets on the calcaneus.

Proximal to the head is the neck of the talus. The superior surface of the neck of talus is unremarkable while the inferior surface of the neck of talus contains a deep trough known as the **talar sulcus**.

The most proximal and largest part of the talus is the body. The most prominent feature on the superior surface of the body of talus is the **trochlea of talus** which contains the saddle-shaped **superior facet**. The superior facet articulates with the inferior articular surface of the tibia contributing to the formation of the ankle joint. The posterior aspect of the body contains the **posterior process** bearing the medial and lateral tubercles which are separated by the groove for the tendon of flexor hallucis longus muscle.

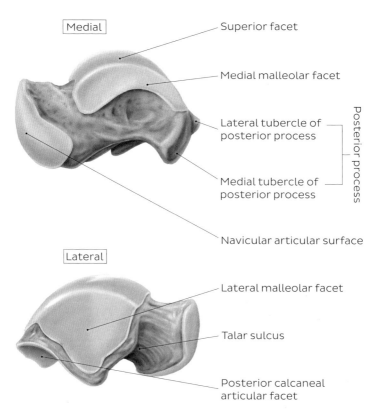

FIGURE 3.21. **Talus (medial and lateral views).** The **navicular articular surface** of the head of talus is best appreciated from the medial aspect of the talus. As its name suggests, it articulates with the articular surface of the navicular bone to form the talonavicular joint.

On the lateral view, the **talar sulcus** of the neck is clearly seen, which forms the tarsal sinus when joined with the calcaneal sulcus of the calcaneus.

On the medial and lateral sides of the body, the talus bears a **medial** and **lateral malleolar facet** that serve as articular surfaces for the medial and lateral malleoli, respectively. The lateral malleolar facet is a concave, triangular area that encloses the trochlea laterally. The medial malleolar facet is a smooth crescent shaped area that encloses the trochlea medially. The **medial** and **lateral tubercles** of the posterior process of the body of the talus provide attachment sites for the medial and posterior talocalcaneal ligaments and the posterior talofibular ligament.

Key points about the talus	
Surfaces	Superior, inferior, medial, lateral, posterior
Bony landmarks and articular surfaces	**Head of talus**: navicular articular surface
	Neck of talus: talar sulcus, tarsal sinus
	Body of talus: trochlea of talus, posterior process of talus, medial tubercle, lateral tubercle, groove for tendon of flexor hallucis longus muscle of talus, medial malleolar surface, lateral malleolar surface
Articulations	**Ankle/talocrural joint**: talus ↔ tibia, fibula
	Subtalar joint: talus ↔ calcaneus
	Talonavicular joint: talus ↔ navicular bone
Articular surfaces	**Ankle joint**: lateral malleolar surface of talus, medial malleolar surface of talus
	Subtalar joint: anterior, middle and posterior facets for calcaneus
	Talonavicuar joint: navicular articular surface

CALCANEUS

The calcaneus, also known as the heel bone, is the largest of the foot bones that sits just below the talus. It articulates with two bones, the talus and cuboid bone, forming the subtalar and calcaneonavicular joints, respectively.

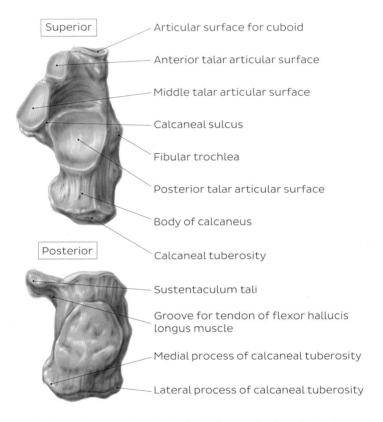

Superior

Articular surface for cuboid

Anterior talar articular surface

Middle talar articular surface

Calcaneal sulcus

Fibular trochlea

Posterior talar articular surface

Body of calcaneus

Posterior

Calcaneal tuberosity

Sustentaculum tali

Groove for tendon of flexor hallucis longus muscle

Medial process of calcaneal tuberosity

Lateral process of calcaneal tuberosity

FIGURE 3.22. **Calcaneus (superior and posterior views).** The superior view of the calcaneus presents with a number of articular surfaces which participate in the formation of the joints of the foot and ankle. One of them is the **posterior talar articular surface**, located along the dorsal surface of the calcaneus. It represents one of the three surfaces on the calcaneus that articulate with the talus, with the other two being the **anterior** and **middle talar articular surfaces**, which can be observed anteromedially.

The large **calcaneal tuberosity** forms the heel of the foot and is the attachment site for the long calcaneal tendon. The inferior aspect of the calcaneal tuberosity presents with a **medial** and **lateral process**, which are important attachment points for the muscles of the foot. From the posterior view, the **sustentaculum tali** can also be observed. This is a large shelf-like projection found along the posteromedial aspect of the calcaneus. It supports the head of the talus and contains the **groove for the flexor hallucis longus muscle** on its inferior surface.

LOWER LIMB

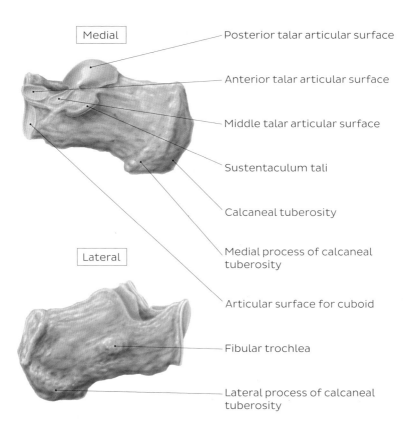

Medial

Posterior talar articular surface

Anterior talar articular surface

Middle talar articular surface

Sustentaculum tali

Calcaneal tuberosity

Lateral

Medial process of calcaneal tuberosity

Articular surface for cuboid

Fibular trochlea

Lateral process of calcaneal tuberosity

FIGURE 3.23. **Calcaneus (medial and lateral views).** On the medial view, the anterior process of the calcaneus features the **cuboid articular surface**, which articulates with the cuboid bone to form the calcaneocuboid joint. The **anterior and middle talar articular surfaces** articulate with their calcaneal counterparts and contribute to the formation of the talocalcaneonavicular joint of the tarsus. Posterior to the anterior talar articular surface is the aforementioned **sustentaculum tali**.

Along the lateral surface of the calcaneus is a small prominence known as the **fibular trochlea**. It is typically located between the tendons of the fibularis longus and brevis muscles and serves as a second pulley for the fibularis tendons.

Key points about the calcaneus	
Surfaces	Superior, medial, lateral, inferior
Bony landmarks	Calcaneal sulcus, sustentaculum tali, groove for the tendon of flexor hallucis longus, fibular trochlea, calcaneal tuberosity, medial and lateral process of calcaneal tuberosity, anterior process of calcaneus
Articulations	**Subtalar joint**: talus ↔ calcaneus **Calcaneocuboid joint**: calcaneus ↔ cuboid bone
Articular surfaces	Anterior/middle/posterior articular surface, articular surface for cuboid

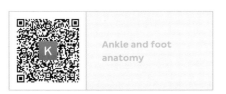

Ankle and foot anatomy

Learning strategies/ use these bones of the foot quizzes to master your identification skills

ANKLE JOINT

The **ankle joint** (a.k.a. talocrural joint) is formed by the articular surfaces of the distal parts (malleoli) of the tibia and fibula and the body of the talus and is classified as a type of synovial hinge joint. It is supported by a complex set of strong ligaments providing it with stabilization to manage the entire body weight against the ground forces below.

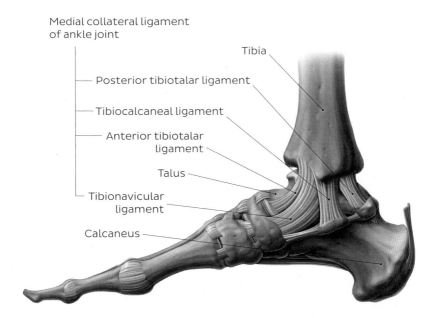

Medial collateral ligament of ankle joint

Posterior tibiotalar ligament

Tibiocalcaneal ligament

Anterior tibiotalar ligament

Tibionavicular ligament

Calcaneus

Tibia

Talus

FIGURE 3.24. Ankle joint (medial view). Considering its role in bearing the entire weight of the body, it is not surprising that the ankle joint has quite a few ligaments that stabilize it during movement. The ligaments are divided into two groups: The medial (tibial) and lateral (fibular) collateral ligaments. The **medial collateral ligament**, also known as the **deltoid ligament**, is a strong band that reinforces the medial aspect of the joint and prevents dislocations of the ankle joint. The ligament has a proximal attachment on the medial malleolus of the tibia, and fans out from there to insert onto the navicular bone, calcaneus, and talus. Consequently, the medial collateral ligament consists of 4 parts: The **tibionavicular ligament**, extending from the tibia to the navicular bone, the **tibiocalcaneal ligament** stretching from the tibia to the calcaneus, and **anterior** and **posterior tibiotalar ligaments**, extending from the tibia to the talus.

The ankle joint

Joints and ligaments of the foot

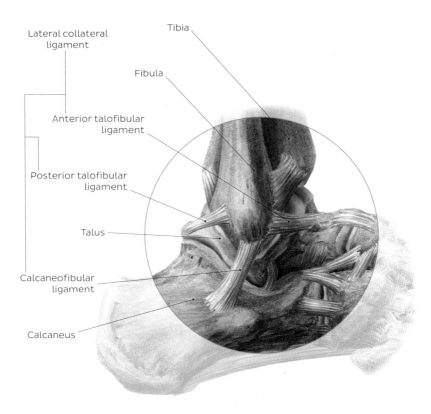

Lateral collateral ligament

Tibia

Fibula

Anterior talofibular ligament

Posterior talofibular ligament

Talus

Calcaneofibular ligament

Calcaneus

FIGURE 3.25. Ankle joint (lateral view). Similarly to the medial collateral ligament, the **lateral collateral ligament** is a strong compound ligament that reinforces the lateral aspect of the ankle joint. The ligament has a proximal attachment on the fibula and a distal attachment on the talus and calcaneus. The lateral collateral ligament is comprised of three distinct bands: The **anterior talofibular** and **posterior talofibular ligaments**, that extend between the fibula and talus, as well as the **calcaneofibular ligament**, that extends between the fibula and calcaneus.

Key points about the ankle joint	
Joint type	Synovial hinge joint; uniaxial
Articulating surfaces	Articular facet of medial malleolus **(tibia)**; articular facet of lateral malleolus **(fibula)**; trochlea, medial/lateral malleolar facets **(talus)**
Ligaments	**Medial collateral (deltoid)**: tibionavicular, tibiocalcaneal, anterior tibiotalar, posterior tibiotalar ligaments
	Lateral collateral: anterior talofibular, posterior talofibular, calcaneofibular ligaments
Movements	Dorsiflexion, plantar flexion

JOINTS AND LIGAMENTS OF THE FOOT

The foot has a complex structure with many bones and joints which require its numerous ligaments and supporting structures to help stabilize and enable optimal movement of the foot. The ligaments of the foot are categorized according to their associated joints, with each joint of the foot containing two or more ligaments. Conveniently, most ligaments are named according to their position relative to the joint they support e.g., dorsal, plantar and interosseous cuboideonavicular ligaments.

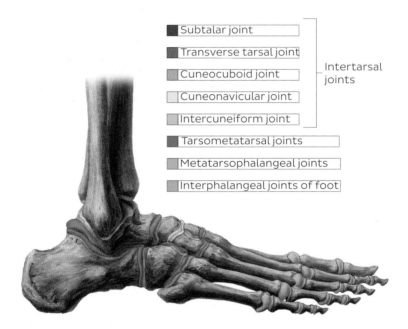

Subtalar joint	
Transverse tarsal joint	
Cuneocuboid joint	Intertarsal joints
Cuneonavicular joint	
Intercuneiform joint	
Tarsometatarsal joints	
Metatarsophalangeal joints	
Interphalangeal joints of foot	

FIGURE 3.26. Joints of the foot (right foot, lateral view). The anatomical **subtalar joint** (a.k.a. talocalcaneal joint) is formed between the inferior surface of the body of the talus and posterior articular surface of the calcaneus. The **transverse tarsal joint** (a.k.a. midtarsal joint) is an S-shaped joint which connects the hindfoot and midfoot. It is a compound joint composed of two smaller joints, the talocalcaneonavicular and calcaneocuboid joints.

Distally, there are a number of smaller **intertarsal joints** between the cuboid, navicular and cuneiform bones, namely the cuboideonavicular, cuneocuboid, cuneonavicular and intercuneiform joints.

There are three **tarsometatarsal joints**: A medial joint involving the medial cuneiform and first metatarsal bones, a middle joint formed by intermediate and lateral cuneiform bones with the second and third metatarsal bones, and a lateral joint between the cuboid and fourth and fifth metatarsal bones. The joints between the heads of the metatarsal bones and bases of the proximal phalanges of the toes are known as **metatarsophalangeal joints**, while those found between contiguous phalanges are termed **interphalangeal joints**.

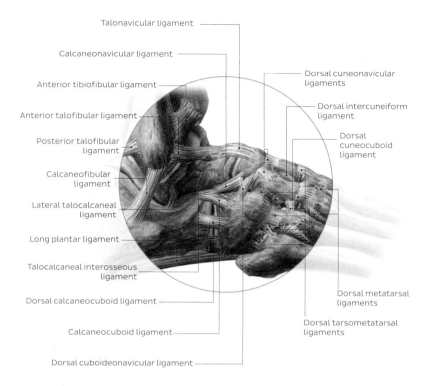

Talonavicular ligament

Calcaneonavicular ligament

Anterior tibiofibular ligament

Anterior talofibular ligament

Posterior talofibular ligament

Calcaneofibular ligament

Lateral talocalcaneal ligament

Long plantar ligament

Talocalcaneal interosseous ligament

Dorsal calcaneocuboid ligament

Calcaneocuboid ligament

Dorsal cuboideonavicular ligament

Dorsal cuneonavicular ligaments

Dorsal intercuneiform ligament

Dorsal cuneocuboid ligament

Dorsal metatarsal ligaments

Dorsal tarsometatarsal ligaments

FIGURE 3.27. Ligaments of the foot (lateral view). The joints of the foot are supported by several plantar, dorsal and interosseous ligaments.

From this lateral perspective, several notable ligaments can be identified:

The lateral, anterior and interosseous **talocalcaneal ligaments** provide support to the subtalar joint, while dorsally, the transverse tarsal joint is supported by the calcaneonavicular and calcaneocuboid ligaments (which collectively are referred as the **bifurcate ligament**) as well as the talonavicular and dorsal calcaneocuboid ligaments. Several additional ligaments can be seen supporting the dorsal aspect of the joints of the midfoot and tarsometatarsal joints.

Ankle and foot anatomy

Joints and ligaments of the foot

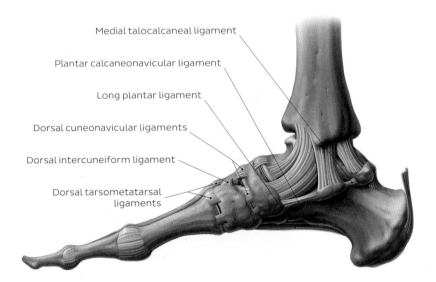

Medial talocalcaneal ligament

Plantar calcaneonavicular ligament

Long plantar ligament

Dorsal cuneonavicular ligaments

Dorsal intercuneiform ligament

Dorsal tarsometatarsal ligaments

FIGURE 3.28. Ligaments of the foot (medial view). From this medial perspective, the **plantar calca-neonavicular ligament** (a.k.a. spring ligament) is of particular interest. It extends between the sustentaculum tali and medioplantar margin of the posterior surface of the navicular bone, filling a wedge-shaped gap between these structures. It functions to stabilize the medial longitudinal arch of the foot and supports the head of the talus within the talocalcaneonavicular joint.

Also visible is the **long plantar ligament** which extends from the plantar surface of the calcaneus to the cuboid and second-fourth/fifth metatarsal bones. It supports the transverse tarsal joint and longitudinal arches of the foot.

Key points about the joints and ligaments the foot	
Talocalcaneal joint	Medial, lateral, posterior, interosseous and anterior talocalcaneal ligaments
Talocalcaneo-navicular joint	[Dorsal] talonavicular ligament, plantar calcaneonavicular ligament
Calcaneocuboid joint	Calcaneocuboid, dorsal calcaneocuboid, plantar calcaneocuboid, long plantar ligaments
Cuboideonavicular joint	Dorsal cuboideonavicular, plantar cuboideonavicular, interosseous cuboideonavicular ligaments
Cuneonavicular joint	Dorsal cuneonavicular (3), plantar cuneonavicular (3), medial cuneonavicular ligaments
Cuneocuboid joints	Dorsal cuneocuboid, plantar cuneocuboid, interosseous cuneocuboid ligaments
Intercuneiform joints	Dorsal (2), interosseous (2) and plantar intercuneiform ligaments (1 or 2)

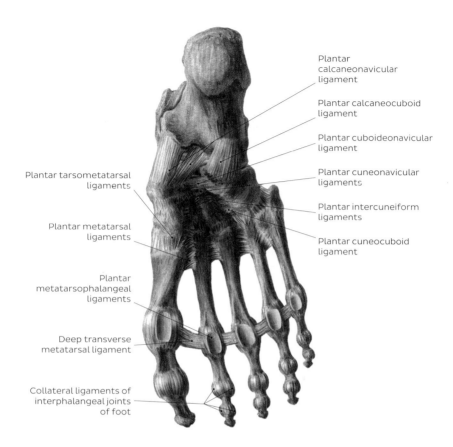

Plantar calcaneonavicular ligament

Plantar calcaneocuboid ligament

Plantar cuboideonavicular ligament

Plantar cuneonavicular ligaments

Plantar intercuneiform ligaments

Plantar cuneocuboid ligament

Plantar tarsometatarsal ligaments

Plantar metatarsal ligaments

Plantar metatarsophalangeal ligaments

Deep transverse metatarsal ligament

Collateral ligaments of interphalangeal joints of foot

FIGURE 3.29. Ligaments of the foot (plantar view). Right foot with long plantar ligament removed. The **major plantar ligaments** are the plantar calcaneonavicular ligament, the long plantar ligament and plantar calcaneocuboid ligament (a.k.a short plantar ligament). The latter of these extends between the anterior part of the plantar surface of the calcaneus to the plantar surface of the cuboid bone. It functions to stabilize the calcaneocuboid part of the transverse tarsal joint and supports the lateral longitudinal arch of the foot. Several **smaller plantar intertarsal ligaments** can be seen between the cuboid, navicular and cuneiform bones. **Plantar tarsometatarsal ligaments** stabilize the articulations between the cuneiform and cuboid bones with the bases of the metatarsal bones. The metatarsophalangeal and interphalangeal joints are strengthened by tight **collateral ligaments**, which prevent excessive range of movement in these joints.

Key points about the joints and ligaments the foot	
Tarsometatarsal joint	Dorsal and plantar tarsometatarsal, cuneometatarsal interosseous ligaments
Intermetatarsal joints	Dorsal, plantar and interosseous metatarsal ligaments
Metatarsophalangeal joints	Plantar and collateral metatarsophalangeal, deep transverse metatarsal ligaments
Interphalangeal joints of foot	Plantar and collateral interphalangeal ligaments

MUSCLES OF THE FOOT

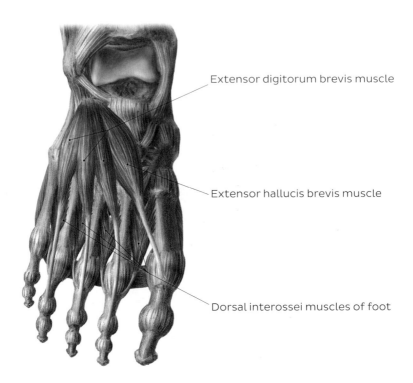

Extensor digitorum brevis muscle

Extensor hallucis brevis muscle

Dorsal interossei muscles of foot

FIGURE 3.30. **Dorsal muscles of the foot.** The dorsal muscles of the foot are composed of two muscles: The **extensor hallucis brevis** and **extensor digitorum brevis**. Both muscles originate from the superolateral surface of the calcaneus and extend distally across the dorsum of the foot, lateral to the tendons of their 'longus' counterparts.

The **dorsal interossei** are part of the fourth layer of plantar muscles of the foot, but are best viewed from this dorsal perspective. They are located between the metatarsal bones and consist of four bipennate muscles which arise from opposing surfaces of adjacent bones. The first (most medial) dorsal interosseous muscle inserts into the medial aspect of the base of the proximal phalanx of the second toe, while the lateral three muscles insert into the lateral aspect of the bases of the proximal phalanges of the toes 2-4.

Dorsal muscles	Origin	Insertion	Innervation	Function
Extensor digitorum brevis	Superolateral surface of calcaneus bone, interosseous talocalcaneal ligament; Stem of inferior extensor retinaculum	Extensor digitorum longus tendons of toes 2–4	Deep fibular nerve (L5,S1)	**Distal interphalangeal joints 2-4**: toe extension
Extensor hallucis brevis	Superolateral surface of calcaneus bone	Proximal phalanx of great toe		**Metatarsophalangeal joint 1**: toe extension

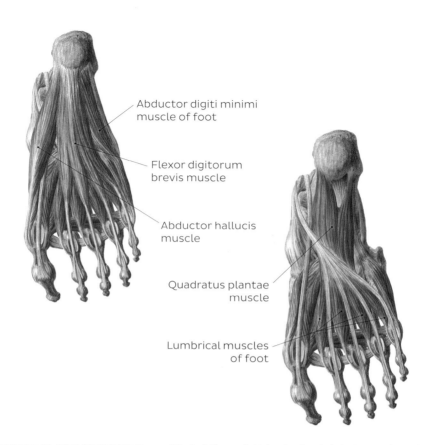

Abductor digiti minimi
muscle of foot

Flexor digitorum
brevis muscle

Abductor hallucis
muscle

Quadratus plantae
muscle

Lumbrical muscles
of foot

FIGURE 3.31. 1st and 2nd plantar layers of the foot. The medial, lateral and central plantar muscles can be alternatively classified according to four muscular layers. The first (left) and second (right) layers can be identified in this image. The **first layer** is composed of three muscles: The abductor hallucis (medial), flexor digitorum brevis (central) and abductor digiti minimi (lateral). All three extend distally from the calcaneal tuberosity to the toes and contribute to the maintenance of the concavity of the foot.

The **second layer** of plantar muscles consist of the quadratus plantae muscle and four lumbrical muscles, both of which belong to the central muscle group of the foot. Tendons of the flexor hallucis longus and flexor digitorum longus muscles run within the same plane as these muscles. The quadratus plantae muscle arises by a medial and lateral head from the calcaneus and inserts onto the lateral aspect of the tendon of the flexor digitorum longus muscle as it passes through this region.

The **four lumbrical muscles** arise from the tendons of the flexor digitorum longus muscle at their angles of separation, and insert onto the medial aspect of the extensor expansions of toes 2–5.

Dorsal muscles of the
foot

Central muscles of
the sole of the foot

Lateral muscles of
the sole of the foot

Medial muscles of the
sole of the foot

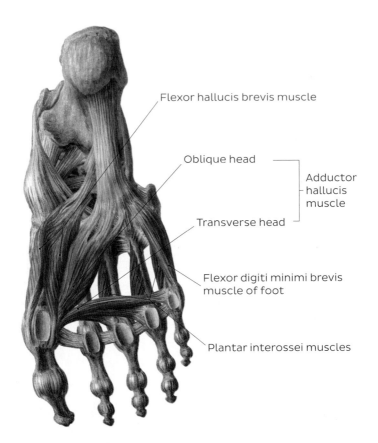

Flexor hallucis brevis muscle

Oblique head

Adductor hallucis muscle

Transverse head

Flexor digiti minimi brevis muscle of foot

Plantar interossei muscles

FIGURE 3.32. **3rd and 4th plantar layers of the foot.** The **third layer** is composed of the flexor hallucis brevis, adductor hallucis and flexor digiti minimi brevis muscles. The **flexor hallucis brevis** muscle arises from the cuboid via its lateral head and from the tendon of the tibialis posterior muscle and medial intermuscular septum via its medial head. Both heads run anteromedially towards the great toe, inserting onto each side of the base of the proximal phalanx of the hallux. The **adductor hallucis** muscle similarly arises by way of two heads: An oblique and transverse head. It's oblique head originates from the bases of metatarsal bones 2-4, cuboid, lateral cuneiform bones and the tendon of fibularis longus, while it's transverse head extends from the plantar metatarsophalangeal ligaments of toes 3-5 and deep transverse metatarsal ligaments to reach and attach onto the base of the proximal phalanx of the great toe. The **flexor digiti minimi brevis** muscle is part of the lateral muscle group and acts on the fifth toe. It originates from the base of metatarsal 5 and extends to insert onto the proximal phalanx of the little toe.

The **fourth layer** of plantar muscles consist of the plantar and dorsal interossei which are located in the central compartment of the foot. The **dorsal interossei** are best viewed from a dorsal perspective of the foot (see previous image).

The **plantar interossei** are three muscles which arise from the medial plantar aspect of the metatarsals 3-5, respectively and insert onto the medial bases of the proximal phalanges and extensor expansion of toes 3-5.

Medial plantar muscles	Origin	Insertion	Innervation	Function
Abductor hallucis	Medial process of calcaneal tuberosity, Flexor retinaculum, Plantar aponeurosis	Base of proximal phalanx of great toe	Medial plantar nerve (S1-S3)	**Metatarsophalangeal joint 1**: toe abduction, toe flexion; support of longitudinal arch of foot
Flexor hallucis brevis	Tendon of tibialis posterior, Medial cuneiform bone, Lateral cuneiform bone, Cuboid bone	Lateral and medial aspects of base of proximal phalanx of great toe	Medial plantar nerve (S1,S2)	**Metatarsophalangeal joint 1**: toe flexion; support of longitudinal arch of foot

Central plantar muscles	Origin	Insertion	Innervation	Function
Adductor hallucis	**Oblique head**: bases metatarsal bones 2-4, Cuboid bone, Lateral cuneiform bone, Tendon of fibularis longus muscle; **Transverse head**: plantar metatarsophalangeal & deep transverse metatarsal ligaments of toes 3-5	Lateral aspect of base of proximal phalanx of great toe	Lateral plantar nerve (S2,S3)	**Metatarsophalangeal joint 1**: toe adduction, toe flexion; support of longitudinal and transverse arches of foot
Flexor digitorum brevis	Medial process of calcaneal tuberosity, Plantar aponeurosis	Middle phalanges of digits 2-5	Medial plantar nerve (S1-S3)	**Metatarsophalangeal joints 2-5**: toe flexion; supports longitudinal arch of foot
Quadratus plantae	Medial surface of calcaneus bone, Lateral process of calcaneal tuberosity	Tendon of flexor digitorum longus	Lateral plantar nerve (S1-S3)	**Metatarsophalangeal joints 2-5**: toe flexion
Lumbricals (4)	Tendons of flexor digitorum longus	Medial bases of proximal phalanges and extensor expansion of digits 2-5	Lumbrical 1: medial plantar nerve (S2,S3); lumbricals 2-4: lateral plantar nerve (S2-S3)	**Metatarsophalangeal joints 2-5**: toe flexion, toes adduction; **Interphalangeal joints 2-5**: toes extension
Plantar interossei (3)	Medial aspects of metatarsal bones 3-5	Medial bases of proximal phalanges and extensor expansion of digits 3-5		**Metatarsophalangeal joints 3-5**: toe flexion, toes adduction; **Interphalangeal joints 3-5**: toes extension
Dorsal interossei (4)	Opposing sides of metatarsal bones 1-5	**1**: medial base of proximal phalanx of digit 2 **2-4**: lateral bases of proximal phalanges and extensor expansion of digits 2-4	Lateral plantar nerve (S2-S3)	**Metatarsophalangeal joints 2-4**: toe flexion, toe abduction; **Interphalangeal joints 2-4**: toe extension

LOWER LIMB

Lateral plantar muscles	Origin	Insertion	Innervation	Function
Abductor digiti minimi	Calcaneal tuberosity, Plantar aponeurosis	Base of proximal phalanx of digit 5, Metatarsal bone 5	Lateral plantar nerve (S1-S3)	**Metatarsophalangeal joint 5**: toe abduction, toe flexion; supports longitudinal arch of foot
Flexor digiti minimi brevis	Base of metatarsal bone 5, Long plantar ligament	Base of proximal phalanx of digit 5	Lateral plantar nerve (S2-S3)	**Metatarsophalangeal joint 5**: toe flexion
Opponens digiti minimi	Long plantar ligament, Base of metatarsal bone 5, Tendon sheath of fibularis longus	Lateral border of metatarsal bone 5	Lateral plantar nerve (S2-S3)	**Metatarsophalangeal joint 5**: toe abduction, toe flexion

The plantar muscles of the foot can also be organized into four layers:

Plantar muscles: layers	
First layer	Abductor hallucis
	Flexor digitorum brevis
	Abductor digiti minimi
Second layer	Quadratus plantae
	Lumbricals
Third layer	Flexor hallucis brevis
	Adductor hallucis
	Flexor digiti minimi brevis
Fourth layer	Plantar and dorsal interossei

LOWER LIMB

NEUROVASCULATURE OF THE HIP AND THIGH

The blood supply for the hip and thigh mainly arises from the **internal iliac** and **femoral arteries**. The internal iliac artery gives rise to the superior gluteal, inferior gluteal and obturator arteries. They mainly supply the gluteal region, but some of their branches also supply the thigh area. The femoral artery is a continuation of the external iliac artery after it enters the femoral triangle and is the main supplier of the structures of the thigh. The region is drained mainly by the **femoral vein** with its two main tributaries: The **deep femoral** and **great saphenous veins**. Both muscular and cutaneous innervation of the hip and thigh comes from the nerves of the **lumbar** (L1-L4) and **sacral** (L4-S4) plexuses.

LOWER LIMB

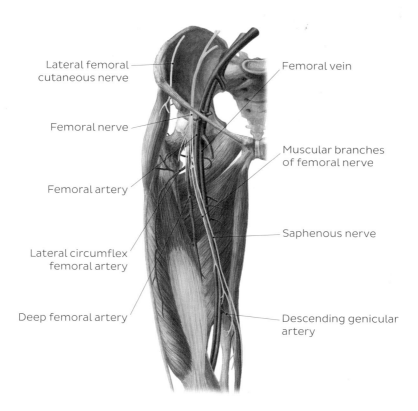

Lateral femoral cutaneous nerve

Femoral nerve

Femoral artery

Lateral circumflex femoral artery

Deep femoral artery

Femoral vein

Muscular branches of femoral nerve

Saphenous nerve

Descending genicular artery

FIGURE 3.33. Anterior view. The main supplier of arterial blood to the thigh and leg is the **femoral artery**. This artery starts at the level of the inguinal ligament, descending through the femoral triangle and along the anteromedial thigh. Once reaching the distal thigh it passes through the adductor canal and then passes through the adductor hiatus to take a posterior position in the popliteal fossa, where it becomes the popliteal artery. A major branch of the femoral artery is the **deep femoral artery**, also sometimes termed the deep artery of thigh or profundus femoris artery. It descends alongside the femoral artery, giving off many smaller branches which supply the hip region (circumflex arteries) and muscles of the posterior and medial thigh (perforating femoral arteries).

Traveling alongside the femoral artery is the **femoral vein**, which drains blood received from the popliteal vein, great saphenous vein, deep femoral vein and their respective tributaries throughout the thigh. Also traveling alongside the femoral artery is the **femoral nerve** which provides muscular and cutaneous innervation to the hip and anterior thigh. The medial thigh is predominantly supplied by the obturator nerve.

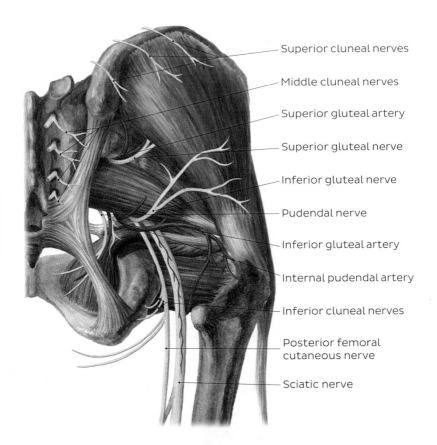

Superior cluneal nerves

Middle cluneal nerves

Superior gluteal artery

Superior gluteal nerve

Inferior gluteal nerve

Pudendal nerve

Inferior gluteal artery

Internal pudendal artery

Inferior cluneal nerves

Posterior femoral cutaneous nerve

Sciatic nerve

FIGURE 3.34. Posterior view. Arterial supply to the lower limb starts in the pelvis with the common iliac artery. This quickly splits into two divisions, the external iliac artery and the internal iliac artery. The internal iliac artery provides branches to the pelvic and gluteal regions, as seen here with the **superior and inferior gluteal arteries**, while the external iliac artery continues to descend into the thigh as the femoral artery. The hip itself is supplied by a periarticular anastomosis, formed by branches of the femoral artery (the medial and lateral circumflex femoral arteries), and branches of the internal iliac artery (the obturator, superior gluteal and inferior gluteal arteries). The posterior thigh is supplied by branches of the femoral artery, specifically by **perforating arteries**, which branch from the deep femoral artery.

Innervation to the posterior hip and thigh regions is supplied either by direct branches from the sacral plexus (such as the posterior femoral cutaneous nerve and the gluteal nerves) or by muscular branches of the **sciatic nerve**, which arise before its bifurcation into the common fibular nerve and tibial nerve. The sciatic nerve does not provide any cutaneous innervation to the posterior thigh;, instead this is provided solely by cutaneous nerves, the **posterior femoral cutaneous nerve** (sacral plexus) and by the anterior and lateral femoral cutaneous nerves (lumbar plexus).

Key points about neurovasculature of the hip and thigh	
Arteries	**External iliac artery**: deep circumflex iliac artery, femoral artery, superficial epigastric artery, superficial circumflex iliac artery, deep femoral artery, medial circumflex femoral artery, lateral circumflex femoral artery, descending genicular artery
	Internal iliac artery: obturator artery, superior gluteal artery, inferior gluteal artery
Veins (tributaries)	**Superficial**: great saphenous vein, accessory saphenous vein
	Deep: femoral vein, deep femoral vein, medial/lateral circumflex femoral veins

Key points about neurovasculature of the hip and thigh	
Nerves	**Lumbar plexus**: lateral femoral cutaneous nerve, accessory obturator nerve, obturator nerve, femoral nerve (saphenous nerve), superior cluneal nerves
	Sacral plexus: superior gluteal nerve, inferior gluteal nerve, posterior femoral cutaneous nerve (inferior cluneal nerves), sciatic nerve (tibial nerve, common fibular nerve), medial cluneal nerves

Muscular innervation

Femoral nerve	Quadriceps femoris, pectineus, sartorius
Sciatic nerve	Biceps femoris, semimembranosus, semitendinosus and ischiocondylar part of adductor magnus
Obturator nerve	Adductor brevis, adductor longus, gracilis, obturator externus, adductor part of adductor magnus
Superior gluteal nerve	Tensor fasciae latae, gluteus minimus, gluteus medius
Inferior gluteal nerve	Gluteus maximus

Cutaneous innervation

Femoral nerve	Anterior and medial thigh (anterior cutaneous branches)
Saphenous nerve	Area over course of saphenous vein; articular branches to hip and knee joints
Lateral femoral cutaneous nerve	Lateral thigh
Posterior femoral cutaneous nerve	Lower border of gluteus maximus, posterior and medial thigh
Obturator nerve	Proximal part of medial thigh
Superior cluneal nerves	Superolateral buttocks
Medial cluneal nerves	Medial buttocks
Inferior cluneal nerves	Inferior buttocks

Lower extremities arteries and nerves

Hip and thigh anatomy

FEMORAL ARTERY AND ITS BRANCHES

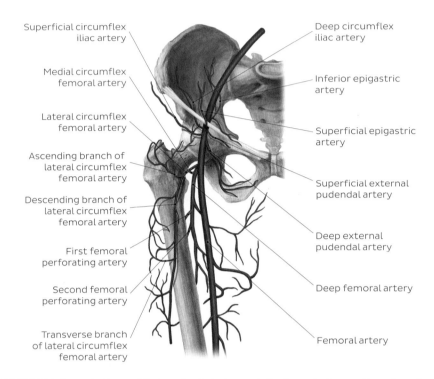

Superficial circumflex iliac artery

Medial circumflex femoral artery

Lateral circumflex femoral artery

Ascending branch of lateral circumflex femoral artery

Descending branch of lateral circumflex femoral artery

First femoral perforating artery

Second femoral perforating artery

Transverse branch of lateral circumflex femoral artery

Deep circumflex iliac artery

Inferior epigastric artery

Superficial epigastric artery

Superficial external pudendal artery

Deep external pudendal artery

Deep femoral artery

Femoral artery

FIGURE 3.35. **Femoral artery and its branches (anterior view).** The femoral artery continues from the external iliac artery after it passes the inguinal ligament. It gives off several branches, including the superficial epigastric, superficial circumflex iliac, superficial external pudendal, deep external pudendal, deep femoral and the descending genicular artery. The **deep femoral artery** in turn gives off the lateral and medial circumflex femoral arteries as well as the perforating femoral arteries. The femoral artery continues into the leg as the **popliteal artery**.

Key points about the femoral artery	
Pathway of the femoral artery	**Origin**: continuation of the external iliac artery after inguinal ligament
	Pathway: descends the anterior thigh
	Termination: popliteal artery
Main branches of the femoral artery	Superficial epigastric, superficial circumflex iliac, superficial external pudendal, deep external pudendal, deep femoral, lateral circumflex artery of the thigh, medial circumflex artery of the thigh, descending genicular artery

Femoral artery

Sciatic nerve

SCIATIC NERVE AND ITS BRANCHES

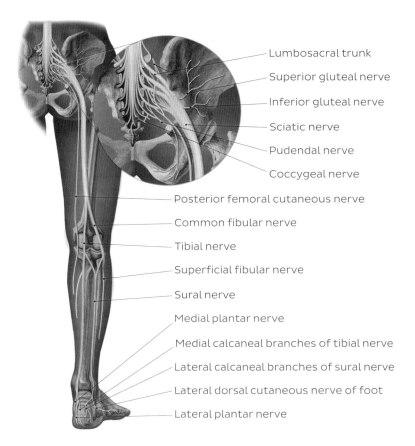

- Lumbosacral trunk
- Superior gluteal nerve
- Inferior gluteal nerve
- Sciatic nerve
- Pudendal nerve
- Coccygeal nerve
- Posterior femoral cutaneous nerve
- Common fibular nerve
- Tibial nerve
- Superficial fibular nerve
- Sural nerve
- Medial plantar nerve
- Medial calcaneal branches of tibial nerve
- Lateral calcaneal branches of sural nerve
- Lateral dorsal cutaneous nerve of foot
- Lateral plantar nerve

FIGURE 3.36. **Overview of the sciatic nerve.** The sciatic nerve is formed within the pelvis from the **anterior rami of spinal nerves L4–S3**. It enters the lower limb by traveling through the greater sciatic foramen of the posterior pelvis and inferior to, or occasionally through, the piriformis muscle. After passing into the free lower limb, the sciatic nerve passes down the posterior thigh supplying innervation to the hip joint, hamstring muscles and ischiocondylar part of the adductor magnus muscle. Just above the level of the knee, the sciatic nerve divides into its two **terminal branches**: The tibial nerve and the common fibular/peroneal nerve.

The **tibial nerve** supplies motor and sensory innervation to the posterior leg and foot. The major branches of the tibial nerve are the sural nerve and the medial and lateral plantar nerves. The **common fibular nerve** quickly divides into the deep fibular nerve and the superficial fibular nerve; these nerves provide motor and sensory supply to the anterolateral aspects of the leg and the dorsum of the foot.

Key points about the sciatic nerve	
Pathway of the sciatic nerve	**Origin**: spinal nerves L4–S3
	Pathway: enters thigh between ischial tuberosity and greater trochanter of femur, descends through posterior compartment of thigh
	Termination: tibial nerve, common fibular nerve
Main branches of the sciatic nerve	**Common fibular nerve**: superficial fibular nerve, deep fibular nerve
	Tibial nerve: sural nerve, medial calcaneal branches, lateral calcaneal branches (of sural nerve), medial and lateral plantar nerves

NEUROVASCULATURE OF THE LEG AND KNEE

The neurovasculature of the knee and leg can be organized around three main structures:

- The **popliteal artery** is the major contributor to arterial supply of this region giving off several branches to the leg (e.g. anterior tibial artery, posterior tibial artery, sural arteries) and genicular arteries around the region of the knee joint.
- The **popliteal vein** drains this region as far as up as the adductor canal. It receives the anterior and posterior tibial veins and other vessels such as the small saphenous vein that carries blood from the lateral surface of the leg. The great saphenous vein drains the medial surface of the leg.
- The **tibial and common fibular nerves** (terminal branches of the sciatic nerve) and their branches provide most of the motor and sensory supply to the leg. (Additional cutaneous innervation is also provided by the saphenous nerve, a terminal branch of the femoral nerve).

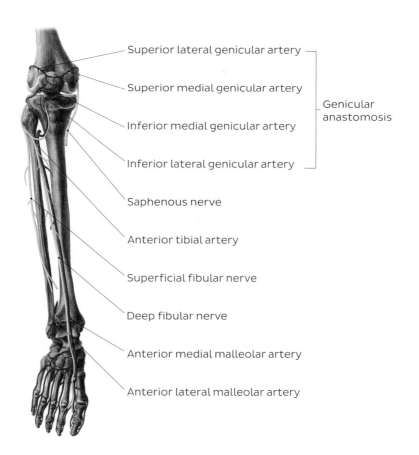

Superior lateral genicular artery ⎤

Superior medial genicular artery

Inferior medial genicular artery ⎬ Genicular anastomosis

Inferior lateral genicular artery ⎦

Saphenous nerve

Anterior tibial artery

Superficial fibular nerve

Deep fibular nerve

Anterior medial malleolar artery

Anterior lateral malleolar artery

FIGURE 3.37. The **anterior tibial artery** and its branches supply arterial blood to the anterior aspect of the leg. Arising from the popliteal artery, it passes from the posteriorly located popliteal fossa to the

LOWER LIMB

anterior leg via an oval aperture in the proximal part of the interosseous membrane, medial to the head of the fibula. The anterior tibial artery continues along the anterior aspect of the interosseous membrane between the tibia and fibula. In the region of the ankle joint, it gives off anterior medial and anterior lateral malleolar branches for supply of the ankle joint, terminating in the foot as the dorsalis pedis artery. The knee is supplied by a network of interlacing branches of the femoral and popliteal arteries, collectively this network is called the **genicular anastomosis**.

Venous drainage occurs via the dual action of deep and superficial venous systems, with the **anterior tibial veins** draining deep structures of the anterior leg and the great and short saphenous veins draining superficial structures. All lower limb veins eventually empty into the femoral vein.

The **common fibular nerve** along with its two branches, the superficial and deep fibular nerves, provides innervation to the lateral and anterior compartments of the leg, respectively. The common fibular is the smaller terminal branch of the sciatic nerve, the larger terminal branch being the tibial nerve.

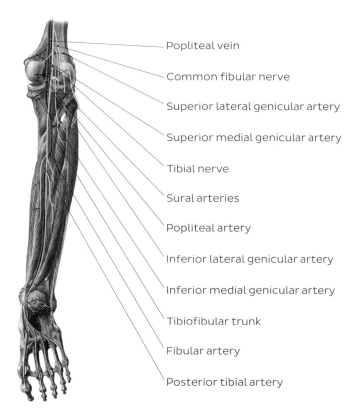

Popliteal vein

Common fibular nerve

Superior lateral genicular artery

Superior medial genicular artery

Tibial nerve

Sural arteries

Popliteal artery

Inferior lateral genicular artery

Inferior medial genicular artery

Tibiofibular trunk

Fibular artery

Posterior tibial artery

FIGURE 3.38. Posterior leg and popliteal fossa, with the **popliteal artery** and genicular anastomosis supplying the knee joint and related structures. Arterial blood to the posterior leg is provided by the **posterior tibial artery**, a continuation of the popliteal artery which gives off the fibular artery as it descends. It enters the foot by passing posterior to the medial malleolus, after which it terminates as the medial and lateral plantar arteries.

Accompanying the posterior tibial artery is the **tibial nerve**. This large terminal branch of the sciatic nerve descends the popliteal fossa and passes into the posterior leg to sit deep to the gastrocnemius and soleus muscles, supplying all the muscles in the posterior compartment of the leg. The tibial nerve then travels just posterior to the medial malleolus to terminate in the foot as plantar nerves. The great and small saphenous veins ascend the posteromedial and lateral aspects, respectively, these work alongside the deep and centrally located posterior tibial veins to drain venous blood from the leg.

Key points about neurovasculature of the knee and leg	
Arteries	**Genicular anastomosis (knee)**: five genicular branches of popliteal artery (superior and inferior medial, superior and inferior lateral, middle genicular arteries), anterior and posterior tibial recurrent arteries, descending branches of femoral and lateral circumflex arteries, circumflex fibular branch of posterior tibial artery **Leg**: popliteal artery, anterior tibial artery, posterior tibial artery, fibular artery
Veins	Popliteal vein, anterior tibial veins, posterior tibial veins, fibular veins, small saphenous vein, great saphenous vein
Nerves	**Femoral nerve**: saphenous nerve **Sciatic nerve**: tibial nerve, common fibular nerve (superficial and deep fibular nerves, lateral sural cutaneous nerve), sural nerve (medial sural cutaneous nerve)

Muscular innervation

Superficial fibular nerve	Fibularis longus, fibularis brevis muscle
Deep fibular nerve	Tibialis anterior, extensor digitorum longus, fibularis tertius, extensor hallucis longus
Tibial nerve	Gastrocnemius, popliteus, soleus, plantaris, tibialis posterior, flexor digitorum longus, flexor hallucis longus

Cutaneous innervation

Saphenous nerve	Anteromedial aspect of knee, medial aspect of leg
Lateral sural cutaneous nerve	Proximal posterolateral aspect of leg
Superficial fibular nerve	Distal lateral aspect of leg
Sural nerve	Posterior aspect of leg

Arteries of the leg and foot

Veins of the lower limb

ARTERIES AND NERVES OF THE FOOT

The arterial supply to the foot can be divided into a dorsal and plantar component, that are connected through the pedal arches:

- The **anterior tibial artery** gives off a number of branches to supply the dorsum of the foot.
- The **posterior tibial artery**, provides the branches for the plantar portion of the foot.

Five major nerves provide innervation to the foot; these are the tibial, sural, deep fibular, superficial fibular and saphenous nerves.

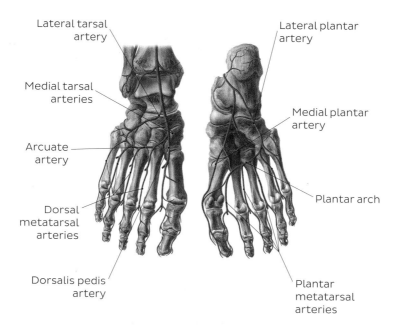

Lateral tarsal artery

Lateral plantar artery

Medial tarsal arteries

Medial plantar artery

Arcuate artery

Dorsal metatarsal arteries

Plantar arch

Dorsalis pedis artery

Plantar metatarsal arteries

FIGURE 3.39. Arteries of the foot. This image demonstrates the arterial network of the foot (dorsum of the foot on the left, sole of the foot on the right), formed by the branches of the two main arteries: **Dorsalis pedis artery** (branch of the anterior tibial artery) and medial and lateral **plantar arteries** (branches of the posterior tibial artery). Notice the anastomoses and arterial arches that these vessels form in order to supply the foot.

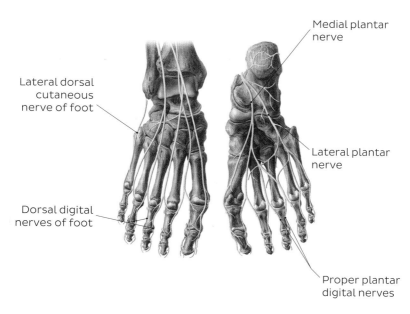

Medial plantar nerve

Lateral dorsal cutaneous nerve of foot

Lateral plantar nerve

Dorsal digital nerves of foot

Proper plantar digital nerves

FIGURE 3.40. Nerves of the foot. At first glance, the trajectory of the neural network seems similar to the arterial one. The difference is that all these branches come from as many as 5 nerves. Notice how the dorsum of the foot (image on the left) is supplied mainly by the branches of the **superficial and deep fibular, tibial** and **sural nerves**. The cutaneous innervation of this area is supplied by the **saphenous nerve**.

Finally, the sole of the foot (image on the right) is mainly innervated by the branches of the tibial nerve (medial and lateral plantar nerves).

Key points about arteries and nerves of the foot	
Arteries	**Dorsalis pedis artery**: lateral and medial tarsal artery, arcuate artery, deep plantar artery
	Posterior tibial artery: medial plantar artery, lateral plantar artery
	Deep plantar arch: lateral plantar artery, deep plantar artery
	Superficial plantar arch: lateral plantar artery, superficial branch of medial plantar artery
Nerves	**Superficial fibular nerve**: medial dorsal cutaneous nerve of foot, intermediate dorsal cutaneous nerve of foot
	Deep fibular nerve: dorsal digital branches
	Tibial nerve: sural, medial calcaneal and medial and lateral plantar nerves

Muscular innervation

Tibial nerve	Flexor digitorum longus and flexor hallucis longus muscles
Medial plantar nerve	Flexor hallucis brevis, flexor digitorum brevis, abductor hallucis and lumbrical muscles
Lateral plantar nerve	Flexor digiti minimi brevis, quadratus plantae, abductor digiti minimi, dorsal and plantar interossei muscles, adductor hallucis and lumbrical muscles
Deep fibular nerve	Extensor digitorum longus, extensor hallucis longus and extensor digitorum brevis muscles

Cutaneous innervation

Dorsum of foot	Saphenous, superficial fibular, sural, deep fibular and lateral plantar nerves
Sole of foot	Saphenous, medial plantar, lateral plantar, sural and tibial nerves

Lower extremities arteries and nerves

Arteries of the leg and foot

Arterial anastomoses of the lower extremity

LOWER LIMB

SPINE AND BACK

4

REGIONS OF THE BACK AND BUTTOCKS

The back and the buttocks comprise the posterior aspect of the trunk. Like the rest of the body, the back and the buttocks are divided into several regions, which help clinicians localize, describe and communicate various diseases and injuries clearly and accurately.

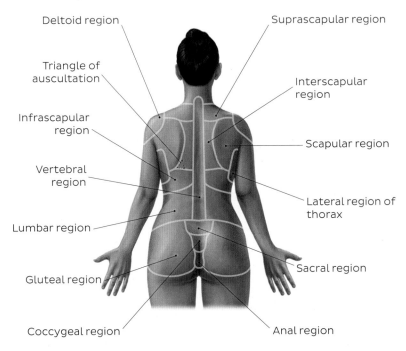

Deltoid region

Triangle of auscultation

Infrascapular region

Vertebral region

Lumbar region

Gluteal region

Coccygeal region

Suprascapular region

Interscapular region

Scapular region

Lateral region of thorax

Sacral region

Anal region

FIGURE 4.1. Regions of the back and buttocks. The back and buttocks present several distinct topographical regions named according to their relations with underlying structures. The nine regions of the back are the deltoid, suprascapular, scapular, interscapular, infrascapular, vertebral, lumbar and sacral regions and the triangle of auscultation. The buttocks can be similarly classified into gluteal, anal and coccygeal regions.

Anatomy of the back

Body regions learn with quizzes and labeled diagrams

SPINE AND BACK

VERTEBRAL COLUMN

The vertebral column (spine) is composed of 33–35 vertebrae, 24 of which are separated by intervertebral discs; the remaining vertebrae are usually fused to compose two respective bones, the sacrum and coccyx. The vertebral column is divided into five regions: (from superior to inferior) the cervical, thoracic, lumbar, sacral and coccygeal regions. The vertebrae articulate with each other by connecting their bodies and their arches via intervertebral joints. These joints are present throughout the whole spine, while some regions have region-specific joints (e.g., the thoracic spine with the ribs).

When observed from the lateral aspect, the vertebral column presents four curvatures: Two concavities and two convexities. The curvatures that are concave anteriorly are called the thoracic and sacral **kyphoses**. The curvatures that are convex anteriorly are known as the cervical and lumbar **lordoses**.

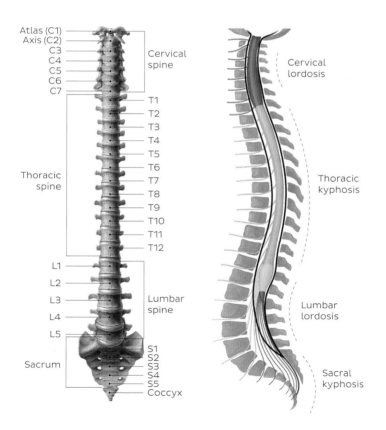

FIGURE 4.2. **Vertebral column (anterior and lateral views).**

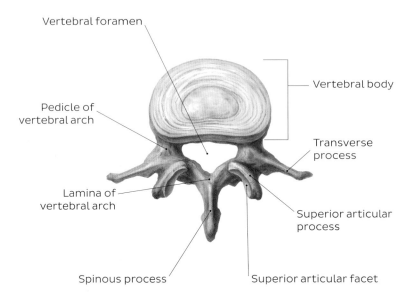

Vertebral foramen

Vertebral body

Pedicle of
vertebral arch

Transverse
process

Lamina of
vertebral arch

Superior articular
process

Spinous process

Superior articular facet

FIGURE 4.3. Anatomy of a typical vertebra. The vertebrae of each region have common anatomical features which help in distincting them one from another. Nevertheless, all vertebrae share a number of common/general features. The large cylindrical part located anteriorly is the vertebral **body**; it is separated above and below from adjacent vertebral bodies by fibrocartilaginous structures known as intervertebral discs. The posterior part of the vertebra is the vertebral **arch**, which is formed by two **pedicles** (one on either side) and two **laminae** that complete the arch posteriorly. The body and arch of each vertebra enclose a space called the **vertebral foramen**. Several projections, or **processes**, extend from the arch. Each vertebra has a spinous process extending posteriorly on the midline, two transverse processes extending laterally, as well as two superior and two inferior articular processes. Each articular process bears an articular facet for articulation with a contiguous vertebra.

Key points about the vertebral column		
Main regions	Cervical spine (7)	
	Thoracic spine (12)	
	Lumbar spine (5)	
	Sacrum (5)	
	Coccyx (3–5)	
Curvatures	Cervical lordosis (C2–T2)	
	Thoracic kyphosis (T2–T12)	
	Lumbar lordosis (T12—sacrovertebral angle)	
	Sacral kyphosis (sacrovertebral articulation—coccyx)	
Movements	Flexion, extension, lateral flexion, rotation (torsion)	
Functions	Movement, stabilization and support of the trunk; protection of the spinal cord	

Key points about the structure of a typical vertebra	
Main components	Vertebral body
	Vertebral arch
	Vertebral foramen
Bony landmarks of vertebral arch	Pedicles
	Laminae
	Vertebral processes: spinous process, transverse processes, superior articular processes (with superior articular facets) and inferior articular processes (with inferior articular facets)

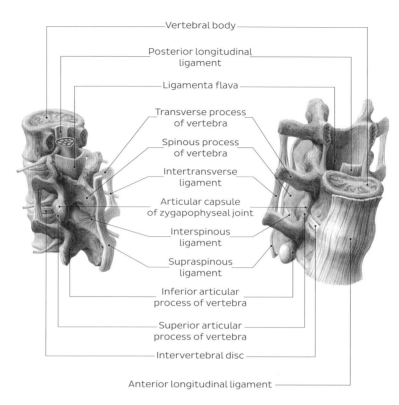

Vertebral body

Posterior longitudinal ligament

Ligamenta flava

Transverse process of vertebra

Spinous process of vertebra

Intertransverse ligament

Articular capsule of zygapophyseal joint

Interspinous ligament

Supraspinous ligament

Inferior articular process of vertebra

Superior articular process of vertebra

Intervertebral disc

Anterior longitudinal ligament

FIGURE 4.4. Joints of the vertebral bodies and arches. Intervertebral joints are articulations between adjacent vertebrae of the spine.

An **intervertebral symphysis** is the articulation of two contiguous vertebral bodies and the intervening intervertebral disc. It is classified as a secondary cartilaginous joint or symphysis (fibrocartilage composition). Vertebral bodies in the cervical region also articulate at uncovertebral joints (of Luschka). These comprise four pairs of plane synovial joints present between the vertebrae C3-C7, along the lateral borders of their vertebral bodies. A **zygapophyseal joint (facet joint)** is a synovial joint formed by the articular processes of neighboring vertebrae. Both intervertebral disc and zygapophyseal joints extend between the levels of the axis (C2) and sacrum (S1). The intervertebral joints are reinforced and supported by numerous ligaments.

The anterior and posterior longitudinal ligaments extend along the anterior and posterior surfaces of the vertebral bodies and interposed intervertebral discs, respectively. The ligamenta flava can be seen on the posterior surface of the vertebral canal, extending between adjacent laminae. The inferior articular processes of each vertebra articulates with the superior articular processes of its neighbor below, forming two zygapophyseal (facet) joints at each vertebral level; each is surrounded by an articular capsule. Other ligaments extend between different bony processes of the adjacent vertebrae, namely the intertransverse ligament (between transverse processes) and interspinous and supraspinous ligaments (between spinous processes).

Key points about the joints of the vertebral bodies and arches	
Joints	Intervertebral symphysis: inferior vertebral plateau of superior vertebral body and superior vertebral plateau of inferior vertebral body
	Zygapophyseal joints: superior articular facets of inferior vertebra and inferior articular facets of superior vertebra
	Uncovertebral joints: uncinate processes of inferior vertebra and inferolateral surfaces of superior vertebral body
Ligaments	**Main ligaments**
	Anterior longitudinal ligament: anterior aspect of vertebral bodies and intervertebral discs
	Posterior longitudinal ligament: posterior aspect of vertebral bodies and intervertebral discs
	Accessory ligaments
	Ligamenta flava: posterior surface of vertebral canal, along adjacent laminae
	Interspinous ligaments: adjacent spinous processes
	Supraspinous ligament: extremities of spinous processes
	Intertransverse ligaments: adjacent transverse processes
	Nuchal ligament: external occipital protuberance to spinous process of C7
Movements	Flexion, extension, lateral flexion, rotation

Vertebral column

Curvature and movements of the vertebral column

CERVICAL SPINE

The cervical spine consists of seven vertebrae named sequentially in a supero-inferior direction, C1–C7.

There are three atypical vertebrae in the cervical spine. The first (C1) and second (C2) cervical vertebrae are known as the atlas and axis, while the seventh vertebra (C7) is named the vertebra prominens, due its elongated spinous process. The rest of the cervical vertebrae, C3–C6, all have a similar anatomical structure and are therefore classified as typical vertebrae.

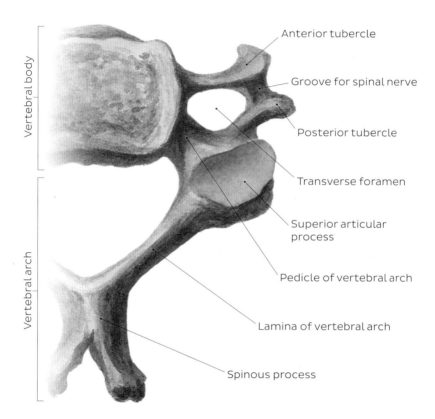

FIGURE 4.5. A typical cervical vertebrae (C3–C6) consists of a body and arch. The vertebral **body** is smaller than that of its thoracic and lumbar counterparts due to the fact that it supports less weight. The **vertebral arch** projects from the posterior side of the body, initially as paired **pedicles** which represent the root of the arch. The pedicles are connected by a pair of **laminae** which enclose the **vertebral foramen**. The spinous process may be bifid, something only seen in cervical vertebrae.

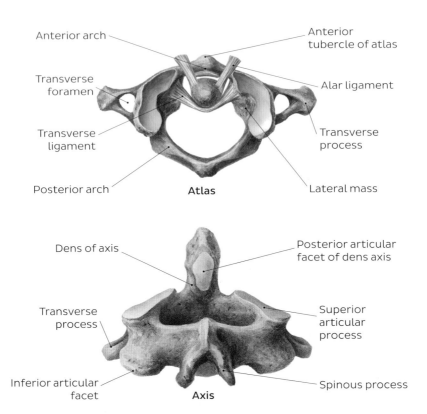

Anterior arch

Anterior tubercle of atlas

Transverse foramen

Alar ligament

Transverse ligament

Transverse process

Posterior arch

Atlas

Lateral mass

Dens of axis

Posterior articular facet of dens axis

Transverse process

Superior articular process

Inferior articular facet

Axis

Spinous process

FIGURE 4.6. Superior view of atlas (C1), posterior view of axis (C2). The **atlas (C1)** is a ring-shaped vertebra, devoid of vertebral body and spinous process. It consists of the anterior and posterior arches which are connected via a lateral mass on each side, together enclosing the vertebral canal through which the spinal cord passes. Each **lateral mass** features articular facets on its superior and inferior surface and a single transverse process that projects laterally.

The anterior and posterior **arches** feature several bony landmarks that provide the attachment points for the ligaments of the cervical spine. Moreover, the anterior arch contains an articular surface that participates in formation of the median atlantoaxial joint, a joint between atlas and axis. The superior and inferior **articular facets** of the lateral masses participate in the atlantooccipital and lateral atlantoaxial joints, respectively. The former is a joint between the atlas and the occipital bone, while the latter is a three-part joint between the atlas and axis. The transverse processes that stem from the lateral masses feature a small foramen called **foramen transversarium**. This foramen exists in vertebrae C1-C6 and it is traversed by the vertebral artery.

The **axis (C2)** primarily differs from a typical vertebra by its prominent bony projection known as the dens (odontoid process). As a whole, the axis consists of anterior and posterior parts. The anterior part is formed by the body and dens, while the posterior part consists of two pedicles, two transverse processes, two laminae and a spinous process. The **body** of the axis is small and inferiorly elongated so that it overlaps the vertebra C3. It serves as an attachment point to several muscles and ligaments of the neck. The **dens of axis** projects from the superior surface of the body. It features an anterior articular facet which articulates with atlas at the median atlantoaxial joint and a posterior articular facet over which runs the transverse ligament of atlas. Either side of the dens, the body of the axis features **superior and inferior articular facets** which are located on its superior and inferior surfaces, respectively. The former participate in the lateral atlantoaxial joints, while the latter articulate with vertebra C3 via specialized zygapophyseal joints, which are sometimes collectively referred to as the vertebroaxial joint.

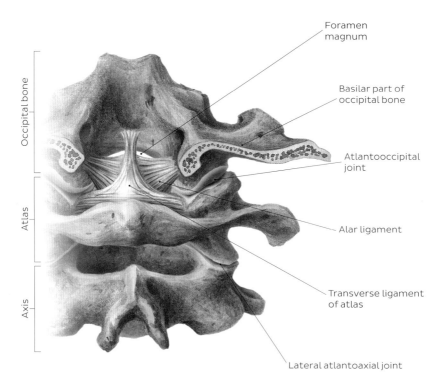

Foramen
magnum

Basilar part of
occipital bone

Atlantooccipital
joint

Alar ligament

Transverse ligament
of atlas

Occipital bone

Atlas

Axis

Lateral atlantoaxial joint

FIGURE 4.7. Atlantooccipital and atlantoaxial joints. The atlas articulates with the occipital bone at the **atlantooccipital joint**, which presents the primary connection of the head with the trunk. This is a synovial joint formed by the occipital condyles and superior articular facets of the atlas. The joint is secured by the anterior and posterior atlantooccipital membranes and allows for flexion and extension of the head, as well as a limited degree of lateral flexion.

The atlas and axis articulate via a complex **atlantoaxial joint**. This joint consists of three synovial components: A single median atlantoaxial joint and paired lateral atlantoaxial joints. The main movement of this complex joint is the axial rotation of the head, but it also allows limited flexion, extension and lateral flexion.

The **median atlantoaxial joint (a.k.a. atlantodental joint)** is formed by the dens of axis, anterior arch of the atlas and transverse ligament of the atlas. It is composed of two elements: An articulation between the anterior articular facet of the dens axis and facet for dens located on the internal surface of the anterior arch of the atlas, as well as a second articulation between the posterior articular facet of the dens axis and the anterior surface of the transverse ligament of atlas. The joint is primarily reinforced by the cruciform ligament complex, which consists of the transverse ligament of atlas, superior and inferior longitudinal bands of cruciform ligament. The additional support is provided by the tectorial membrane, alar ligaments, apical ligament of dens, anterior and posterior atlantoaxial membranes.

The left and right **lateral atlantoaxial joints** are formed by the inferior articular surfaces of the lateral masses of the atlas with the superior articular surfaces of the axis. They are reinforced by several ligaments e.g. the accessory atlantoaxial ligament, anterior/posterior atlantoaxial membranes, tectorial membrane etc.

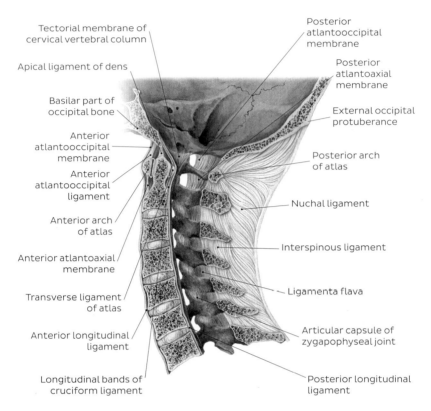

Tectorial membrane of cervical vertebral column

Apical ligament of dens

Basilar part of occipital bone

Anterior atlantooccipital membrane

Anterior atlantooccipital ligament

Anterior arch of atlas

Anterior atlantoaxial membrane

Transverse ligament of atlas

Anterior longitudinal ligament

Longitudinal bands of cruciform ligament

Posterior atlantooccipital membrane

Posterior atlantoaxial membrane

External occipital protuberance

Posterior arch of atlas

Nuchal ligament

Interspinous ligament

Ligamenta flava

Articular capsule of zygapophyseal joint

Posterior longitudinal ligament

FIGURE 4.8. Craniovertebral ligaments (midsagittal view). Midsagittal section through the base of the skull and cervical vertebrae. The dynamic craniovertebral joints are stabilized by a number of ligaments which can be identified in this image. The anterior and posterior atlantooccipital membranes prevent excessive movement at the atlantooccipital joint, and are further stabilized by the anterior and lateral atlantooccipital ligaments. The anterior atlantooccipital ligament is a median thickening of the anterior atlantooccipital membrane while the lateral atlantooccipital ligaments (not shown) develop as a thickening of the articular capsule of the joint. Connecting the axis to the base of the cranium are the apical ligament of dens, the transverse occipital ligament (not shown), the alar ligaments and the tectorial membrane. The median atlantoaxial joint is stabilized by a series of ligaments known as the anterior atlantoaxial membrane, the anterior atlantodental ligament (not shown) and the cruciform ligament.

Key points about the cervical spine	
Structure	**Seven cervical vertebrae**
	Typical: C3–C6
	Atypical: C1, C2, C7
Typical vertebra	Body, arch (pedicles and laminae), spinous process, transverse processes, superior and inferior articular processes and their articular facets
Atypical vertebra	**Atlas (C1)**: anterior arch, posterior arch, lateral mass, transverse process, vertebral canal
	Axis (C2): vertebral body, dens axis, pedicle (x2), transverse process (x2), lamina (x2), spinous process
	Vertebra prominens (C7): all features as in typical vertebra, except that the spinous process is longer and not bifid and the body is larger

Key points about the cervical spine

Joints	**Atlantooccipital joint**: atlas (C1) and occipital bone
	Atlantoaxial joints: atlas (C1) and axis (C2)
	Intervertebral symphyses: bodies of contiguous vertebrae
	Zygaopophyseal joints: superior and inferior articular processes of contiguous vertebrae
	Uncovertebral joints: uncinate processes of the superior surface of vertebral body with inferior surface of vertebral body above

Key points about the atlantooccipital joint

Type	Synovial ellipsoid joint; biaxial
Articular surfaces	Occipital condyles, superior articular facets of atlas
Ligaments	Posterior atlantooccipital ligament, anterior atlantooccipital ligament
Movements	Principal movement; Flexion – extension
	Limited lateral flexion

Key points about the atlantoaxial joint

Type	Atlantoaxial joint complex: synovial joint; biaxial
Articular surfaces	Median atlantoaxial joint: dens of axis (C2), osteoligamentous ring (anterior arch of atlas [C1], transverse ligament of atlas)
	Lateral atlantoaxial joints: inferior articular surface of lateral mass for atlas, superior articular facet of axis
Ligaments	Cruciform ligament (transverse ligament of atlas, superior and inferior longitudinal bands), tectorial membrane, alar ligaments, apical ligament of dens
Movements	Principal movement; axial rotation,
	Limited flexion, extension, lateral flexion

 Vertebral column

 Cervical spine

 Atlantooccipital joint

 Atlantoaxial joint

THORACIC SPINE

The thoracic spine consists of 12 vertebrae, designated T1–T12 from superior to inferior. Eight thoracic vertebrae, T2–T9 are the typical vertebrae, while the remaining four are atypical. The exclusive feature of the thoracic vertebrae is that each of them articulates with a pair of ribs, and therefore contain components to accommodate that.

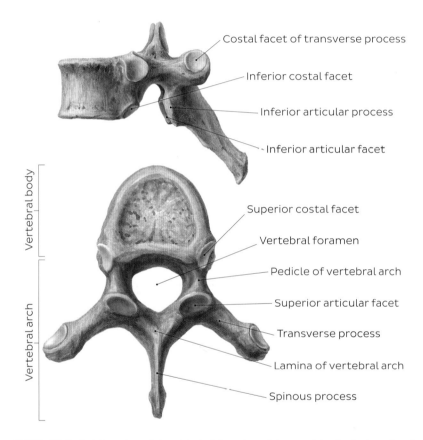

FIGURE 4.9. Typical thoracic vertebra. A typical thoracic vertebra consists of a body, arch, spinous, transverse and superior and inferior articular processes. The body (typically heart-shaped) is larger than those seen in the cervical spine, but smaller than those of lumbar vertebrae. Specific features of thoracic vertebrae are:

- **Costal facets:** Vertebrae T2–T9 bear superior and inferior '**demifacets**' which are located on the superior and inferior margins of the lateral sides of each vertebral body (therefore, articulation with the head of one rib is shared between adjacent vertebrae. Vertebra T1 features a demifacet along its inferolateral margins, and a whole facet on its superolateral surfaces. Vertebrae T10–T12 features a single whole costal facet on each side of their body.

- **Vertebral arch:** More circular and smaller than that in cervical vertebrae.

- **Spinous process:** Elongated, the angle between the spinous process and the body becomes more acute in lower levels.

- **Transverse processes:** Feature costal facets for articulation with the tubercle of the ipsilateral numerically equivalent rib (exception: Vertebrae T11/T12).

- **Superior and inferior articular processes:** Superior processes face backward (and slightly lateral/ upwards), inferior process are oriented forward (and slightly medial/downward)

Key points about the thoracic spine

Structure	**12 thoracic vertebrae** **Typical**: T2–T9 **Atypical**: T1, T10–T12
Typical vertebra	Body, arch, costal facets, spinous process, transverse processes, superior and inferior articular processes
Atypical vertebra	**T1**: features one demifacet and one full facet on each side **T10**: single costal facets on each side **T11, T12**: single costal facets on each side, no costotransverse joints
Joints	**Intervertebral symphyses**: between bodies of contiguous vertebrae **Zygapophyseal joints**: between articular processes of contiguous vertebrae **Costocorporeal joints**: between costal facets/demifacets of vertebral bodies and head of ribs **Costotransverse joints**: between costal facets on transverse processes and tubercles of ribs

Key points about costovertebral joints

Articular surfaces	**Costocorporeal joint**: costal demifacets on vertebrae T1–T9, full costal facets on vertebrae T1, T10, T11, T12; heads of ribs 1–12 **Costotransverse joint**: tubercle of ribs 1–10, transverse costal facets on transverse processes of numerically equivalent vertebra
Ligaments	**Costocorporeal joint**: fibrous capsule, radiate, intraarticular ligaments (only joints 2–9) **Costotransverse joint**: fibrous capsule, costotransverse, superior costotransverse, lateral costotransverse, accessory ligament (sometimes absent)
Movements	**Costocorporeal joints**: internal rotation and elevation of head of rib **Costotransverse joints 1–6**: internal rotation of neck of rib **Costotransverse joints 7–10**: posteromedial translation of neck of rib

 Thoracic vertebrae

 Thoracic cage

 Learn anatomy of the spine diagrams and interactive vertebrae quizzes

LUMBAR SPINE

The lumbar spine consists of five lumbar vertebrae, designated L1–L5. They are the largest and sturdiest examples of all vertebrae due to their role in supporting the weight of the upper body. Like their cervical and thoracic counterparts, the lumbar vertebrae articulate with each other via the intervertebral symphyses and zygapophyseal joints. The inferiormost lumbar vertebra, L5, articulates with the sacrum via the **lumbosacral joint**, which is morphologically similar to the more superior intervertebral joints.

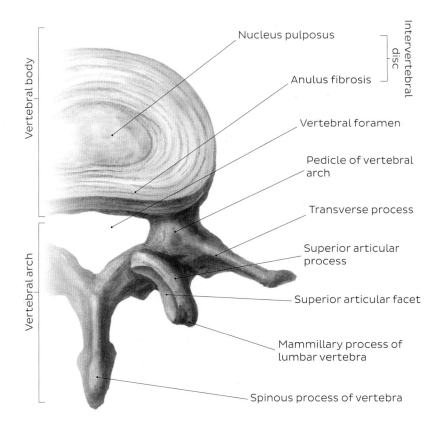

Nucleus pulposus

Anulus fibrosis

Intervertebral disc

Vertebral body

Vertebral arch

Vertebral foramen

Pedicle of vertebral arch

Transverse process

Superior articular process

Superior articular facet

Mammillary process of lumbar vertebra

Spinous process of vertebra

FIGURE 4.10. **Typical lumbar vertebra.** A typical lumbar vertebra bears a large and ellipsoid vertebral **body** which increases in size from L1 to L5. The lumbar vertebral **arches** are noticeably smaller, therefore enclosing a relatively narrow vertebral canal. The **spinous process** is thick and short and nearly horizontally oriented. The **transverse processes** are more slender than those in the upper segments of the spine and are devoid of any articular surfaces. The superior processes are concave and face medially, whereas the inferior processes are convex and are laterally oriented towards the superior processes of the next vertebra.

The distinguishing components of the lumbar vertebrae are the accessory and mammillary processes, which serve as the attachment sites for the deep muscles of the back; the **accessory processes** projects from the roots of the transverse processes (not shown), while the **mammillary processes** project from the posterior surfaces of the superior articular processes.

Key points about the lumbar spine	
Structure	**Five lumbar vertebrae (L1-L5)**
Typical vertebra	Vertebral body, vertebral arch, spinous process, transverse processes, accessory process, mammillary processes
Joints	Intervertebral symphyseal joints: between the bodies of the contiguous vertebrae
	Lumbosacral joint: intervertebral and zygapophyseal joints between L5 and sacrum

Key points about the lumbosacral joint	
Type	Anterior intervertebral joint: symphysis
	Facet joints: synovial plane joints
Articular surfaces	Anterior intervertebral joint: inferior surface of L5 vertebral body, superior surface of S1 vertebral body
	Facet joints: superior articular processes of the S1, inferior articular processes of L5
Ligaments	Iliolumbar ligament, lateral lumbosacral ligament
Movements	Flexion, extension, lateral flexion

Lumbar vertebrae

SPINE AND BACK

SACRUM AND COCCYX

The sacrum is a triangular bone comprising five fused sacral vertebrae, S1–S5. It articulates with the iliac components of the hip bones via the sacroiliac joint, therefore contributing to the pelvic girdle and playing an important role in stabilization of the pelvis. Superiorly, it articulates with the inferiormost lumbar vertebra (L5) to form the lumbosacral joint. Inferiorly, it articulates with the coccyx to form the sacrococcygeal joint.

The coccyx is the most inferior part of the spine and consists of three to five fused rudimentary coccygeal vertebrae.

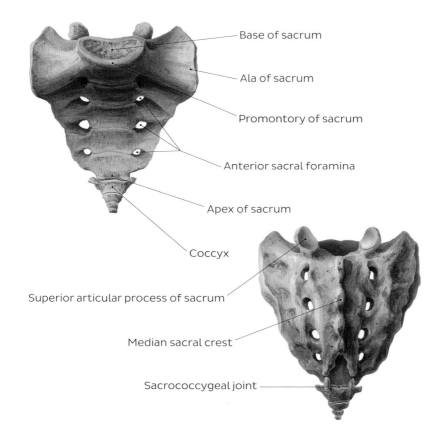

Base of sacrum

Ala of sacrum

Promontory of sacrum

Anterior sacral foramina

Apex of sacrum

Coccyx

Superior articular process of sacrum

Median sacral crest

Sacrococcygeal joint

FIGURE 4.11. Overview of sacrum and coccyx (anterior and posterior views). The sacrum consists of a base, paired lateral parts and apex. It is convex anteriorly and features dorsal and pelvic surfaces. The dorsal surface is vertically ridged due to the presence of the following crests: A single median sacral crest (fusion of spinous processes), as well as bilateral/paired intermediate and lateral sacral crests (fusion of articular and transverse processes, respectively). The intermediate crests terminate inferiorly as the sacral horns. Between the intermediate and lateral ridges are four posterior sacral foramina. The pelvic surface is relatively smooth, except for four transverse ridges located between the bodies of vertebrae S1-S5. Four anterior sacral foramina are also present, as well as a large anterior projection of the base, known as the sacral promontory. The lateral parts of sacrum represent the fused expansions of the transverse processes as well as vestiges of the sacral ribs. The lateral aspects of the sacrum each feature a rough articular surface, known as the auricular surface, at which the sacrum articulates with ilium forming the sacroiliac joints.The apex of the sacrum articulates with the base of coccyx, forming at the sacrococcygeal joint. The vertebral foramina of fused sacral vertebrae together form a vertebral canal that passes through the sacrum, transmitting the distal parts of the cauda equina and the filum terminale.

The coccyx is the most inferior/caudal part of the spine and consists of three to five fused coccygeal vertebrae (Co1-5). It consists of three parts: A base, a pair of horns and an apex. The base of coccyx articulates with the sacrum, while the apex faces inferiorly and represents the termination of the vertebral column. The coccygeal horns project superiorly from the posterior margin of the base to articulate with the sacral horns.

Key points about the sacrum	
Structure	Five fused sacral vertebrae (S1–S5)
Parts	Dorsal surface: median crest, intermediate crests, lateral crests, four pairs of posterior sacral foramina, sacral horns
	Pelvic surface: transverse ridges, sacral promontory, four pairs of anterior sacral foramina
	Lateral (auricular) surface: articulates with ilium
	Base: articulates with L5
	Apex: articulates with coccyx
Joints	Lumbosacral joint: between the superior auricular process of sacrum and inferior articular facets of L5
	Sacrococcygeal joint: between the apex of the sacrum and the base of the coccyx
	Sacroiliac joint: between lateral sacral surface and iliac articulation surface

Key points about the coccyx	
Structure	**3-5 fused coccygeal vertebrae**
Parts	Apex, base, coccygeal horns
Joints	Sacrococcygeal joint: between the apex of the sacrum and the base of the coccyx

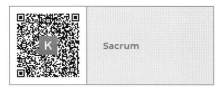

Sacrum

ARTERIES OF THE VERTEBRAL COLUMN

Each vertebra is supplied by a number of spinal, periosteal, pre/postcentral and pre/postlaminar l vessels which arise from larger parent arteries. The vertebrae of the cervical region primarily receive their arterial supply from the vertebral and ascending cervical arteries. The posterior intercostal and subcostal arteries supply vertebrae of the thoracic region, the lumbar arteries supply vertebrae of the lumbar region, while the vertebrae of the sacral region receive their blood supply from the iliolumbar and lateral and medial sacral arteries.

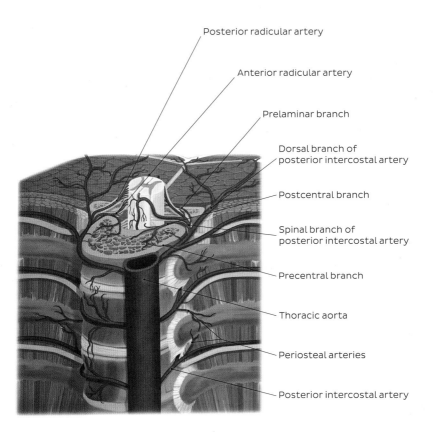

Posterior radicular artery

Anterior radicular artery

Prelaminar branch

Dorsal branch of posterior intercostal artery

Postcentral branch

Spinal branch of posterior intercostal artery

Precentral branch

Thoracic aorta

Periosteal arteries

Posterior intercostal artery

FIGURE 4.12. Blood supply of thoracic vertebrae. The thoracic aorta descends along the anterior surface of the vertebral bodies giving off multiple paired posterior intercostal arteries. Small precentral and periosteal branches arise directly from the posterior intercostal arteries along the anterolateral aspect of the vertebral bodies. The spinal arterial branches arise either directly from the posterior intercostal artery or from one of its major branches, the dorsal branch of the posterior intercostal artery. The segmental spinal branch travels with the spinal nerve in the intervertebral foramen towards the vertebral foramen, where it branches into postcentral (anterior), prelaminar (posterior) and radicular arteries. The postcentral and prelaminar arteries give off branches to supply the vertebral body and the lamina respectively, and anastomose with arteries of adjacent vertebral levels. The radicular arteries supply the spinal nerves and meninges of the spinal cord.

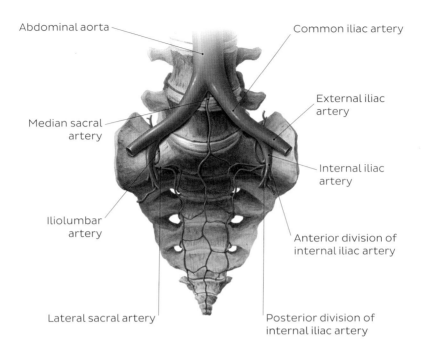

Abdominal aorta

Common iliac artery

External iliac artery

Median sacral artery

Internal iliac artery

Iliolumbar artery

Anterior division of internal iliac artery

Lateral sacral artery

Posterior division of internal iliac artery

FIGURE 4.13. Arteries of the sacrum and coccyx (anterior view). The abdominal aorta terminates by bifurcating into the left and right common iliac arteries anterior to the body of L4, each of which in turn divide into internal and external iliac arteries. Arising from the posterior division of the internal iliac artery is the iliolumbar artery, a small vessel which runs superolaterally along the anterior surface of the ala of the sacrum supplying structures within this region. Also arising from the posterior division of the internal iliac artery are the lateral sacral arteries. The paired lateral sacral arteries descend anterior to the anterior sacral foramina and anterior rami of the sacral spinal nerves and give off several spinal branches which travel through the sacral foramina to supply structures of the spinal cord. Arising from the posterior aspect of the abdominal aorta, just proximal to the bifurcation is the median sacral artery. This is an unpaired artery which runs along the anterior surface of the last two lumbar vertebrae and the length of the sacrum and coccyx. As this artery passes over the sacral promontory it gives off small transverse branches which anastomose with the right and left lateral sacral arteries.

Key points about the arteries of the vertebral column	
Parent arteries by region	Cervical: vertebral and ascending cervical arteries
	Thoracic: posterior intercostal arteries
	Lumbar: L1-L4: subcostal and lumbar arteries L5: iliolumbar and median sacral arteries
	Sacrum: iliolumbar and lateral and median sacral arteries
Arteries of isolated vertebra	Periosteal branches, equatorial branches, nutrient branches, segmental spinal branches, prelaminar arterial branch, postcentral arterial branch, radicular arteries

Lumbar arteries

VEINS OF THE VERTEBRAL COLUMN

The vertebral column is drained by four venous plexuses: The anterior external, anterior internal, posterior internal and posterior external vertebral venous plexuses. These plexuses communicate with each other through the intervertebral foramina and drain the external and internal regions of each vertebra.

Intervertebral veins drain the vertebral venous plexuses and travel through the intervertebral foramina to empty into the vertebral veins (cervical), the posterior intercostal veins (thoracic), the lumbar veins and the sacral veins.

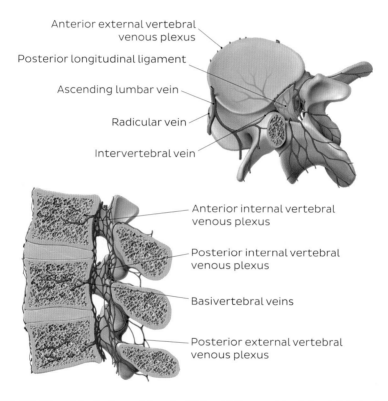

Anterior external vertebral venous plexus
Posterior longitudinal ligament
Ascending lumbar vein
Radicular vein
Intervertebral vein
Anterior internal vertebral venous plexus
Posterior internal vertebral venous plexus
Basivertebral veins
Posterior external vertebral venous plexus

FIGURE 4.14. Veins of the lumbar vertebrae (sagittal and left superolateral views). Spinal veins form internal and external vertebral venous plexuses along the vertebral column. Each of these plexuses can be further divided into an anterior and a posterior plexus. Within the trabecular bone of the vertebral body are the basivertebral veins. These veins emerge on the posterior aspect of each vertebral body and drain into the anterior external and anterior internal venous plexuses. The intervertebral veins are located on the superior surface of the pedicle of each vertebra and drain regions of the spinal cord and vertebral plexuses. The intervertebral veins travel through the intervertebral foramina of the vertebral column to drain into the vertebral veins of the neck and segmental veins of the trunk.

SPINE AND BACK

Key points about the veins of the vertebral column	
Collecting veins by region	Cervical: vertebral veins
	Thoracic: intercostal veins
	Lumbar: lumbar veins → Ascending lumbar veins
	Sacrum: sacral veins
Veins of isolated vertebra	Anterior and posterior external vertebral venous plexuses, anterior and posterior internal vertebral venous plexuses, basivertebral veins, intervertebral veins

Veins of the vertebral column

MUSCLES OF THE BACK

The back muscles are divided into two large groups:

- The **superficial (extrinsic) back muscles,** which lie most superficially on the back. These muscles are also called *immigrant muscles,* since they actually represent muscles of the upper limb that have migrated to the back during fetal development. These muscles are divided into superficial and intermediate layers.
- The **deep (intrinsic) back muscles**, which are also called *true back muscles.* They are located deep to the extrinsic muscles, from which they are separated by the thoracolumbar fascia. Their primary function is to produce movements of the vertebral column. These muscles are divided into superficial, deep, and deepest layers.

Superficial muscles of the back

The superficial muscles are located beneath the skin and superficial fascia of the back and extend between the vertebral column and bones of the pectoral girdle and arm. Their principal function is to support and move the upper limb through movement of the scapula and humerus.

They are divided into two different groups consisting of a:

- Superficial layer: Trapezius, latissimus dorsi, levator scapulae, rhomboid major and minor muscles
- Intermediate layer: Serratus posterior superior and serratus posterior inferior muscles

Overview of back muscles

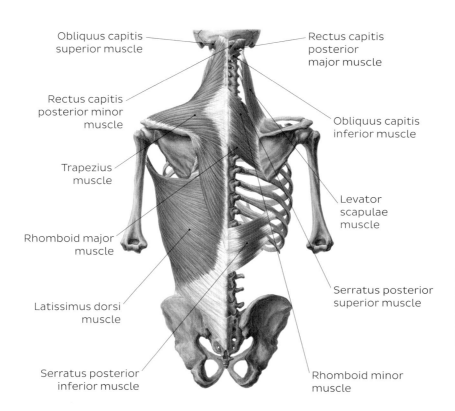

Obliquus capitis superior muscle

Rectus capitis posterior major muscle

Rectus capitis posterior minor muscle

Obliquus capitis inferior muscle

Trapezius muscle

Levator scapulae muscle

Rhomboid major muscle

Latissimus dorsi muscle

Serratus posterior superior muscle

Serratus posterior inferior muscle

Rhomboid minor muscle

FIGURE 4.15. Overview of the superficial muscles of the back. Overview of the superficial muscles of the back showing their attachment points on the bones of the trunk and upper limb. The trapezius and latissimus dorsi muscles are the largest members of this group and cover most of the back with the exception of the scapular region. Deep to them are the smaller members of the superficial layer (levator scapulae, rhomboid major and minor muscles). The serratus posterior superior and inferior muscles belong to the intermediate layer. In addition, a few of the suboccipital muscles can also be observed along the occipitocervical junction.

SPINE AND BACK

SPINE AND BACK

Superficial layer	Origin	Insertion	Innervation	Function
Trapezius	**Descending part**: medial third of superior nuchal line, External occipital protuberance, Spinous processes of cervical vertebrae/Nuchal ligament	**Descending part**: lateral third of clavicle	**Motor**: accessory nerve (CN XI) **Sensory**: anterior rami of spinal nerves C3-C4 (via cervical plexus)	**Descending part**: *scapulothoracic joint*: draws scapula superomedially; *atlantooccipital joint/upper cervical vertebrae*: extension of head and neck, lateral flexion of head and neck (ipsilateral); *altantoaxial joint*: rotation of head (contralateral)
	Transverse part: broad aponeurosis at spinous processes of vertebrae T1-T4 (or C7-T3)	**Transverse part**: medial aspect of acromion, Superior crest of spine of scapula		**Transverse part**: *scapulothoracic joint*: draws scapula medially
	Ascending part: spinous processes of vertebrae T5-T12 (or T2-T12)	**Ascending part**: medial end of spine of scapula		**Ascending part**: *scapulothoracic joint*: draws scapula inferomedially (All parts support scapula)
Levator scapulae	Transverse processes of vertebrae C1-C4	Medial border of scapula (from superior angle to root of spine of scapula)	Anterior rami of spinal nerves C3-C4, Dorsal scapular nerve (C5)	**Scapulothoracic joint**: draws scapula superomedially, rotates glenoid cavity inferiorly; **Cervical joints**: lateral flexion of neck (ipsilateral)
Rhomboid major	Spinous process of vertebrae T2-T5	Medial border of scapula (from inferior angle to root of spine of scapula)	Dorsal scapular nerve (C5)	**Scapulothoracic joint**: draws scapula superomedially, rotates glenoid cavity inferiorly; supports position of scapula
Rhomboid minor	Nuchal ligament, Spinous processes of vertebrae C7-T1	Root (medial end) of spine of scapula		
Latissimus dorsi	**Vertebral part**: spinous processes of vertebrae T7-T12, Thoracolumbar fascia **Iliac part**: posterior third of crest of ilium **Costal part**: ribs 9-12 **Scapular part**: inferior angle of scapula	Intertubercular sulcus of humerus	Thoracodorsal nerve (C6-C8)	**Shoulder joint**: arm internal rotation, arm adduction, arm extension; assists in respiration

Intermediate layer	Origin	Insertion	Innervation	Function
Serratus posterior superior	Nuchal ligament, spinous processes of vertebrae C7-T3	Superior borders of ribs 2-5	2nd-5th Intercostal nerves	Elevates ribs
Serratus posterior inferior	Spinous processes of vertebrae T11-L2	Inferior borders of ribs 9-12	Anterior rami of spinal nerves T9-T12 (a.k.a. 9th-11th intercostal nerves + subcostal nerve)	Depresses ribs/ Draws ribs inferoposteriorly

Deep muscles of the back

The deep (intrinsic) muscles of the back extend along the length of either side of the vertebral column, deep to the thoracolumbar fascia. Their main functions include maintaining the body posture as well as facilitating the movements of the vertebral column.

They can be subdivided into four groups, or layers:

- Superficial layer: Splenii muscles
- Intermediate layer: Erector spinae muscles
- Deep layer: Transversospinal muscles
- Deepest layer: Segmental muscles

The majority of the deep back muscles are innervated by the segmental branches of the posterior rami of spinal nerves. The blood supply comes from branches of the occipital, deep and transverse cervical, vertebral, posterior intercostal, subcostal, lumbar and lateral sacral arteries.

SPINE AND BACK

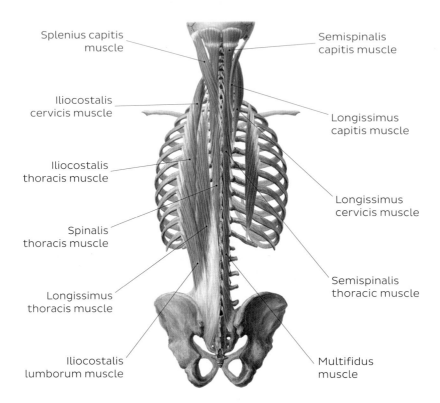

Splenius capitis muscle

Iliocostalis cervicis muscle

Iliocostalis thoracis muscle

Spinalis thoracis muscle

Longissimus thoracis muscle

Iliocostalis lumborum muscle

Semispinalis capitis muscle

Longissimus capitis muscle

Longissimus cervicis muscle

Semispinalis thoracic muscle

Multifidus muscle

FIGURE 4.16. Superficial and intermediate deep back muscles. The superficial layer of deep back muscles consists of the two splenii muscles: Splenius capitis and cervicis (not labeled). The intermediate layer consists of the erector spinae muscle group which is composed of three muscle columns: The iliocostalis, longissimus and spinalis muscles. They are regionally divided into lumbar, thoracic, cervical, and capital components.

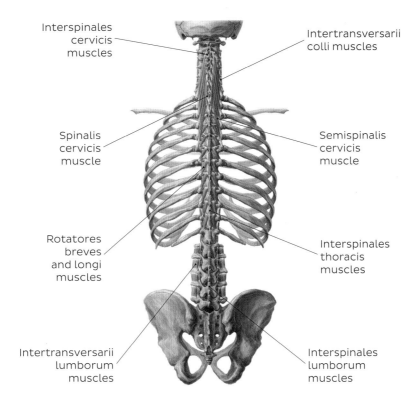

Interspinales
cervicis
muscles

Intertransversarii
colli muscles

Spinalis
cervicis
muscle

Semispinalis
cervicis
muscle

Rotatores
breves
and longi
muscles

Interspinales
thoracis
muscles

Intertransversarii
lumborum
muscles

Interspinales
lumborum
muscles

FIGURE 4.17. **Deep and deepest deep back muscles.** The deep and deepest layers of the deep back muscles consist of several smaller muscle groups. Broken down simply, the deep layer consists of a muscle group called transversospinal muscles, subdivided into the semispinalis, multifidus and rotatores muscles. These subgroups are further broken down into regional components, with the exception of the rotatores that are divided based on their length into the short and long rotatores breves and longi.

The deepest layer consists of three muscle groups: Levatores costarum, interspinales and intertransversarii muscles. They are often referred to as the segmental or minor back muscles given their small size and limited role in the back movements.

Suboccipital muscles	Origin	Insertion	Innervation	Function
Rectus capitis posterior minor	Posterior tubercle of atlas (C1)	Medial part of inferior nuchal line	Posterior ramus of spinal nerve C1 (suboccipital nerve)	**Atlantooccipital joint**: head extension
Rectus capitis posterior major	Spinous process of axis (C2)	Lateral part of inferior nuchal line		Bilateral contraction— **Atlantooccipital joint**: head extension Unilateral contraction— **Atlantoaxial joint**: head rotation (ipsilateral)
Obliquus capitis inferior	Spinous process of axis (C2)	Transverse process of atlas		
Obliquus capitis superior	Transverse process of atlas (C1)	Occipital bone (between superior and inferior nuchal lines)		Bilateral contraction— **Atlantooccipital joint**: head extension Unilateral contraction— **Atlantoaxial joint**: head lateral flexion (ipsilateral)

Superficial layer	Origin	Insertion	Innervation	Function
Splenius capitis	Spinous processes of vertebrae C7-T3, nuchal ligament	Lateral superior nuchal line of occipital bone, Mastoid process of temporal bone	Lateral branches of posterior rami of spinal nerves C2-C3	Bilateral contraction— Extends head/ neck Unilateral contraction— Lateral flexion and rotation of head (ipsilateral)
Splenius cervicis	Spinous processes of vertebrae T3-T6	Transverse processes of vertebrae C1-C3	Lateral branches of posterior rami of lower cervical spinal nerves	Bilateral contraction— Extends neck Unilateral contraction— Lateral flexion and rotation of neck (ipsilateral)

SPINE AND BACK

Superficial layer	Origin	Insertion	Innervation	Function
Iliocostalis	**Iliocostalis cervicis**: angle of ribs 3-6 **Iliocostalis thoracis**: angle of ribs 7-12 **Iliocostalis lumborum**: lateral crest of sacrum, medial end of iliac crest, thoracolumbar fascia	**Iliocostalis cervicis**: transverse processes of vertebrae C4-C6 **Iliocostalis thoracis**: angles of ribs 1-6, Transverse process of vertebra C7 **Iliocostalis lumborum**: angle of ribs 5-12, Transverse processes of vertebrae L1-L4 (+ Adjacent thoracolumbar fascia)	Lateral branches of posterior rami of spinal nerves	Bilateral contraction— Extension of spine Unilateral contraction— Lateral flexion of spine (ipsilateral)
Longissimus	**Longissimus capitis**: transverse processes of vertebrae C4-T5 **Longissimus cervicis**: transverse processes of vertebrae T1-T5 **Longissimus thoracis**: **Lumbar part**: lumbar intermuscular aponeurosis, medial part of sacropelvic surface of ilium, posterior sacroiliac ligament **Thoracic part**: spinous and transverse processes of vertebrae L1-L5, median sacral crest, posterior surface of sacrum, posterior iliac crest	**Longissimus capitis**: mastoid process of temporal bone **Longissimus cervicis**: transverse processes of vertebrae C2-C6 **Longissimus thoracis**: lumbar part: accessory and transverse processes of vertebrae L1-L5 **Thoracic part**: transverse process of vertebrae T1-T12, Angles of ribs 7-12		Entire muscle: Bilateral contraction— Extension of spine Unilateral contraction— Lateral flexion of spine (ipsilateral) Longissimus capitis only: Bilateral contraction— Extension of head and neck Unilateral contraction— Lateral flexion and rotation of head (ipsilateral)

Deep layer (transversospinales)	Origin	Insertion	Innervation	Function
Semispinalis	**Semispinalis capitis**: articular processes of vertebrae C4-C7, Transverse processes of vertebrae T1-T6 **Semispinalis cervicis**: transverse processes of vertebrae T1-T6 **Semispinalis thoracis**: transverse processes of vertebrae T6-T10	**Semispinalis capitis**: between superior and inferior nuchal lines of occipital bone **Semispinalis cervicis**: spinous processes of vertebrae C2-C5 **Semispinalis thoracis**: spinous processes of vertebrae C6-T4	**Semispinalis capitis**: descending branches of greater occipital nerve (C2) and spinal nerve C3 **Semispinalis cervicis/ thoracis**: medial branches of posterior rami of spinal nerves	Bilateral contraction— Extension of head, cervical and thoracic spine Unilateral contraction— Lateral flexion of head, cervical and thoracic spine (ipsilateral), rotation of head, cervical and thoracic spine (contralateral)
Multifidus	**Multifidus cervicis**: superior articular processes of vertebrae C4-C7 **Multifidus thoracis**: transverse process of thoracic vertebrae **Multifidus lumborum**: mammillary processes of lumbar vertebrae, posterior aspect of sacrum, posterior superior iliac spine (PSIS) of ilium, posterior sacroiliac ligament	Lateral aspect and tips of spinous processes of vertebrae 2-5 levels above origin	Medial branches of posterior rami of spinal nerves	Bilateral contraction— Extension of spine Unilateral contraction— Lateral flexion of spine (ipsilateral), rotation of spine (contralateral)
Rotatores breves and longi	**Rotatores breves**: transverse processes of vertebrae T2-T12 **Rotatores longi**: transverse processes of thoracic vertebrae	**Rotatores breves**: laminae/Spinous process of vertebra (1 level above origin) **Rotatores longi**: laminae/Spinous process of vertebra (2 levels above origin)		Bilateral contraction— Extension of thoracic spine Unilateral contraction— Rotation of thoracic spine (contralateral)

Deepest layer	Origin	Insertion	Innervation	Function
Interspinales	**Interspinales cervicis**: superior aspect of spinous processes of vertebrae C3-T1	**Interspinales cervicis**: inferior aspect of spinous processes of vertebrae C2-C7	Posterior rami of spinal nerves	Extension of cervical and lumbar spine
	Interspinales thoracis: superior aspect of spinous process of vertebrae T2, T11 & T12 (variable)	**Interspinales thoracis**: inferior aspect of spinous processes of vertebrae T1, T10 & T11		
	Interspinales lumborum: superior aspects of spinous processes of vertebrae L2-L5	**Interspinales lumborum**: inferior aspects of spinous processes of vertebrae L1-L4		
Intertransversarii	**Anterior/ posterior cervical intertransversarii**: superior border of transverse processes of vertebrae C2-T1	**Anterior/ posterior cervical intertransversarii**: inferior border of transverse process of superior adjacent cervical vertebra	**Anterior/ posterior cervical intertransversarii**: anterior and posterior rami of cervical spinal nerves	Assists in lateral flexion of spine; stabilizes spine
	Medial lumbar intertransversarii: accessory processes of vertebrae L1-L4	**Medial lumbar intertransversarii**: mammillary process of succeeding vertebra		
	Lateral lumbar intertransversarii: transverse and accessory processes of vertebrae L1-L4	**Lateral lumbar intertransversarii**: transverse process of succeeding vertebra	**Lumbar intertransversarii**: anterior rami of lumbar spinal nerves	
Levatores costarum	Transverse process of vertebrae C7-T11	Superior border/ external surface of rib (one level below origin)	Posterior rami of spinal nerves T1-T12	Elevation of ribs; rotation of thoracic spine

Intrinsic back muscles

Overview of back muscles

NEUROVASCULATURE OF THE BACK

The arterial supply of the back is primarily derived via the posterior intercostal and lumbar arteries, which arise directly from the aorta. Additional supply is delivered by cutaneous branches of arteries supplying the superficial (extrinsic) muscles of the back (e.g. transverse cervical artery) as well as those forming the scapular anastomosis. Venous drainage is achieved via similar patterns however these vessels empty into the brachiocephalic veins, azygos venous system and inferior vena cava. The skin of the back is primarily innervated by the posterior rami of most of spinal nerves, specifically the medial branches of these rami in the cervical and thoracic regions (C2–C5, T2–T12) and the lateral branches of the posterior rami in the lumbar region (L1–L3). The superficial back muscles are mainly innervated by branches of the cervical and brachial plexuses, and intercostal nerves. Most of the deep muscles of the back are innervated by the posterior rami of cervical, thoracic and lumbar spinal nerves.

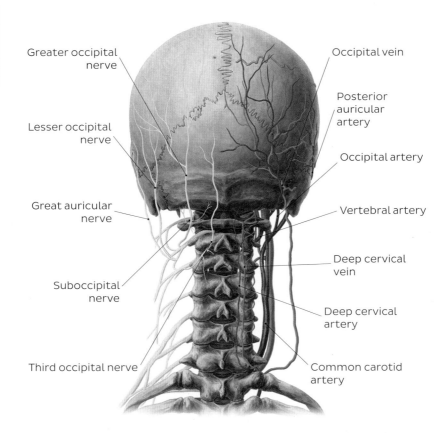

FIGURE 4.18. **Neurovasculature of the dorsal neck.**

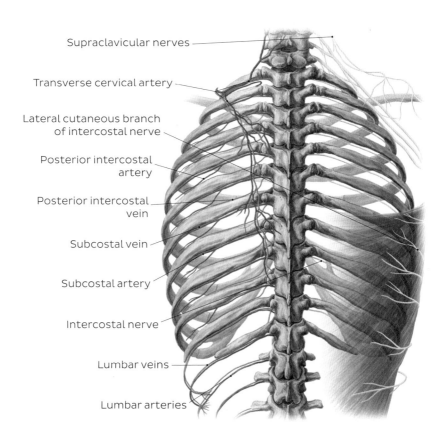

Supraclavicular nerves

Transverse cervical artery

Lateral cutaneous branch of intercostal nerve

Posterior intercostal artery

Posterior intercostal vein

Subcostal vein

Subcostal artery

Intercostal nerve

Lumbar veins

Lumbar arteries

FIGURE 4.19. Neurovasculature of the back. The arterial supply of the back is primarily derived via the posterior intercostal and lumbar arteries which arise directly from the aorta. Additional supply is delivered by cutaneous branches of arteries supplying the superficial (extrinsic) muscles of the back (e.g. transverse cervical artery) as well as those forming the scapular anastomosis. Venous drainage is achieved via similar patterns however these vessels empty into the brachiocephalic veins, azygos venous system and inferior vena cava. The skin of the back is primarily innervated by the posterior rami of most of spinal nerves, specifically the medial branches of these rami in the cervical and thoracic regions (C2-C5, T2-T12) and the lateral branches of the posterior rami in the lumbar region (L1-L3). The superficial back muscles are mainly innervated by branches of the cervical and brachial plexus, and intercostal nerves. Most of the deep muscles of the back are innervated by the posterior rami of cervical, thoracic and lumbar spinal nerves.

Arteries of the back and dorsal neck	
Occipital artery	Back of scalp, sternocleidomastoid muscle, deep muscles of back and neck
Deep cervical artery	Deep muscles of neck
Transverse cervical artery	Trapezius muscle, sternocleidomastoid muscle
Posterior intercostal arteries	Muscles and skin of the thoracic region
Subcostal artery	Subcostal region
Lumbar arteries	Muscles and skin in lumbar region, contents of vertebral canal, abdominal wall

Motor innervation of the back and dorsal neck	
Superficial (extrinsic) muscles of back	All muscles innervated by branches of cervical/brachial plexus or intercostal nerves except for the trapezius muscle (accessory nerve [CN XI])
Deep (intrinsic) muscles of back	Almost all muscles innervated by posterior rami of cervical/thoracic/lumbar spinal nerves
Suboccipital muscles	Suboccipital nerve (C1)

Cutaneous innervation of the back and dorsal neck	
Cervical region	Posterior rami of spinal nerves C2–C4/5, greater/lesser/third occipital nerves (C2–C3)
Thoracic region	Posterior rami of spinal nerves T2–T12, lateral cutaneous branches of 2nd–11th intercostal nerves/subcostal nerve
Lumbar region	Posterior rami of spinal nerves L1–L2/3

 Muscles of the neck: An overview

 Overview of back muscles

 Anatomy of the back: Spine and back muscles

 Intrinsic back muscles

SPINE AND BACK

THORAX

5

STERNUM

The **sternum** is a flat, elongated bone located centrally in the anterior thoracic wall. It's made up of three main parts: The manubrium, body and xiphoid process. It articulates with the clavicles at the **sternoclavicular joints** and with the cartilages of the first seven pairs of ribs through the **sternochondral/sternocostal joints**. The sternum anchors the right and left ribs to stabilize the rib cage, and has various functions including the protection of the heart and lungs from mechanical damage.

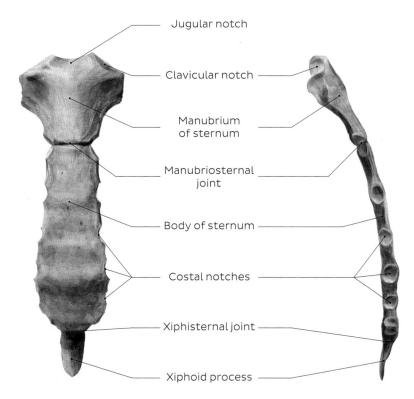

Jugular notch

Clavicular notch

Manubrium of sternum

Manubriosternal joint

Body of sternum

Costal notches

Xiphisternal joint

Xiphoid process

FIGURE 5.1. Anterior and lateral perspectives of the sternum. The **manubrium** articulates with the body of the sternum at the manubriosternal joint, and the body of the sternum with the **xiphoid process** at the xiphisternal joint. On the manubrium, the **jugular/suprasternal notch** is located centrally along its superior border and is flanked either side by the **clavicular notches** which accommodate the sternal end of each clavicle.

Directly below the clavicular notch and along the length of the manubrium and body of the sternum are seven paired **costal notches** which receive the cartilages of the true ribs. It's important to note that the sternum articulates with the costal cartilages and not directly with the ribs, through the **sternochondral joints**. These joints allow slight movement of the thoracic cavity and expansion when breathing.

THORAX

Key points about sternum	
Parts	Manubrium, body of sternum, xiphoid process
Bony landmarks	**Manubrium:** jugular notch, clavicular notch, 1st costal notch, 2nd costal notch **Body of sternum:** 2nd–7th costal notches **Xiphoid process**
Joints	**Sternoclavicular joint:** articulation between manubrium and clavicle **Sternochondral joints:** articulation between sternum and costal cartilages of 1st–7th ribs **Manubriosternal joint:** articulation between manubrium and body of sternum **Xiphisternal joint:** articulation between body of sternum and xiphoid process
Function	Provides an anchoring point for the costal cartilages; Protection of heart and lungs from mechanical damage.

Sternum

RIBS

The ribs are arc-shaped, flat bones that form the majority of the thoracic cage. There are **12 pairs of ribs**, articulating posteriorly with the thoracic vertebrae. They serve to protect the thoracic organs such as the heart and lungs, and provide attachment points to muscles of the back, chest and proximal upper limb. In addition, ribs have an important role in breathing where they move during chest expansion to enable lung inflation.

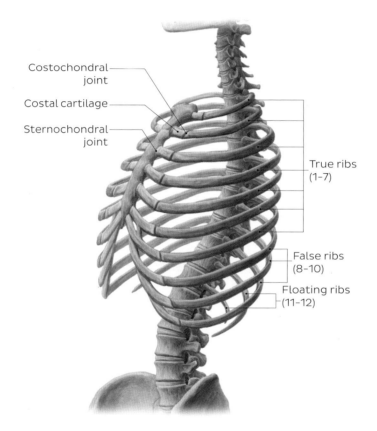

Costochondral joint

Costal cartilage

Sternochondral joint

True ribs (1-7)

False ribs (8-10)

Floating ribs (11-12)

FIGURE 5.2. Ribs (lateral-left view). The ribs can be divided into groups based on which structure they articulate with anteriorly. The first seven pairs of ribs articulate directly with the sternum through their costal cartilages and are known as the **true ribs** or vertebrosternal ribs. The joints between the ribs and their cartilages are called **costochondral joints**, while the joints between the cartilages and sternum are called the **sternochondral joints**.

The 8th-10th ribs unite anteriorly via their costal cartilages and articulate indirectly with the sternum via the 7th rib; they are known as **false ribs** or vertebrocostal ribs. The 11th and 12th ribs are known as **floating ribs** as they do not attach to the sternum in any manner and are particularly short and have no necks nor tubercles.

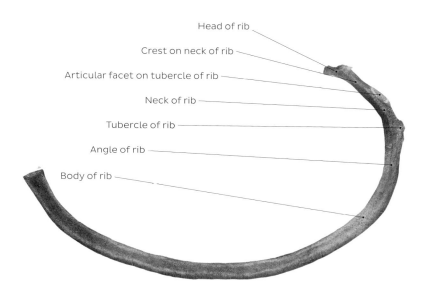

Head of rib
Crest on neck of rib
Articular facet on tubercle of rib
Neck of rib
Tubercle of rib
Angle of rib
Body of rib

FIGURE 5.3. Typical rib (superior view). The seventh rib is shown as a representative of all typical ribs (3rd-9th). The typical ribs all present a **head**, **neck**, **tubercle** and **body**. From a superior perspective, the crest of the neck, angle and external surface are visible. Each typical rib has a head with **two articular facets**, separated crest of the head (not labeled): For articulation with the superior costal facet of its corresponding vertebral body, and the other for articulation with the inferior costal facet of the superior vertebra.

Inferiorly, the internal surface is shown medial to where the costal groove is located; this groove contains the intercostal artery, vein and nerve. The distal end of a typical rib is continuous with a costal cartilage which articulates directly, or indirectly, with the sternum.

Key points about ribs	
Classifications	**True ribs:** 1st-7th (vertebrosternal ribs)
	False ribs: 8th-12th
	(vertebrocostal ribs: 8th-10th, floating ribs: 11th-12th)
	Typical ribs: 3rd-9th
	Atypical ribs: 1st, 2nd, 10th-12th
Parts & landmarks (typical ribs)	**Head:** facet divided into two by crest of head of rib
	Neck: crest of neck of rib
	Body: tubercle, costal groove, angle
	External and internal surfaces
	Round superior border, sharp inferior border
	Proximal (vertebral) and distal (sternal) ends
Function	Provide attachment points to muscles of the back, thorax and proximal upper limb
	Protect thoracic organs such as heart and lungs

THORAX

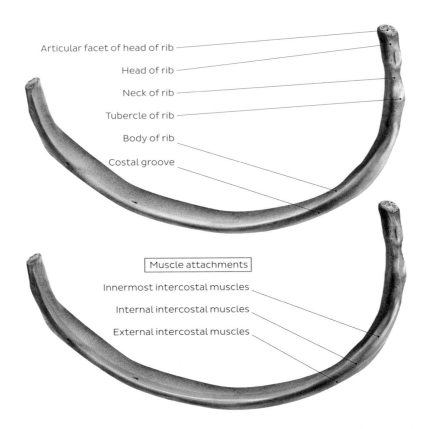

Articular facet of head of rib
Head of rib
Neck of rib
Tubercle of rib
Body of rib
Costal groove

Muscle attachments
Innermost intercostal muscles
Internal intercostal muscles
External intercostal muscles

FIGURE 5.4. Typical rib (inferior view). The 5th rib is shown from an inferior view. This perspective allows the appreciation of the **costal groove** which is traversed by the intercostal vessels and intercostal nerve. The order of these structures from superior to inferior is vein, artery, nerve.

The inferior surface of the rib provides the attachment sites for the intercostal muscles. The external and internal intercostal muscles attach to the anterior margin of the groove, while the innermost intercostal muscles attach to the posterior margin.

Ribs

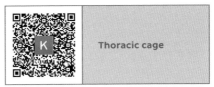

Thoracic cage

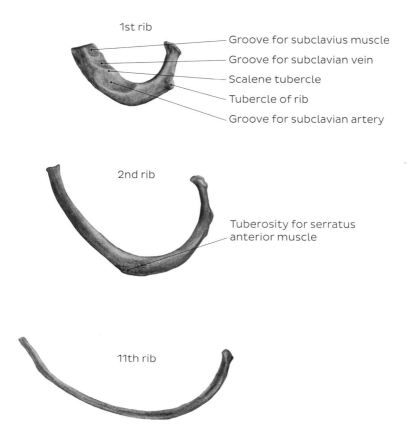

1st rib

Groove for subclavius muscle

Groove for subclavian vein

Scalene tubercle

Tubercle of rib

Groove for subclavian artery

2nd rib

Tuberosity for serratus anterior muscle

11th rib

FIGURE 5.5. Atypical ribs (superior view). The ribs 1, 2 and 11 are shown as representatives of atypical ribs. The atypical ribs (1st, 2nd, 10th-12th) also have a head, neck and body, however, they differ in their morphology and/or unique landmarks. For example, the **1st rib** features attachment points for subclavius/scalene muscles and grooves for subclavian vessels, while the **2nd rib** contains the tuberosity for serratus anterior muscle. The **11th** and **12th** ribs are more slender than the other ribs and lack several of the typical landmarks seen on typical ribs. For example, these ribs don't have a neck or tubercule, while only having one facet on their heads, and as such articulating with only one vertebra.

Key points about ribs	
Atypical ribs	**Rib 1:** shortest true rib, single facet on head; lacks angle and costal groove, has two grooves for subclavian vessels, scalene tubercle
	Rib 2: tuberosity for serratus anterior muscle
	Rib 10: single facet on head
	Rib 11: single facet on head; short neck, lacks tubercle, has a slight costal groove
	Rib 12: single facet on head; lacks tubercle, angle, costal groove

COSTOVERTEBRAL JOINTS

The **costovertebral joints** refer to the articulations between the proximal ends of the ribs and their corresponding vertebrae. A costovertebral joint comprises two groups of synovial plane joints:

- **Joint of head of rib** (also sometimes referred to as costocorporeal joint)
- **Costotransverse joint**

In most cases, each rib articulates with its numerically equivalent vertebra and the vertebra immediately superior to it. Exceptions to this are the costovertebral joints related to the 1st rib and the ribs 10-12, which only articulate with one vertebra.

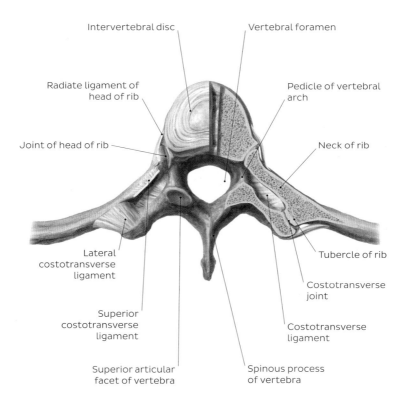

FIGURE 5.6. Costotransverse joints (superior view). The **costotransverse joints** are articulations between the articular facets of the tubercles of the ribs and the costal facets on the transverse processes of the corresponding vertebrae. These joints have a small **synovial cavity** that is surrounded by a weak articular capsule. The capsule is reinforced and strengthened by the **costotransverse**, **lateral costotransverse** and **superior costotransverse ligaments**. These joints are only present in the **ribs 1-10**.

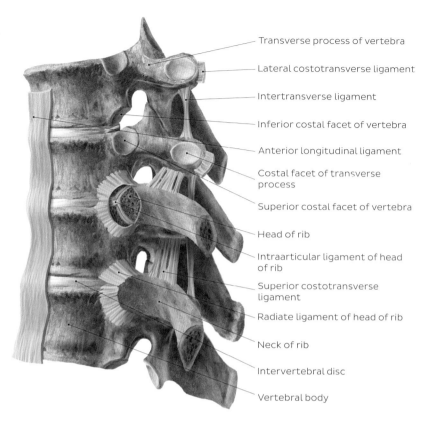

Transverse process of vertebra

Lateral costotransverse ligament

Intertransverse ligament

Inferior costal facet of vertebra

Anterior longitudinal ligament

Costal facet of transverse process

Superior costal facet of vertebra

Head of rib

Intraarticular ligament of head of rib

Superior costotransverse ligament

Radiate ligament of head of rib

Neck of rib

Intervertebral disc

Vertebral body

FIGURE 5.7. Joint of head of rib (lateral view). The **joint of head of rib** (costocorporeal joint), connects the head of a rib to the body/bodies of adjacent thoracic vertebrae. The **articulating surfaces** of the 2nd to 9th ribs consist of a superior and an inferior costal facet, that articulate with the bodies of two adjacent vertebrae: The vertebra of the same number and the vertebra above. An **intervertebral disc** is positioned between these facets.

A short horizontally oriented **intraarticular ligament** extends from the anterior surface of the head of the rib to the intervertebral disc, which helps to delineate an **upper** and a **lower joint cavity**. These cavities are covered by a single articular capsule, which becomes thickened anteriorly to form the **radiate ligament**. The heads of the 1st, 10th, 11th and 12th ribs each articulate with only one vertebra; thus, these joints only have a single cavity.

THORAX

MUSCLES OF THE THORACIC WALL

The **muscles of the thoracic wall** are defined as muscles attached to the bony framework of the thoracic cage. They maintain the **stability** of the thoracic wall, and play a role in **respiration**. The muscles of the thoracic wall are divided into two groups: Intrinsic and extrinsic.

The **intrinsic muscles** of the thoracic wall originate and insert onto the thoracic cage and contribute to its structure. This group of muscles generally work together to facilitate breathing movements through the elevation and depression of the lateral shaft of each rib and are therefore also known as the **muscles of respiration**. Intrinsic muscles of the thoracic wall include the: Serratus posterior, levatores costarum, intercostal, subcostal and transversus thoracis muscles, as well as the variably present sternalis muscle.

The **extrinsic muscles** of the thoracic wall usually have one attachment to the thoracic cage and are functionally related to the neck, abdomen, back and/or upper limbs. Although these muscles can be classified as thoracic muscles and are involved in movement of the rib cage for respiration, their primary functions relate to movement of the pectoral girdle and/or the arm and are therefore also known as the **anterior axioappendicular muscles**. As a secondary function these muscles contribute to movements during breathing and include the subclavius, pectoralis major and minor muscles as well as the inferior portion of the serratus anterior muscle.

Extrinsic muscles	Origin	Insertion	Innervation	Function
Subclavius	Costal cartilage, Sternal end of rib 1	Anteroinferior surface of middle third of clavicle	Subclavian nerve (C5–C6)	**Sternoclavicular joint:** anchors and depresses clavicle
Pectoralis major	**Clavicular head:** anterior surface of clavicle (medial half) **Sternocostal head:** anterior surface of sternum, Costal cartilages of ribs 1–6 **Abdominal (rectus) head:** anterior layer of rectus sheath	Crest of greater tubercle of humerus (all heads)	**Clavicular head:** lateral pectoral nerve (C5–C7) **Sternocostal head:** medial pectoral nerve (C8–T1) **Abdominal (rectus) head:** medial pectoral nerve (C8–T1)	**Shoulder joint:** arm adduction, arm internal rotation, arm flexion (clavicular head), arm extension (sternocostal head);
Pectoralis minor	Anterior surface, Costal cartilages of ribs 3–5	Coracoid process of scapula	Lateral and medial pectoral nerves (C5–T1)	**Scapulothoracic joint:** draws scapula anteroinferiorly, stabilizes scapula on thoracic wall
Serratus anterior	**Superior part:** ribs 1–2, Intercostal fascia **Middle part:** ribs-3–6 **Inferior part:** ribs 7–8/9/10 (+ external oblique muscle)	**Superior part:** anterior surface of superior angle of scapula **Middle part:** anterior surface of medial border of scapula **Inferior part:** anterior surface of inferior angle of scapula	Long thoracic nerve (C5–C7)	**Scapulothoracic joint:** draws scapula anterolaterally, Suspends scapula on thoracic wall, rotates scapula (draws inferiorly angle laterally)

THORAX

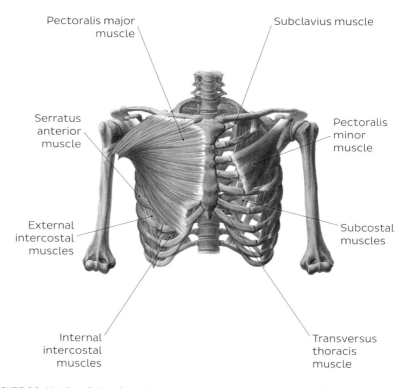

Pectoralis major muscle

Subclavius muscle

Serratus anterior muscle

Pectoralis minor muscle

External intercostal muscles

Subcostal muscles

Internal intercostal muscles

Transversus thoracis muscle

FIGURE 5.8. Muscles of thoracic wall (anterior view). Intrinsic muscles evident from this anterior view include the intercostal, subcostal and transversus thoracis muscles. Lying beneath the large extrinsic muscles of the thoracic wall are the **intercostal muscles** (external, internal and innermost intercostal muscles). These muscles are located within the intercostal spaces and function to elevate, stabilize or depress the thoracic cage and therefore facilitate breathing movements. The **subcostal muscles** are bands of muscle located on the internal surface of the lower ribs, sharing a plane with the innermost intercostals. They support the intercostal spaces and thoracic cage, and depress the ribs during forced expiration. Also located along the internal aspect of the thoracic cage is the **transversus thoracis muscle**. This is a weak muscle of the rib cage which assists in expiration.

The **extrinsic muscles** of the thoracic wall include the subclavius, pectoralis major and minor and serratus anterior muscles. The short, triangular **subclavius muscle** is located beneath the clavicle and mainly functions in anchoring and depressing the bone. The large **pectoralis major muscle** arises from three heads (clavicular, sternocostal and abdominal) which unite before inserting into the intertubercular sulcus of the humerus. Deep to the pectoralis major muscle, is the smaller **pectoralis minor muscle**. The pectoralis major primarily flexes, adducts and internally rotates the arm at the shoulder joint on contraction, while the pectoralis minor muscle stabilizes and draws the scapula anteroinferiorly.

Located along the anterolateral aspect of the thoracic wall is the large fan shaped **serratus anterior muscle**. This muscle primarily functions to rotate and draw the scapula anterolaterally. All of the extrinsic muscles of the thoracic wall participate in elevation of the rib cage during forced inspiration as a secondary function.

THORAX

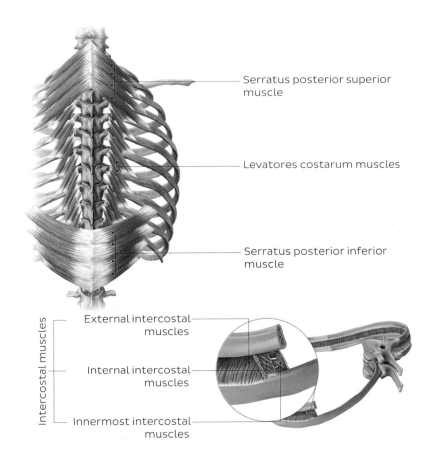

Serratus posterior superior muscle

Levatores costarum muscles

Serratus posterior inferior muscle

Intercostal muscles

External intercostal muscles

Internal intercostal muscles

Innermost intercostal muscles

FIGURE 5.9. Muscles of thoracic wall (posterior view). The **intrinsic muscles** of the posterior thoracic wall can be better appreciated from this view. The **serratus posterior superior** and **inferior** muscles are two paired muscles located in the upper and lower back. Their main function is to facilitate the act of respiration; the serratus posterior superior muscle elevates the ribs, while the serratus posterior inferior muscle depresses the ribs. The **levatores costarum** consists of 12 small triangular bilateral muscles that connect the thoracic vertebrae with the adjacent ribs. This group of muscles function in elevating the ribs to facilitate forced inspiration and produce rotation and lateral flexion of the thoracic vertebrae.

The external, internal and innermost intercostal muscles can also be appreciated from a posterolateral view of the thoracic cage. The **external intercostal muscles** are the most superficial intercostal muscles; their fibers are oriented in an inferomedial direction. The **internal intercostal muscles** form the middle layer of the intercostal musculature; their fibers course inferolaterally. The **innermost intercostals** are the deepest intercostal muscles and course in the same manner as the internal intercostal muscles. All three intercostal muscles are accessory respiratory muscles that participate in the process of forced breathing.

Intrinsic muscles	Origin	Insertion	Innervation	Function
Serratus posterior superior	Nuchal ligament, spinous processes of vertebrae C7-T3	Superior borders of ribs 2-5	2nd-5th Intercostal nerves	Elevates ribs
Serratus posterior inferior	Spinous processes of vertebrae T11-L2	Inferior borders of ribs 9-12	Anterior rami of spinal nerves T9-T12 (9th-11th Intercostal nerves + subcostal nerve)	Depresses ribs/ Draws ribs inferoposteriorly
External intercostals	Inferior border of ribs	Superior border of immediate rib below	Intercostal nerves	Elevate ribs during forced inspiration; Supports intercostal spaces and thoracic cage
Internal intercostals	Costal groove of ribs			Depresses ribs during forced expiration; Supports intercostal spaces and thoracic cage
Innermost intercostals	Costal groove of ribs			Depresses ribs during forced expiration; Supports intercostal spaces and thoracic cage
Subcostal muscles	Internal surface of ribs (near angle of rib)	Internal surface of rib (2-3 levels below origin)		Depresses ribs during forced expiration; Supports intercostal spaces and thoracic cage
Transversus thoracis	Sternal ends of costal cartilages of ribs 4-7, Inferoposterior surface of body of sternum and xiphoid process	Internal surface of costal cartilages of ribs 2-6		Depresses costal cartilages

Thorax

Muscles of the trunk

Intercostal muscles

THORACIC SURFACE OF THE DIAPHRAGM

The **diaphragm** is a large, dome-shaped, musculotendinous structure that separates the thoracic cavity from the abdominal cavity. Contraction of this large muscle is vital for respiration, as it flattens the dome-like structure of the diaphragm and thus expands the thoracic cavity, allowing air to flow into the lungs.

The diaphragm is innervated by the left and right phrenic nerves, which arise from spinal nerves C3 to C5. There are a number of apertures, or openings, which allow structures to pass through the diaphragm and enter or leave the thoracic cavity. The three major openings are named after the structures that pass through them: The aortic hiatus, esophageal hiatus and caval foramen.

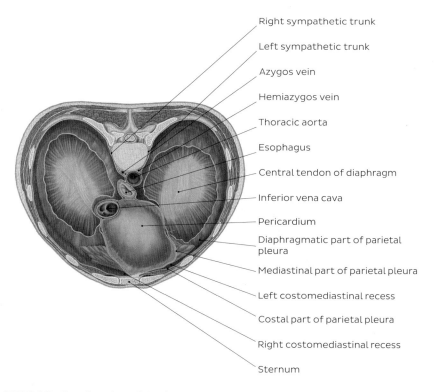

Right sympathetic trunk

Left sympathetic trunk

Azygos vein

Hemiazygos vein

Thoracic aorta

Esophagus

Central tendon of diaphragm

Inferior vena cava

Pericardium

Diaphragmatic part of parietal pleura

Mediastinal part of parietal pleura

Left costomediastinal recess

Costal part of parietal pleura

Right costomediastinal recess

Sternum

FIGURE 5.10. Thoracic surface of the diaphragm (superior view). The diaphragm is the large muscular structure, which separates the thoracic cavity from the abdominal cavity and allows for the passage of several important structures, including the aorta, inferior vena cava and esophagus. Directly covering the diaphragm is a layer of the parietal pleura of the lungs called the **diaphragmatic part of the parietal pleura**. In this illustration, the parietal pleura is partially removed on both sides, to reveal the left and right **central tendons** of the diaphragm beneath.

The **pericardium** also lies directly on the diaphragm and encloses the heart. The muscle fibers of the diaphragm radiate outwards from the central tendons and attach peripherally to the circumference of the inferior thoracic aperture (vertebra T12, 11th and 12th ribs, costal cartilages of 7th-10th ribs and xiphoid process of the sternum). The domed shape of the diaphragm accommodates several **pleural recesses** along its border - the left and right costomediastinal recesses, located between the thoracic surface of the diaphragm and the anterior wall of the rib cage, as well as the costodiaphragmatic recesses, located between the diaphragm and lateral wall of the rib cage.

Key points about the thoracic surface of the diaphragm	
Parts	Skeletal muscle (sternal, costal and lumbar parts), central tendon
Function	Main muscle responsible for respiration; increases abdominal pressure to expel feces, vomit and urine; applies pressure on the esophagus to prevent acid reflux
Relations	Parietal pleura, pericardium
Openings (apertures)	**Aortic hiatus:** aorta, azygos vein, thoracic duct
	Esophageal hiatus: esophagus, branches of the left gastric artery and vein, anterior and posterior vagal trunks
	Caval foramen: inferior vena cava, branches of the right phrenic nerve
Innervation	Left and right phrenic nerves (C3-C5)

Diaphragm

Anatomy of breathing

NEUROVASCULATURE OF THE THORACIC WALL

The thoracic wall has a rich **arterial supply** via branches that arise from three main sources: The subclavian artery, axillary artery and the thoracic aorta. The **veins** of the thoracic wall initially follow a similar course to that of their arterial counterparts, however, most of them terminate by draining into the azygos venous system. Lastly, the **nervous supply** to the thoracic wall mainly stems from the anterior rami of the spinal nerves T1-T12 (intercostal/subcostal nerves). Additional nervous supply to the thoracic wall stems from a small number of preterminal branches of the brachial plexus (e.g., medial and lateral pectoral nerves, long thoracic nerve).

THORAX

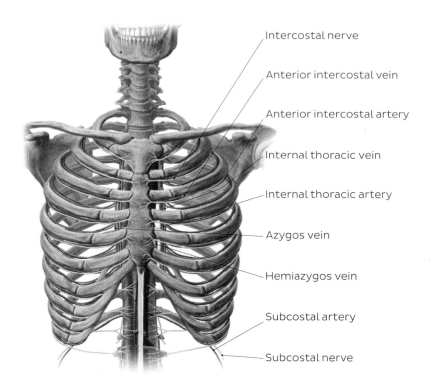

Intercostal nerve

Anterior intercostal vein

Anterior intercostal artery

Internal thoracic vein

Internal thoracic artery

Azygos vein

Hemiazygos vein

Subcostal artery

Subcostal nerve

FIGURE 5.11. Arteries, veins and nerves of the thoracic wall. The main arteries of the thoracic wall are the internal thoracic, anterior intercostal, posterior intercostal and subcostal arteries. The **internal thoracic artery** arises from the subclavian artery, and distally terminates by splitting into the musculophrenic and superior epigastric arteries.

The **anterior intercostal arteries** are a set of nine arteries that supply the anterior part of intercostal spaces of the ribs 1-10. The upper six anterior intercostal arteries arise from the internal thoracic artery, while the rest are branches of the musculophrenic artery. The **posterior intercostal arteries** are a set of eleven arteries that supply the posterior intercostal spaces. The first and second arise from the supreme intercostal artery, while the rest arise from the thoracic aorta. Finally, the **subcostal artery** arises from the thoracic aorta and supplies the subcostal region below the 12th rib.

The venous drainage of the thoracic wall is accommodated by **intercostal veins** that accompany the intercostal arteries. Most of the posterior intercostal veins (4th-11th) drain directly into the **azygos venous system**. The 1st posterior intercostal vein, called the supreme intercostal vein drains directly into the ipsilateral brachiocephalic vein. Additionally, the 2nd and 3rd posterior intercostal veins merge to form a superior intercostal vein on each side. The left superior intercostal vein goes on to drain into the left brachiocephalic vein, while the right one drains into the azygos vein.

The anterior rami of spinal nerves T1–T11 (1st-11th thoracic nerves) form the **intercostal nerves** that course within the intercostal spaces. The anterior ramus of spinal nerve T12 (12th thoracic nerve) forms the **subcostal nerve** that runs below the rib cage. The pectoral muscles of the thoracic wall also receive innervation from the medial and lateral pectoral nerves, which arise from the medial and lateral cords of the brachial plexus, respectively.

THORAX

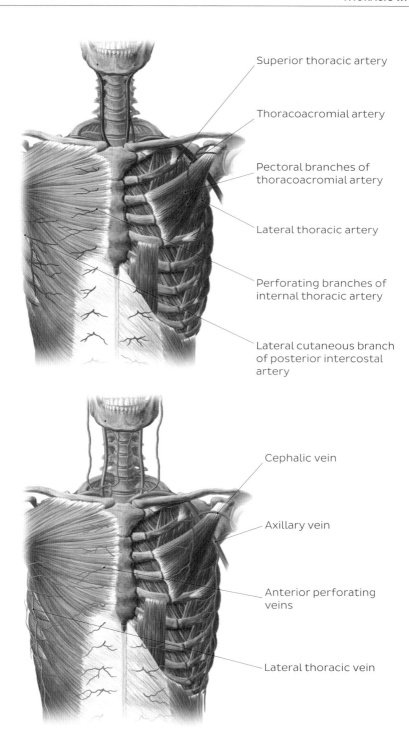

Superior thoracic artery

Thoracoacromial artery

Pectoral branches of thoracoacromial artery

Lateral thoracic artery

Perforating branches of internal thoracic artery

Lateral cutaneous branch of posterior intercostal artery

Cephalic vein

Axillary vein

Anterior perforating veins

Lateral thoracic vein

THORAX

FIGURE 5.12. Top image: Arteries of the thoracic wall. This image depicts the cutaneous and perforating branches of the main thoracic vessels supplying the skin and muscles of the thoracic wall. **Bottom image: Veins of the thoracic wall.** This image depicts the cutaneous and muscular tributaries to the veins of the thoracic wall.

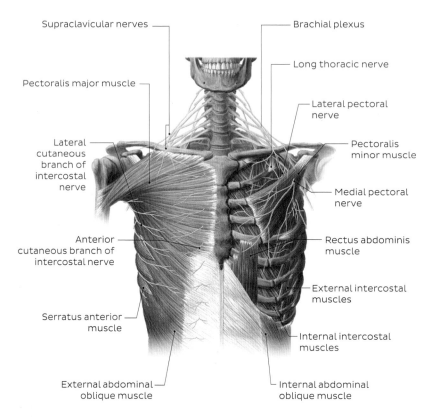

Supraclavicular nerves

Brachial plexus

Pectoralis major muscle

Long thoracic nerve

Lateral pectoral nerve

Lateral cutaneous branch of intercostal nerve

Pectoralis minor muscle

Medial pectoral nerve

Anterior cutaneous branch of intercostal nerve

Rectus abdominis muscle

External intercostal muscles

Serratus anterior muscle

Internal intercostal muscles

External abdominal oblique muscle

Internal abdominal oblique muscle

FIGURE 5.13. Nerves of the thoracic wall. This image depicts the cutaneous and muscular branches supplying the skin and musculature of the thoracic wall.

Key points about the neurovasculature of the thoracic wall	
Arteries	Internal thoracic artery (origin: subclavian artery)
	Superior thoracic artery (origin: axillary artery)
	Lateral thoracic artery (origin: axillary artery)
	Anterior intercostal arteries (origin: internal thoracic artery (upper 6), musculophrenic artery (lower 3))
	Posterior intercostal arteries (origin: supreme intercostal artery (upper 2), thoracic aorta (lower 10))
	Subcostal artery (origin: thoracic aorta)
Veins	Anterior intercostal veins (drain into: internal thoracic vein)
	Posterior intercostal veins:
	• Supreme intercostal vein drains into: brachiocephalic vein
	• Superior intercostal vein drains into: azygos vein (right), left brachiocephalic vein (left)
	• Right 4th–11th drain into: azygos vein
	• Left 4th–7th drain into: accessory hemiazygos vein
	• Left 8th–11th drain into: hemiazygos vein
	• Subcostal vein drains into: azygos vein (right), hemiazygos vein (left)

Key points about the neurovasculature of the thoracic wall	
Nerves	**Thoracic nerves:** Anterior rami of spinal nerves T1-T11 = intercostal nerves Anterior ramus of spinal nerve T12 = subcostal nerve **Brachial plexus:** Long thoracic nerve (C5, C6, C7) Lateral pectoral nerve (C5, C6, C7) Medial pectoral nerve (C8, T1)

 Intercostal arteries and veins

 Intercostal spaces

NEUROVASCULATURE OF THE INTERCOSTAL SPACE

Intercostal spaces are anatomical spaces which lie between adjacent ribs. They are occupied by three layers of **intercostal muscles** as well as neurovascular bundles of intercostal vessels and nerves. Each neurovascular bundle lies within the costal groove, along the inferior margin of the superior rib, and passes in the plane between the inner and innermost layers of muscles. From superior to inferior, they are arranged as vein, artery and then nerve. Smaller collateral branches of each nerve, artery and vein run along the superior aspect of the lower rib.

Key points about the neurovasculature of the intercostal space	
Arteries	**Anterior intercostal arteries** Origin: internal thoracic artery (upper six intercostal spaces), musculophrenic artery (lower three intercostal spaces) Branches: collateral branch **Posterior intercostal arteries** Origin: supreme intercostal artery (upper two), descending thoracic aorta (lower nine) Branches: dorsal branch, collateral branch, lateral cutaneous branch
Veins	**Anterior intercostal veins** Drain into: internal thoracic vein **Posterior intercostal veins** Supreme intercostal vein (1st) → drains into brachiocephalic vein Right 2nd-3rd (form right superior intercostal vein) → drains into azygos vein Left 2nd-3rd (form left superior intercostal vein) → drains into left brachiocephalic vein Right 4th-11th → drain into azygos vein Left 4th-8th → drain into accessory hemiazygos vein Left 9th-11th → drain into hemiazygos vein
Nerves	Anterior rami of spinal nerves T1-T11 = Intercostal nerves Branches: collateral branch, lateral cutaneous branch, anterior cutaneous branch (muscular branches)

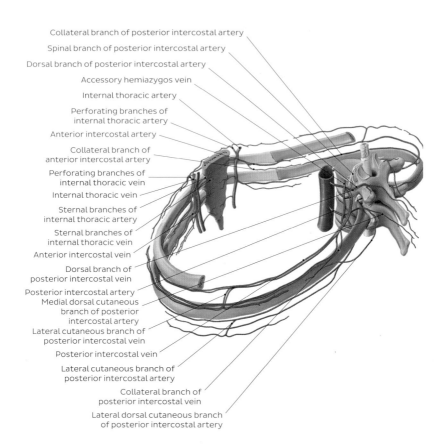

Collateral branch of posterior intercostal artery
Spinal branch of posterior intercostal artery
Dorsal branch of posterior intercostal artery
Accessory hemiazygos vein
Internal thoracic artery
Perforating branches of internal thoracic artery
Anterior intercostal artery
Collateral branch of anterior intercostal artery
Perforating branches of internal thoracic vein
Internal thoracic vein
Sternal branches of internal thoracic artery
Sternal branches of internal thoracic vein
Anterior intercostal vein
Dorsal branch of posterior intercostal vein
Posterior intercostal artery
Medial dorsal cutaneous branch of posterior intercostal artery
Lateral cutaneous branch of posterior intercostal vein
Posterior intercostal vein
Lateral cutaneous branch of posterior intercostal artery
Collateral branch of posterior intercostal vein
Lateral dorsal cutaneous branch of posterior intercostal artery

FIGURE 5.14. Vessels of the intercostal space (superolateral view). The **anterior** and **posterior intercostal arteries** pass around the thoracic wall forming a basket-like pattern of vascular supply around it. These arteries mostly originate from the thoracic aorta and internal thoracic artery, respectively. Venous drainage generally parallels the pattern of arterial supply. The **anterior intercostal veins** drain into the internal thoracic vein, adjacent to the internal thoracic artery. Most of the posterior intercostal veins drain into the azygos venous system which is represented by the accessory hemiazygos vein at this level and left lateral perspective of the thoracic cavity. Collateral vessels are given off towards the lower edge of each intercostal space (superior border of lower rib).

THORAX

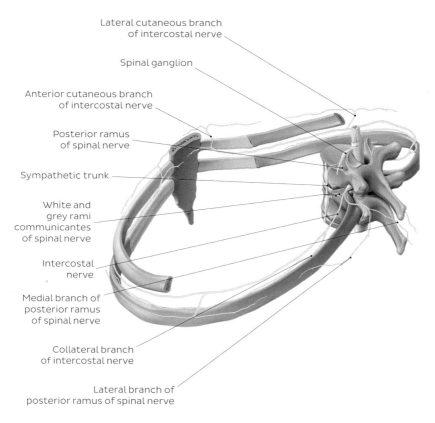

Lateral cutaneous branch
of intercostal nerve

Spinal ganglion

Anterior cutaneous branch
of intercostal nerve

Posterior ramus
of spinal nerve

Sympathetic trunk

White and
grey rami
communicantes
of spinal nerve

Intercostal
nerve

Medial branch of
posterior ramus
of spinal nerve

Collateral branch
of intercostal nerve

Lateral branch of
posterior ramus of spinal nerve

FIGURE 5.15. Nerves of the intercostal space. Intercostal nerves originate as the **anterior rami of spinal nerves T1 to T11**. Each gives rise to a lateral cutaneous branch and terminates anteriorly as anterior cutaneous branches. In addition to these major branches, small collateral branches can be found in the intercostal space running along the superior border of the lower rib.

Intercostal arteries
and veins

Intercostal spaces

Intercostal nerves

THORAX

STRUCTURE OF THE FEMALE BREAST

The female breasts are glandular organs that contain **mammary glands** used in the production of milk for nursing newborns. They are located on the antero-lateral walls of the thoracic cage, extending vertically between the 2nd and 6th ribs and horizontally between the lateral border of the sternum and midaxillary line. A small axillary process may extend towards the axillary fossa.

Between each breast and underlying **pectoral fascia** is a **retromammary space** containing fat and loose connective tissue which allows a degree of movement on the thoracic wall.

Breast size and shape is highly dependent on various genetic, ethnic and dietary factors as well as age, menstrual status and parity. They are frequently asymmetric, variably pendulous and usually conoid or piriform in appearance.

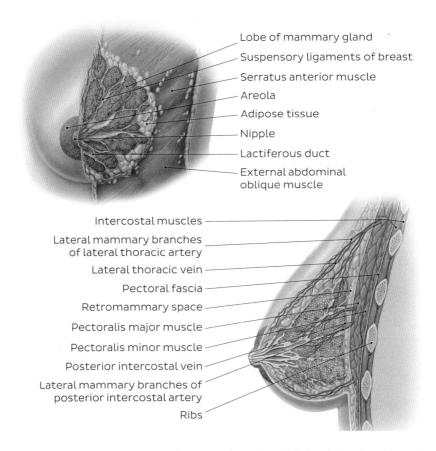

Lobe of mammary gland
Suspensory ligaments of breast
Serratus anterior muscle
Areola
Adipose tissue
Nipple
Lactiferous duct
External abdominal oblique muscle

Intercostal muscles
Lateral mammary branches of lateral thoracic artery
Lateral thoracic vein
Pectoral fascia
Retromammary space
Pectoralis major muscle
Pectoralis minor muscle
Posterior intercostal vein
Lateral mammary branches of posterior intercostal artery
Ribs

FIGURE 5.16. Structure of the female breast (anterior and sagittal views). Each breast comprises 15-20 secretory **lobes** which are separated by fibrous suspensory ligaments which extend between the clavipectoral fascia and dermis of the overlying skin. The secretory lobes contain numerous lobules composed of the tubuloalveolar glands, which are drained by **lactiferous ducts** which converge and open at the nipple. The nipples are surrounded by a pigmented circular region of skin called the **areola**, which

THORAX

becomes more pigmented and prominent during pregnancy. The areola shows small punctual elevations on its surface, which are formed by areolar glands. These are mostly sweat and sebaceous glands which produce an antimicrobial secretion that protects the surface of areola.

 Breast

 Breast cancer development after prophylactic subcutaneous mastectomy

BLOOD VESSELS OF THE FEMALE BREAST

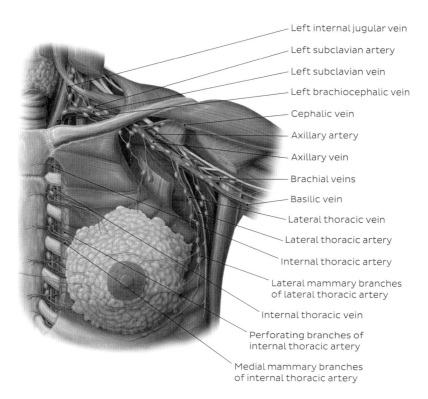

- Left internal jugular vein
- Left subclavian artery
- Left subclavian vein
- Left brachiocephalic vein
- Cephalic vein
- Axillary artery
- Axillary vein
- Brachial veins
- Basilic vein
- Lateral thoracic vein
- Lateral thoracic artery
- Internal thoracic artery
- Lateral mammary branches of lateral thoracic artery
- Internal thoracic vein
- Perforating branches of internal thoracic artery
- Medial mammary branches of internal thoracic artery

FIGURE 5.17. Blood vessels of the female breast. The image shows the left pectoral region of a female, with the skin removed to reveal the breast tissue. The pectoralis major and minor muscles are also partially removed to better expose the blood vessels and lymphatics beneath them.

The arterial supply of the female breast is given by branches of three arteries:

- **Internal thoracic artery** (supply to the medial part of the breast)
    - Main branches to the breast: **Medial mammary branches** [of perforating arteries] and anterior inter-costal arteries
- **Axillary artery** (supply to the superolateral part of the breast)
    - Main branches to the breast: **Lateral mammary branches** of lateral thoracic artery, superior thoracic artery, pectoral branch of thoracoacromial artery

THORAX

- **Posterior intercostal artery** (supply to the lateral part of the breast)
  - Main branches to the breast: Lateral mammary branches of lateral cutaneous branches

The venous drainage of the female breast mostly mimics the arteries. The blood drains mainly into the axillary vein, but there is some drainage into the internal thoracic vein.

Key points about the blood vessels of the female breast	
Arteries of the female breast	**Internal thoracic artery** (supply to the medial part of the breast) → medial mammary branches [of perforating arteries] and anterior intercostal arteries **Axillary artery** (supply to the superolateral part of the breast) → lateral mammary branches of lateral thoracic artery, superior thoracic artery, pectoral branch of thoracoacromial artery **Posterior intercostal artery** (supply to the lateral part of the breast) → lateral mammary branches of lateral cutaneous branches
Veins of the female breast	**Axillary vein:** receives blood from superolateral breast, drains into subclavian vein **Posterior intercostal vein:** receives blood from lateral breast, drains into azygos venous system **Internal thoracic vein:** receives blood from medial breast, drains into brachiocephalic vein

Breast

LYMPHATICS OF THE FEMALE BREAST

In the context of mammary carcinoma/breast cancer, a knowledge of the anatomy of the lymphatics of the female breast is of utmost importance in the staging and treatment of this disease.

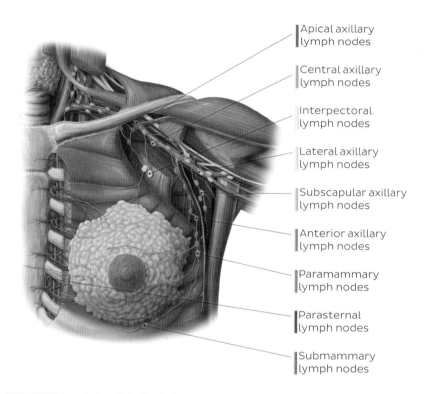

Apical axillary
lymph nodes

Central axillary
lymph nodes

Interpectoral
lymph nodes

Lateral axillary
lymph nodes

Subscapular axillary
lymph nodes

Anterior axillary
lymph nodes

Paramammary
lymph nodes

Parasternal
lymph nodes

Submammary
lymph nodes

FIGURE 5.18. Lymphatics of the female breast. Lymph from the breast tissue and adjacent structures usually take three main routes of drainage:

- Most of the lymph from the nipple, areola and breast lobules (especially those from the lateral quadrants) are drained into a lateral route by the **subareolar lymphatic plexus**. From there, the lymph is carried to the **axillary lymph nodes**. Those are subdivided into **five groups**: Anterior (pectoral), posterior (subscapular), lateral (brachial or humeral), central and apical. Lymphatic vessels draining these large node groups converge to form the **subclavian lymph trunk(s)**. The left and right subclavian lymph trunks usually open independently into the ipsilateral **venous angle** (junction of subclavian and internal jugular veins), but can also join the ipsilateral jugular and/or bronchomediastinal lymph trunk – forming a right lymphatic duct on the right side, or joining the thoracic duct on the left. This route drains over 75% of the lymph from the breast tissue.

- A medial pathway is composed mainly of **parasternal lymph nodes** that drain lymph mostly from the medial quadrants of the breast tissue and enter the **bronchomediastinal lymph trunks**, which usually independently drain into ipsilateral **venous angle**.

A deep pathway drains the deeper portions of the breast tissue to the **subclavicular lymphatic plexus**.

Key points about the lymphatics of the female breast	
Lateral pathway	• Dominant pathway of female breast (nipple, areola, majority of glandular tissue) • Axillary lymph nodes: anterior (pectoral), posterior (subscapular), lateral (brachial or humeral) → central → apical • Drains to the ipsilateral venous angle (sometimes via right lymphatic or thoracic duct)
Medial pathway	• Drain medial quadrants of the breast • Parasternal lymph nodes • Drains to bronchomediastinal lymph trunks
Deep pathway	• Drain deep portions of breast directly to subclavicular lymphatic plexus

Lymphatic drainage of the breast

Axillary lymph nodes

BORDERS, DIVISIONS AND CONTENTS OF THE MEDIASTINUM

The **mediastinum** is a compartment of the thorax located in the midline of the body, that contains most of the thoracic viscera, apart from the lungs. It extends vertically from the superior thoracic aperture to the diaphragm and is bounded laterally by the medial surfaces of the pleura.

The **thoracic plane** (of Ludwig), is an imaginary line extending from the sternal angle, anteriorly, to the T4-T5 intervertebral space, posteriorly. This plane divides the mediastinum into **superior** (above the thoracic plane) and **inferior** (below the thoracic plane) **mediastinal divisions**.

The **inferior division** is further subdivided into anterior, middle and posterior compartments by the pericardial sac. Structures located anterior to the pericardial sac belong to the **anterior mediastinum**, whereas those located posterior to pericardial sac are said to be structures of the **posterior mediastinum**. Those located in and around the pericardial sac belong to the **middle mediastinum**.

These structures course longitudinally through the superior and inferior mediastinum: Esophagus, azygos vein and vagus and phrenic nerves.

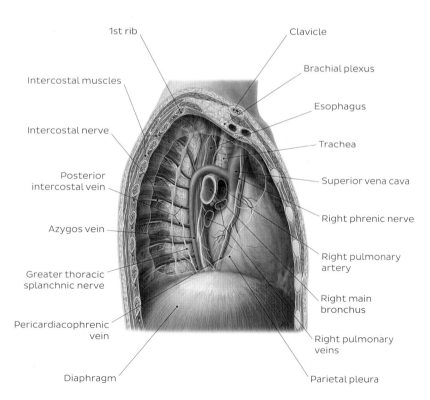

FIGURE 5.19. Overview of the mediastinum (right lateral view). The **esophagus** courses longitudinally throughout the mediastinum, posterior to the trachea and main bronchi and anteromedial to the

azygos vein. The **pericardial sac** can be seen anteriorly, with its contents and adjacent structures forming the middle compartment of the inferior mediastinum. **Pericardiophrenic arteries** and **veins** are also seen abutting the pericardial sac.

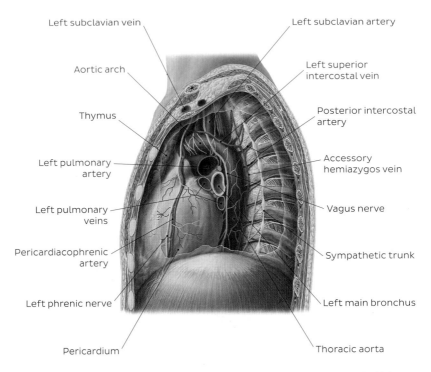

FIGURE 5.20. Overview of the mediastinum (left lateral view). The main structures seen in this image are the **thoracic aorta** (situated anterolateral to the thoracic vertebral bodies and posterior to the pulmonary artery and veins), the **left main bronchus** as well as the **pericardial sac** and its contents. The phrenic and vagus nerves are also shown.

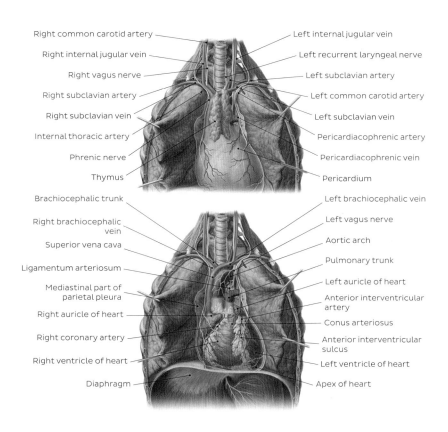

Right common carotid artery

Right internal jugular vein

Right vagus nerve

Right subclavian artery

Right subclavian vein

Internal thoracic artery

Phrenic nerve

Thymus

Brachiocephalic trunk

Right brachiocephalic vein

Superior vena cava

Ligamentum arteriosum

Mediastinal part of parietal pleura

Right auricle of heart

Right coronary artery

Right ventricle of heart

Diaphragm

Left internal jugular vein

Left recurrent laryngeal nerve

Left subclavian artery

Left common carotid artery

Left subclavian vein

Pericardiacophrenic artery

Pericardiacophrenic vein

Pericardium

Left brachiocephalic vein

Left vagus nerve

Aortic arch

Pulmonary trunk

Left auricle of heart

Anterior interventricular artery

Conus arteriosus

Anterior interventricular sulcus

Left ventricle of heart

Apex of heart

THORAX

FIGURE 5.21. Overview of the mediastinum (anterior view). The **thymus** can be seen as the anteriormost structure of the superior mediastinum; posterior to this structure it is possible to partially see the **main supraaortic vessels** (brachiocephalic trunk, left common carotid artery and left subclavian artery), as well as the main venous structures of the superior mediastinum (internal jugular, subclavian, brachiocephalic veins and superior vena cava). The pericardial sac is also shown, with its relation to the adjacent pleural sacs.

Key points about the mediastinum		
Borders	**Superior:** superior thoracic aperture (delineated by the manubrium of the sternum, superior border of the first rib and T1 vertebral body)	
	Inferior: diaphragm	
	Anterior: sternum and costal cartilages of 1st–5th ribs	
	Posterior: vertebral bodies of superior thoracic vertebrae	
	Lateral: parietal pleura of each lung	
Divisions	**Thoracic plane:** extends from sternal angle to vertebrae T4/5 intervertebral space	
	Superior mediastinum: above thoracic plane	
	Inferior mediastinum: below thoracic plane, further subdivided into anterior, middle and posterior compartments, according to relations with pericardial sac	

Key points about the mediastinum	
Contents	**Superior mediastinum:** thymus, trachea, superior part of superior vena cava, aortic arch and its branches (brachiocephalic trunk, left common carotid artery and left subclavian artery, esophagus)
	Anterior mediastinum: thymus
	Middle mediastinum: pericardial sac and heart; roots of superior and inferior vena cava; pulmonary trunk, arteries and veins; root of aorta; main bronchi; pericardiacophrenic arteries and veins
	Posterior mediastinum: descending thoracic aorta and its branches; azygos veins, esophagus

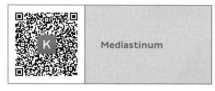

Mediastinum

NEUROVASCULATURE OF THE POSTERIOR MEDIASTINUM

Major vessels in the posterior mediastinum include the **thoracic aorta** and its branches, as well as the **azygos venous system**. The main nerves of the posterior mediastinum include the right and left **vagus nerves**, the **esophageal nerve plexus** and the anterior and posterior **vagal trunks**. The sympathetic trunks and the **thoracic splanchnic nerves**, commonly described as part of the posterior mediastinum, are actually located a bit more laterally, on each side of the thoracic vertebral column.

THORAX

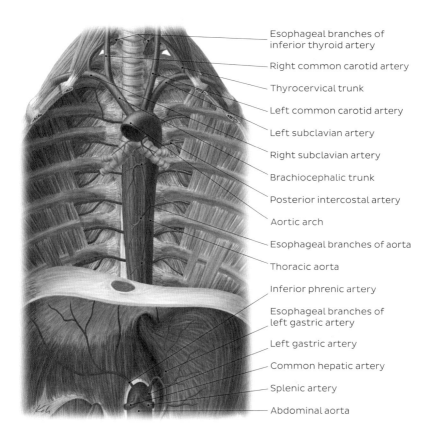

Esophageal branches of
inferior thyroid artery

Right common carotid artery

Thyrocervical trunk

Left common carotid artery

Left subclavian artery

Right subclavian artery

Brachiocephalic trunk

Posterior intercostal artery

Aortic arch

Esophageal branches of aorta

Thoracic aorta

Inferior phrenic artery

Esophageal branches of
left gastric artery

Left gastric artery

Common hepatic artery

Splenic artery

Abdominal aorta

FIGURE 5.22. Arteries of the posterior mediastinum. The main arteries that supply blood to the posterior mediastinum originate from the **thoracic aorta**. In this image, the esophageal branches and the posterior intercostal arteries are visible. Along its course through the posterior mediastinum the thoracic aorta also gives off branches to the pericardium, the bronchi, the mediastinum, and the superior surface of the diaphragm.

THORAX

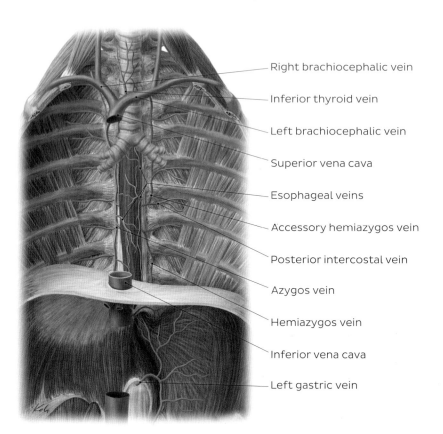

Right brachiocephalic vein

Inferior thyroid vein

Left brachiocephalic vein

Superior vena cava

Esophageal veins

Accessory hemiazygos vein

Posterior intercostal vein

Azygos vein

Hemiazygos vein

Inferior vena cava

Left gastric vein

FIGURE 5.23. Veins of the posterior mediastinum. The venous drainage of the posterior mediastinum is facilitated by the **azygos venous system**. This includes the azygos vein situated on the right aspect of the thoracic cavity, as well as the hemiazygos and accessory hemiazygos veins on the left. These veins receive blood from the esophagus through the esophageal veins and blood from the intercostal spaces drained by the posterior intercostal veins.

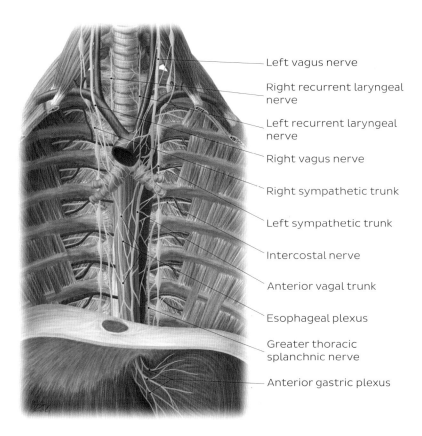

Left vagus nerve

Right recurrent laryngeal nerve

Left recurrent laryngeal nerve

Right vagus nerve

Right sympathetic trunk

Left sympathetic trunk

Intercostal nerve

Anterior vagal trunk

Esophageal plexus

Greater thoracic splanchnic nerve

Anterior gastric plexus

FIGURE 5.24. Nerves of the posterior mediastinum. The posterior mediastinum houses different nervous structures from the autonomic nervous system. The right and left **sympathetic trunks** and their associated ganglia are found on each side of the thoracic vertebral column. The **thoracic splanchnic nerves**, also known as greater, lesser, and least splanchnic nerves, arise from these trunks. Surrounding the esophagus we find the **esophageal plexus**, a wide-meshed autonomic network of nerves mainly derived from the right and left vagus nerves. The fibers of this plexus converge to form the **anterior** and **posterior vagal trunks**. The anterior trunk is constituted mainly from the left vagus nerve and the posterior mainly from the right vagus nerve.

Key points about the neurovasculature of the posterior mediastinum	
Arteries	Thoracic aorta and its branches (pericardial branches, bronchial branches, esophageal branches, mediastinal branches, posterior intercostal arteries, superior phrenic artery, subcostal artery)
Veins	Azygos system of veins (azygos vein, hemiazygos vein, accessory hemiazygos vein), posterior intercostal veins, esophageal veins
Nerves	Sympathetic trunks and thoracic splanchnic nerves, right and left vagi nerves, esophageal plexus, anterior and posterior vagal trunks

Neurovascular supply and lymphatic drainage of the esophagus

Mediastinum

ESOPHAGUS

The **esophagus** is a muscular hollow organ that propels food from the pharynx to the stomach through peristaltic movements. Two muscular rings, the upper and lower **esophageal sphincters**, regulate the passage of food and liquids. The esophagus is located mainly in the mediastinum and is closely related to several surrounding structures. Based on its position, the esophagus can be divided into **three parts**: Cervical, thoracic and abdominal.

The **vascular supply** of the esophagus mainly stems from the inferior thyroid artery, direct branches from the thoracic aorta, as well as the left gastric artery. **Venous drainage** is provided by esophageal veins, which are largely received by the azygos venous system. The esophageal plexus provides **nervous supply** to the esophagus via parasympathetic and sympathetic fibers. **Lymph** is drained to the deep cervical lymph nodes, regional lymph nodes (juxtaoesophageal lymph nodes), paratracheal, superior and inferior tracheobronchial lymph nodes, left gastric and coeliac lymph nodes.

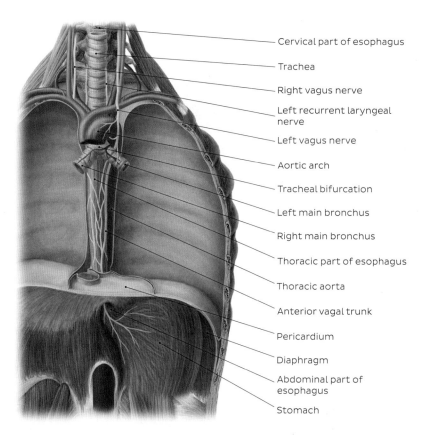

Cervical part of esophagus

Trachea

Right vagus nerve

Left recurrent laryngeal nerve

Left vagus nerve

Aortic arch

Tracheal bifurcation

Left main bronchus

Right main bronchus

Thoracic part of esophagus

Thoracic aorta

Anterior vagal trunk

Pericardium

Diaphragm

Abdominal part of esophagus

Stomach

FIGURE 5.25. Esophagus in situ. The esophagus is located posterior to the trachea and anterior to the vertebral column. On its course, it is closely associated with several structures, such as the thoracic aorta, the left main bronchus, and the left atrium of the heart (not visible here). The **cervical portion** of

THORAX

the esophagus begins at the pharyngoesophageal junction and ends at the entry into the upper thoracic aperture. The **thoracic portion** travels through the superior and posterior mediastinum. It ends at the esophageal hiatus where the esophagus passes through the diaphragm. The **abdominal portion** lies intraperitoneally. It starts where the esophagus passes through the diaphragm and terminates at the cardial orifice of the stomach (esophagogastric junction).

Key points about the esophagus	
Definition	Esophagus is a muscular, tubular part of the gastrointestinal tract, connecting the pharynx to the stomach
Parts	**Cervical part:** between pharyngoesophageal junction and upper thoracic aperture
	Thoracic part: between upper thoracic aperture and esophageal hiatus
	Abdominal part: between esophageal hiatus and gastroesophageal junction
Function	Propel food from pharynx to stomach through peristaltic movements
Neurovascular supply	**Arterial supply:** esophageal branches of inferior thyroid artery, thoracic aorta and left gastric artery
	Venous drainage: esophageal veins drain into inferior thyroid vein, azygos venous system, left gastric vein
	Innervation: via esophageal plexus. Parasympathetic innervation from vagus nerve (CN X), recurrent laryngeal nerve; sympathetic supply from cervical and thoracic sympathetic trunk and thoracic spinal nerves T5–T12
	Myenteric plexus (of Auerbach) and submucosal plexus (of Meissner) embedded in esophageal wall play role in regulating peristalsis
	Lymphatics: deep cervical lymph nodes, juxtaoesophageal lymph nodes, paratracheal, superior and inferior tracheobronchial lymph nodes, left gastric and coeliac lymph nodes
Relations	**Posterior:** vertebral column, distal part of descending thoracic aorta
	Anterior: trachea, left main bronchus, left atrium of heart
	Lateral: proximal part of descending thoracic aorta

 Esophagus

 Neurovascular supply and lymphatic drainage of the esophagus

LYMPHATICS OF THE MEDIASTINUM

The mediastinum contains several aggregations of lymph nodes which can be broadly categorized into **three groups**: Anterior mediastinal, intermediate (tracheobronchial) and posterior. As with all lymph nodes in the body, these node groups are ultimately drained into large thoracic lymphatic vessels (thoracic duct/right lymphatic duct) which terminate at the junction of the subclavian and internal jugular veins.

Given their close proximity and common drainage pathways, the lymph nodes of the thoracic wall (a.k.a. parietal thoracic lymph nodes) will also be evaluated in this section.

THORAX

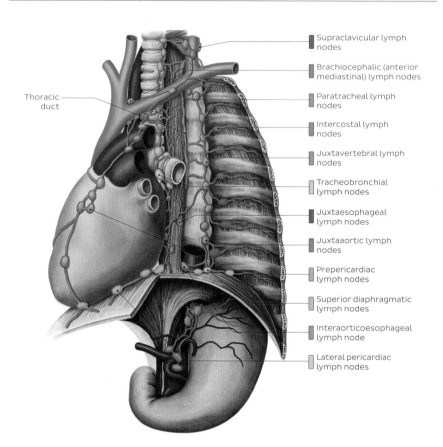

Supraclavicular lymph nodes

Brachiocephalic (anterior mediastinal) lymph nodes

Paratracheal lymph nodes

Intercostal lymph nodes

Juxtavertebral lymph nodes

Tracheobronchial lymph nodes

Juxtaesophageal lymph nodes

Juxtaaortic lymph nodes

Prepericardiac lymph nodes

Superior diaphragmatic lymph nodes

Interaorticoesophageal lymph node

Lateral pericardiac lymph nodes

Thoracic duct

THORAX

FIGURE 5.26. Lymphatics of the mediastinum (anterolateral view, heart displaced). Several groups of visceral lymph nodes are visible. The **brachiocephalic**/anterior **mediastinal lymph nodes** are located in the superior mediastinum in relation to the great vessels. The **tracheobronchial**/intermediate mediastinal lymph nodes surround the bifurcation of the trachea, as well as the superior and inferior aspects of the main bronchi.

The **juxtaesophageal**, **interaorticoesophageal** and **juxtaaortic** lymph nodes are commonly grouped as posterior mediastinal lymph nodes. They drain adjacent organs, vessels and tissues of the posterior mediastinum and send efferents to the paratracheal lymph nodes and right lymphatic/thoracic ducts.

Parietal thoracic lymph nodes visible in this illustration include the **intercostal**, **juxtavertebral** and **superior diaphragmatic** lymph nodes. They collect the lymph from the deep back and intercostal muscles, parietal pleura and vertebral column. Lymph drained from the upper intercostal nodes (approx. levels 1-7) drains into a common intercostal trunk destined for the supraclavicular nodes while the lower intercostal nodes often drain below the diaphragm to the gastric or celiac lymph nodes/cisterna chyli before ultimately reaching the thoracic duct. Efferent vessels of the juxtavertebral nodes may follow a similar drainage pattern and/or alternatively pass via the posterior mediastinal lymph nodes. The **superior diaphragmatic** lymph nodes drain the diaphragm, diaphragmatic portion of the pericardium and diaphragmatic pleura. They usually drain to the parasternal (not shown) or posterior mediastinal lymph nodes.

Below is the summary of the lymphatic drainage of the main lymphatic vessels in the thorax.

Thoracic duct	Drains most of the mediastinal organs via left bronchomediastinal lymphatic trunk (as well as the majority of the body, except for regions received by right lymphatic duct listed below)
Right lymphatic duct	Drains left side of the heart, right lung, lower lobe of left lung, right side of the thorax via right bronchomediastinal lymphatic trunk (as well as right side of the head and neck and right upper limb)

 Lymphatic system of the thoracic cavity and mediastinum

 Lymph nodes of the thorax and abdomen

TRACHEA

The **trachea** (windpipe) is a long fibrocartilaginous respiratory tube that connects the larynx to the main bronchi. As it is located below the larynx, it is
considered part of the lower respiratory tract. The main **function** of this cartilaginous tube is to conduct air from the larynx to the bronchi and vice versa. The
trachea also protects the lungs from potentially harmful external agents with
its immune cells and from particles physically entering the lungs through its
specialized epithelial cells.

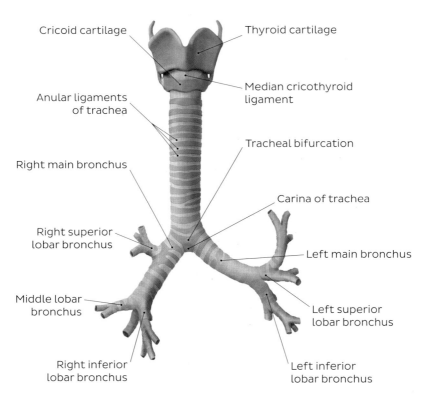

Cricoid cartilage

Thyroid cartilage

Anular ligaments
of trachea

Median cricothyroid
ligament

Right main bronchus

Tracheal bifurcation

Carina of trachea

Right superior
lobar bronchus

Left main bronchus

Middle lobar
bronchus

Left superior
lobar bronchus

Right inferior
lobar bronchus

Left inferior
lobar bronchus

THORAX

FIGURE 5.27. Trachea (anterior view). The trachea is continuous with the larynx at the inferior border
of the cricoid cartilage. Its tubular structure is maintained by 16-20 incomplete/C-shaped **cartilaginous
rings** which comprise its anterolateral wall. These cartilages are interconnected by **anular ligaments**
located between adjacent cartilage rings. The posterior wall of the trachea is occupied by the **trachealis
muscle** (not visible from this perspective). The trachea normally terminates at the level of vertebra **T5** in a
bifurcation giving off two main bronchi.

Key points about the trachea	
Definition	Fibrocartilaginous tube that transports air from the upper respiratory tract to the lungs and vice versa
Structure	Anterolateral wall: 16-20 tracheal cartilages connected by anular ligaments
	Posterior wall: fibromuscular wall (trachealis muscle)
Function	Air conduction, immune and mechanical protection

Trachea

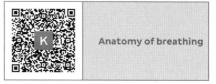

Anatomy of breathing

BRONCHIAL TREE AND ALVEOLI

The **bronchial tree** is a branching tubular structure which conducts air between the trachea and lungs. It comprises the **bronchi** and their subsequent branches (**bronchioles**), which open into **terminal alveolar ducts**. There are **four types of bronchi** including main (primary) bronchi, lobar (secondary) bronchi, segmental (tertiary) and intrasegmental bronchi. All bronchi have an outer layer containing variable amounts of irregularly placed cartilaginous plates.

The airway divisions after the intrasegmental bronchi are called **bronchioles**, which lack cartilage. The last divisions of the bronchial tree are known as **respiratory bronchioles**, which end in small sacs containing alveoli. This is the site of gaseous exchange between the blood and the lungs. The main **function** of the bronchial tree is to provide a passageway for air to move into and out of each lung. In addition, the mucous membrane of these airways protects the lungs by capturing debris and pathogens.

THORAX

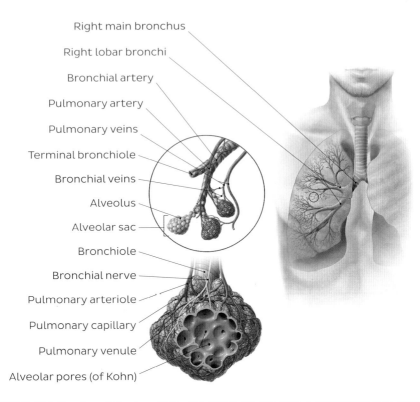

Right main bronchus

Right lobar bronchi

Bronchial artery

Pulmonary artery

Pulmonary veins

Terminal bronchiole

Bronchial veins

Alveolus

Alveolar sac

Bronchiole

Bronchial nerve

Pulmonary arteriole

Pulmonary capillary

Pulmonary venule

Alveolar pores (of Kohn)

FIGURE 5.28. Overview of the bronchioles and alveoli. On the right, a macroscopic view shows the branching of the bronchial tree. On the left, the respiratory bronchioles, alveoli and associated neurovasculature are shown. **Bronchioles** arise from the intrasegmental bronchi, lack cartilage and may divide up to 20-25 times. The last divisions of a bronchiole that *does not* contain alveoli (i.e. one whose sole function is gas conduction) are known as **terminal bronchioles**. They subdivide into **respiratory bronchioles** which open into small alveolar sacs containing alveoli via small alveolar ducts.

Each **alveolus** opens up internally in the **alveolar sac**, while externally it is surrounded by a nest of blood capillaries supplied by small branches of the pulmonary and bronchial arteries.

Key points about the bronchial tree and alveoli	
Definition	Bronchial tree is a term used to describe the multiple bronchi that conduct air from the trachea to alveoli
Branching	Bronchial tree: • Main (primary) bronchi • Lobar (secondary) bronchi • Segmental (tertiary) bronchi • Intrasegmental bronchi • Bronchioles • Terminal bronchioles • Respiratory bronchioles • Alveolar duct → alveolar sac → alveolus
Function	Airway conduction, protection against pathogens and debris

THORAX

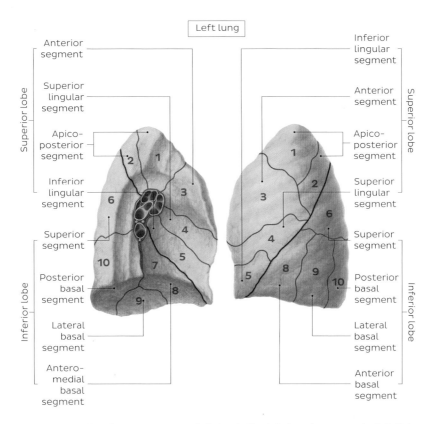

FIGURE 5.29. Bronchopulmonary segments (left lung). The left lung is composed of **8–10 bron-chopulmonary segments** (depending on classification) which can be identified from both medial and lateral views. Each bronchopulmonary segment has its own tertiary bronchus and segmental branch of the pulmonary artery (of the same name).

The superior lobe of the left lung is formed by four main bronchopulmonary segments: The **apicoposterior** (1, 2), **anterior** (3), **superior lingular** (4) and **inferior lingular segments** (5) which are situated at the lingula of the left lung. The inferior lobe is composed of **superior** (6) and **basal segments**. The latter are further divided into the **anteromedial basal** (7, 8), **lateral basal** (9) and **posterior basal** (10) segments.

Key points about the bronchial tree and alveoli	
Segmental bronchi/ bronchopulmonary segments	**Left lung:** • Superior lobe (Apicoposterior segment (1,2), anterior segment (3), superior lingular segment (4), inferior lingular segment (5)) • Inferior lobe (Superior segment (6), anteromedial basal segment (7,8), lateral basal segment (9), posterior basal segment (10)) **Right lung:** • Superior lobe (Apical segment (1), posterior segment (2), anterior segment (3)) • Middle lobe (Lateral segment (4), medial segment (5)) • Inferior lobe (Superior segment (6), medial basal segment (7), anterior basal segment (8), lateral basal segment (9), posterior basal segment (10))

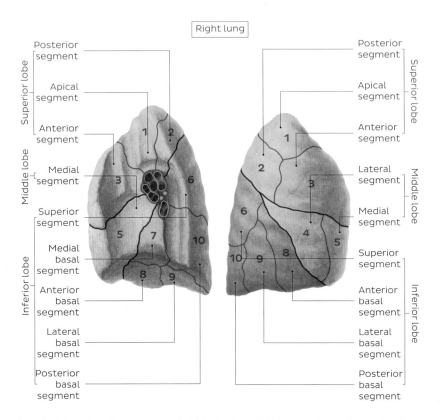

Right lung

Superior lobe
- Posterior segment
- Apical segment
- Anterior segment

Middle lobe
- Medial segment

Inferior lobe
- Superior segment
- Medial basal segment
- Anterior basal segment
- Lateral basal segment
- Posterior basal segment

Superior lobe
- Posterior segment
- Apical segment
- Anterior segment

Middle lobe
- Lateral segment
- Medial segment

Inferior lobe
- Superior segment
- Anterior basal segment
- Lateral basal segment
- Posterior basal segment

FIGURE 5.30. Bronchopulmonary segments (right lung). The right lung consists of **10 bronchopulmonary segments**. Just like in the left lung, each bronchopulmonary segment of the right lung also has its own tertiary bronchus and segmental branch of the pulmonary artery (of the same name).

The superior lobe of the right lung has three bronchopulmonary segments: **Apical** (1), **posterior** (2) and **anterior** (3). The middle lobe of the right lung is formed of the **lateral** (4) and **medial** (5) segments, while the inferior lobe of the right lung is composed of **superior** (6), **medial basal** (7), **anterior basal** (8), **lateral basal** (9) and **posterior basal** (10) segments.

Alveoli

Bronchi

THORAX

OVERVIEW OF THE LUNGS

The **lungs** are paired organs located in the thoracic cavity. They are considered to be central organs of the respiratory system since they are in charge of **gaseous exchange** between the inspired air and blood.

Due to the differences in space in the two sides of the thoracic cavity, the lungs are asymmetrical (the left lung is smaller in size). Each lung has **three borders** (anterior, posterior, and inferior) that marginate **three surfaces** (costal, medial and diaphragmatic).

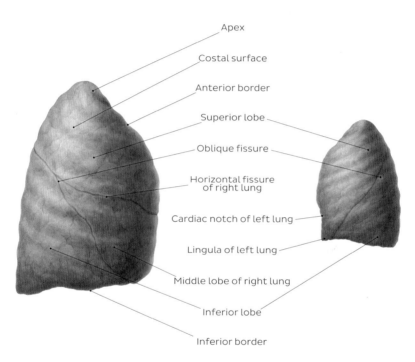

Apex

Costal surface

Anterior border

Superior lobe

Oblique fissure

Horizontal fissure of right lung

Cardiac notch of left lung

Lingula of left lung

Middle lobe of right lung

Inferior lobe

Inferior border

FIGURE 5.31. Lateral views of the lungs. This perspective clearly shows the **anterior** and **inferior borders** of the lungs as well as their costal surfaces. The **costal surface** faces the ribs and is covered by visceral pleura. Due to the 'spongy' nature of the lung parenchyma, the ribs leave defined marks known as **costal impressions** along the entire costal surface.

The lungs are divided into **lobes** by double folds of pleura which form fissures. From the lateral view the fissures are seen as thick lines that extend across the costal surface. The left lung has only one fissure (**oblique fissure of left lung**) which divides it into superior and inferior lobes, while the right lung has two fissures (**oblique** and **horizontal fissures of right lung**) that divide it into superior, middle, and inferior lobes.

THORAX

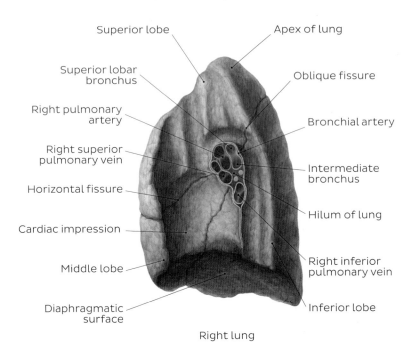

Superior lobe

Apex of lung

Superior lobar
bronchus

Oblique fissure

Right pulmonary
artery

Bronchial artery

Right superior
pulmonary vein

Intermediate
bronchus

Horizontal fissure

Hilum of lung

Cardiac impression

Right inferior
pulmonary vein

Middle lobe

Diaphragmatic
surface

Inferior lobe

Right lung

FIGURE 5.32. Medial view of the right lung. The superior most, pointed portion of each lung is known as the **apex**. Inferior to it on the mediastinal surface is a wedge shaped depression known as the the **hilum** of the lung; the most prominent feature seen from this medial perspective.

Many structures enter or exit the lung via the hilum such as the pulmonary artery and veins and bronchial arteries, the lobar bronchi, lymphatic vessels and bronchopulmonary lymph nodes. **Impressions** seen on the right lung include the smaller cardiac impression and grooves for trachea, esophagus, brachiocephalic and azygos veins, as well as the superior and inferior vena cava.

THORAX

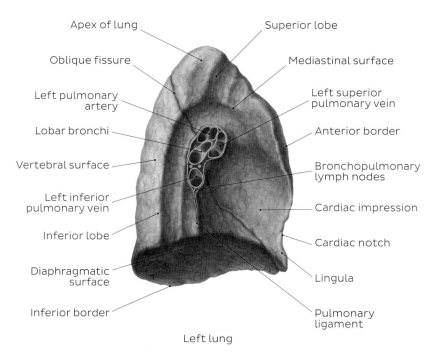

Apex of lung

Oblique fissure

Left pulmonary artery

Lobar bronchi

Vertebral surface

Left inferior pulmonary vein

Inferior lobe

Diaphragmatic surface

Inferior border

Superior lobe

Mediastinal surface

Left superior pulmonary vein

Anterior border

Bronchopulmonary lymph nodes

Cardiac impression

Cardiac notch

Lingula

Pulmonary ligament

Left lung

FIGURE 5.33. Medial view of the left lung. Due to the presence of other organs in the thoracic cavity, on the surfaces of the lungs there are marks or **impressions** by those adjacent organs. The most prominent impression seen on the medial surface of the left lung is the **cardiac impression**, while the smaller impressions include the grooves for the aorta, subclavian artery, 1st rib, trachea and esophagus.

Key points about the medial and lateral views of the lungs	
Lateral view	**Right lung:** apex, costal impressions, oblique fissure, horizontal fissure, superior lobe, medial lobe, inferior lobe
	Left lung: apex, cardiac notch, lingula, superior lobe, inferior lobe
Medial view	**Right lung:** horizontal and oblique fissures, smaller cardiac impression, grooves for trachea, esophagus, brachiocephalic vein, azygos vein, superior vena cava, inferior vena cava
	Left lung: oblique fissure, cardiac impression, grooves for aorta, subclavian artery, 1st rib, trachea, esophagus
Hilum contents	Main bronchus, lobar bronchi (superior, intermediate, inferior), one pulmonary artery, two pulmonary veins, bronchial arteries and veins, pulmonary nervous plexus, lymphatics, bronchopulmonary lymph nodes, areolar tissue

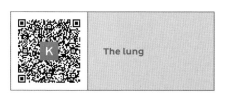

The lung

Bronchopulmonary segments

THORAX

LUNGS *IN SITU*

The lungs are located either side of the mediastinum, surrounded by the thoracic cage and superior to the diaphragm. Hence, each lung has a **mediastinal**, **costal** and **diaphragmatic surface**. Both lungs are enveloped by visceral and parietal **pleura**, between which is a potential space known as the **pleural cavity**.

Inferior and anterior to the lungs are two potential spaces called **pleural recesses** to which the pulmonary tissue does not extend (or extends only during a forced inspiration), called the costodiaphragmatic and costomediastinal recesses, respectively.

Each lung has an apex and a base, as well as anterior, posterior and inferior borders. The **apices** of the lungs project into the superior thoracic aperture, about 2.5 cm above the medial third of the clavicle. The **base** of each lung rests upon the ipsilateral hemidiaphragms; the inferior border is located around the level of the 6th rib at the midclavicular line, 8th rib at the midaxillary line, and 10th rib posteriorly at the scapular line. The **anterior border of right lung** is located deep to the right margin of the sternum, extending between the second and sixth costal cartilages; the **anterior border of the left lung** begins deep to the sternum at the level of the second intercostal space before running inferolaterally to the sixth intercostal space, about 3 cm from the left margin of the sternum.

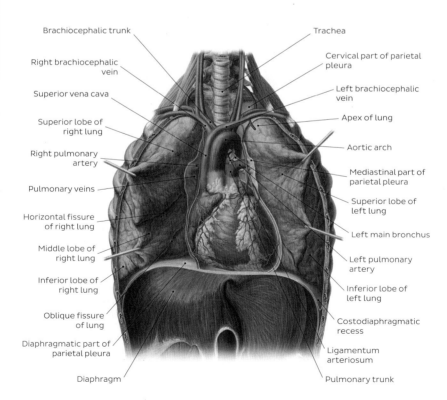

Brachiocephalic trunk

Right brachiocephalic vein

Superior vena cava

Superior lobe of right lung

Right pulmonary artery

Pulmonary veins

Horizontal fissure of right lung

Middle lobe of right lung

Inferior lobe of right lung

Oblique fissure of lung

Diaphragmatic part of parietal pleura

Diaphragm

Trachea

Cervical part of parietal pleura

Left brachiocephalic vein

Apex of lung

Aortic arch

Mediastinal part of parietal pleura

Superior lobe of left lung

Left main bronchus

Left pulmonary artery

Inferior lobe of left lung

Costodiaphragmatic recess

Ligamentum arteriosum

Pulmonary trunk

FIGURE 5.34. Lungs and heart in situ (anterior view). In this image, both the right and the left lungs are slightly retracted so the relations of the lungs with the heart and other mediastinal structures can

THORAX

be seen. The **right lung** lies closely to the superior and inferior venae cavae as well as the azygos vein (not seen), while the **left lung** relates to the ascending and thoracic aorta. Both lungs conform around the shape of the heart. Each lung is suspended from the mediastinum by its root: A pedicle formed by structures entering and exiting the lungs via the hilum (e.g., bronchi, pulmonary/bronchial vasculature, lymphatics and nerves).

Notice the two potential spaces (out of four in total) between the lungs and the parietal pleura, also known as the pleural recesses. The **costodiaphragmatic recess** is located at the inferior most part of the pleural cavity whereas the **costomediastinal recess** lies anteriorly, between the costal and mediastinal layers of parietal pleura. Those recesses are usually empty, so dull percussion sound in those areas as well as positive chest radiograph can indicate a pathological condition.

Surface projections	
Apex of lung	~2.5 cm above the clavicle
Inferior border of lung	6th rib, 8th rib, and 10th rib
Inferior border of pleura	8th rib, 10th rib, and 12th rib
Anterior margin of lung	2nd-6th intercostal spaces (laterally displaced by ~3cm on left side)

 The lung

 The pleural cavity

 Normal chest x-ray

THORAX

LYMPHATICS OF THE LUNGS

The lymphatics of the lung consist of several lymph node groups and lymphatic vessels that drain the superficial and deep regions of both lungs into the **tracheobronchial nodes** surrounding the bifurcation of the trachea and main bronchi. These in turn empty into the right and left **bronchomediastinal trunks** via paratracheal lymph nodes and ultimately into venous circulation.

The **superficial (or subpleural) lymphatics** of the lung drain lymph from the visceral pleura and peripheral lung tissue to the bronchopulmonary lymph nodes at the hilar region of each lung. The **deep (or central) lymphatics** of the lung drain the bronchi and peribronchial parenchyma of the lung via intrapulmonary lymph nodes after which lymph is also ultimately received by the bronchopulmonary lymph nodes. From here, lymph from both the superficial and deep lymphatics of the lungs is passed to the tracheobronchial nodes.

A good understanding of the lymphatic drainage of the lungs is important clinically, particularly in the staging and treatment of lung cancer.

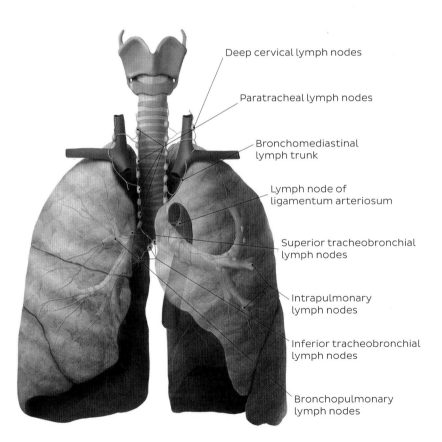

Deep cervical lymph nodes

Paratracheal lymph nodes

Bronchomediastinal lymph trunk

Lymph node of ligamentum arteriosum

Superior tracheobronchial lymph nodes

Intrapulmonary lymph nodes

Inferior tracheobronchial lymph nodes

Bronchopulmonary lymph nodes

FIGURE 5.35. Overview of the lymphatics of the lung (anterior view). Anterior view of the lungs and tracheobronchial tree, showing the thoracic aorta and brachiocephalic veins. Lymph drained from the

THORAX

right superior and **inferior tracheobronchial nodes**, as well as the **left inferior tracheobronchial nodes**, is received by the **right bronchomediastinal trunk**. From here, lymph is carried via paratracheal nodes and returned to venous circulation around the **right venous angle**.

The **left superior tracheobronchial nodes** drain to the **left bronchomediastinal trunk** (also via paratracheal nodes) which empties into the **left venous angle**, sometimes via the thoracic duct.

Key points about the lymphatic drainage of the lungs	
Superficial (subpleural) pathway	Drains visceral pleura and superficial lung parenchyma (tissue) → drains initially into the bronchopulmonary nodes
Deep (central) pathway	Drains bronchi and peribronchial parenchyma → drains initially into the intrapulmonary nodes
Right lung	Intrapulmonary nodes → bronchopulmonary nodes → right inferior tracheobronchial nodes → right superior tracheobronchial nodes → right paratracheal nodes → right bronchomediastinal lymph trunk → right venous angle → venous circulation
Left lung	**Superior lobe:** intrapulmonary nodes → bronchopulmonary nodes → left inferior tracheobronchial nodes → left superior tracheobronchial nodes → left paratracheal nodes → left bronchomediastinal lymph trunk → left venous angle (or thoracic duct) venous circulation **Inferior lobe:** intrapulmonary nodes → bronchopulmonary nodes → left inferior tracheobronchial nodes → right superior tracheobronchial nodes → right paratracheal nodes → right bronchomediastinal lymph trunk → right venous angle → venous circulation

The lung

The lymphatic system of the thoracic cavity and mediastinum

THORAX

HEART *IN SITU*

Exploring the anatomical relations of the heart *in situ* will allow you to better understand its function. The heart is located in the **middle mediastinum**, mostly to the left of the midsagittal plane. The main relations of the hearts are with the thymus and sternum (anteriorly), the lungs (laterally), the diaphragm (inferiorly), and the great vessels (posterosuperiorly).

Usually, the heart has the size of a fist and is positioned roughly along an axis extending from the right shoulder to the left hypochondrium. Its position has often been described as "*a pyramid which has fallen over*" where the **apex** is located on the left midclavicular line, pointing in an anteroinferior direction. Its inferior surface, also known as the **diaphragmatic surface**, sits on the diaphragm and can be located at the level of the 5th-6th intercostal space. The superior border lies at the level of the second costal space, while the posterior part is located at the level of the third costal cartilage.

It's important to know where the heart is located and its orientation in clinical practice when listening for heart sounds with a stethoscope (auscultation) or while performing cardiopulmonary reanimation (CPR) in the case of an emergency.

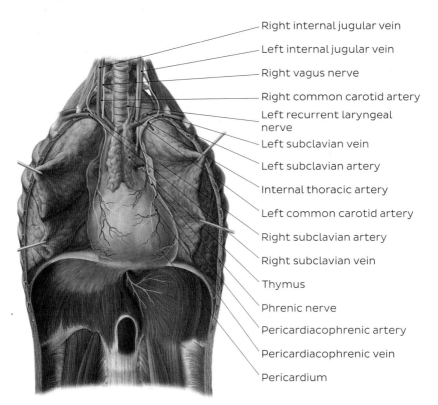

Right internal jugular vein

Left internal jugular vein

Right vagus nerve

Right common carotid artery

Left recurrent laryngeal nerve

Left subclavian vein

Left subclavian artery

Internal thoracic artery

Left common carotid artery

Right subclavian artery

Right subclavian vein

Thymus

Phrenic nerve

Pericardiacophrenic artery

Pericardiacophrenic vein

Pericardium

FIGURE 5.36. Heart *in situ* (anterior view). The heart is separated from other structures of the mediastinum by a double layered fibroserous sac called the **pericardium**. On its surface are important vessels which

THORAX

supply and drain the pericardium and diaphragm, known as the **pericardiacophrenic artery** and **vein**. The right and left phrenic nerves, which innervate the diaphragm, course laterally on either side of the heart. These are clinically important since they can be damaged during surgical interventions to the heart.

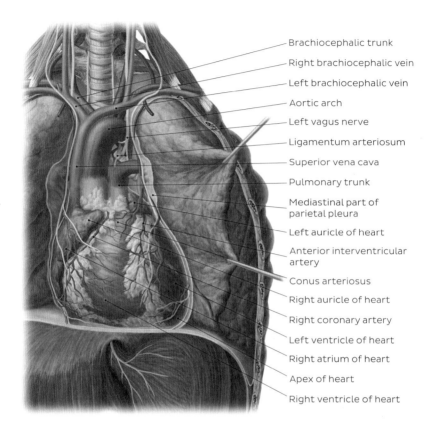

Brachiocephalic trunk

Right brachiocephalic vein

Left brachiocephalic vein

Aortic arch

Left vagus nerve

Ligamentum arteriosum

Superior vena cava

Pulmonary trunk

Mediastinal part of parietal pleura

Left auricle of heart

Anterior interventricular artery

Conus arteriosus

Right auricle of heart

Right coronary artery

Left ventricle of heart

Right atrium of heart

Apex of heart

Right ventricle of heart

THORAX

FIGURE 5.37. Heart *in situ* (anterior pericardium removed). Removing the pericardium allows the appreciation of the relations of the heart with the great vessels. The **great vessels** (venae cavae, aorta and pulmonary trunk) attach to the posterosuperior aspect of the heart, known as the **base** of the heart. The **apex** of the heart is its sharpest point, located at its bottom left portion and angled anteroinferiorly.

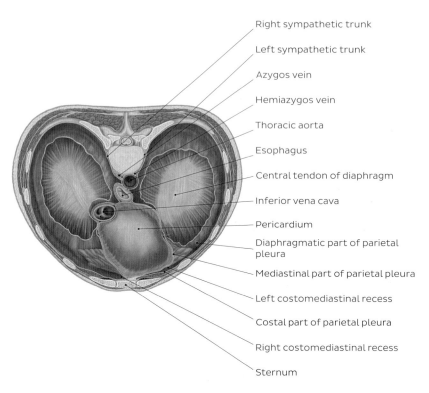

Right sympathetic trunk

Left sympathetic trunk

Azygos vein

Hemiazygos vein

Thoracic aorta

Esophagus

Central tendon of diaphragm

Inferior vena cava

Pericardium

Diaphragmatic part of parietal pleura

Mediastinal part of parietal pleura

Left costomediastinal recess

Costal part of parietal pleura

Right costomediastinal recess

Sternum

THORAX

FIGURE 5.38. Diaphragmatic relations of the heart (superior view). Cross section showing the thoracic surface of the diaphragm. The heart is located anterior to the esophagus, thoracic aorta and thoracic vertebrae. Each lung has a base resting on the diaphragm; the deviation of the apex to the left is clearly visible as an indentation of the left lung known as the cardiac notch.

Key points about the anatomical relations of the heart	
Position	**Location:** middle mediastinum, mostly to the left of the midsagittal plane
	Orientation: positioned in a direction of a plane extending from the right shoulder to left hypochondrium, with the apex leaned towards the left
Visceral relationships	Pericardium (sac surrounding the heart)
	Thymus (anterior)
	Lungs (lateral)
	Diaphragm (inferior)
	Esophagus (posterior)
Surrounding neurovasculature	**Arteries:** aortic arch, brachiocephalic trunk, left and right common carotid arteries, left and right subclavian arteries, internal thoracic artery, pericardiacophrenic artery, pulmonary trunk
	Veins: left and right internal jugular veins, left and right subclavian veins, left and right brachiocephalic veins, superior vena cava, pericardiacophrenic veins
	Nerves: left and right vagus nerves (CN X), left and right phrenic nerves
Blood supply	Left and right phrenic arteries (branches of the abdominal aorta)
Nerves	Left and right phrenic nerves (C3–C5)

Heart

SURFACE ANATOMY OF THE HEART

The heart has **five surfaces**:

- **Anterior (sternocostal)** surface, which lies adjacent to the body of sternum, sternocostal muscles and the third to sixth costal cartilages.
- **Inferior (diaphragmatic)** surface, which sits mainly on the central tendon of the diaphragm.
- **Left** and **right (pulmonary)** surfaces, which face the left and right lungs, respectively. The left surface involves the lateral portion of the left ventricle as well as a small part of the left atrium/auricle, while the right surface is found between the superior vena cava and the intrathoracic part of the inferior vena cava.
- **Posterior surface (base)**, which lies anterior to the principal bronchi and esophagus.

The heart also presents **four borders**:

- The **right border** is a line that runs mainly over the right atrium, extending between the superior and inferior vena cava, and over a small portion of the right ventricle.
- The **left (obtuse) border** separates the left and anterior surfaces, mainly formed by the left ventricle and part of the left auricle.
- The **superior border** is a line that goes over the roots of the aorta and pulmonary trunk and a small portion of the left and right auricle.
- The **inferior (acute) border** extends along the right ventricle and part of the left ventricle at its apex.

THORAX

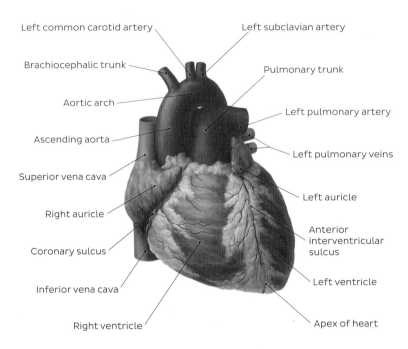

Left common carotid artery

Brachiocephalic trunk

Aortic arch

Ascending aorta

Superior vena cava

Right auricle

Coronary sulcus

Inferior vena cava

Right ventricle

Left subclavian artery

Pulmonary trunk

Left pulmonary artery

Left pulmonary veins

Left auricle

Anterior interventricular sulcus

Left ventricle

Apex of heart

FIGURE 5.39. Anterior view of the heart. The anterior surface of the heart faces anterosuperiorly and bears a profound right convexity compared to the left. The **right ventricle** occupies about two-thirds of its extent, while the **left ventricle** makes up the remaining one-third. The **left atrium** is mainly obscured by the roots of the aorta and pulmonary trunk, with only a small part of the **left auricle** of the heart projecting.

The atria and ventricles are separated by a deep groove called the **coronary** (atrioventricular) **sulcus** that contains the largest of the cardiac vessels; it is interrupted anteriorly by the root of the pulmonary trunk. The anterior surface is marked by another groove, called the **anterior interventricular sulcus**, that separates the left and right ventricles and contains the anterior interventricular artery and vein. In this image one can also visualize the outline of the **right (pulmonary) surface** of the heart, which is longer and more protuberant than the left surface, and is formed by the right atrium superiorly and right ventricle inferiorly.

THORAX

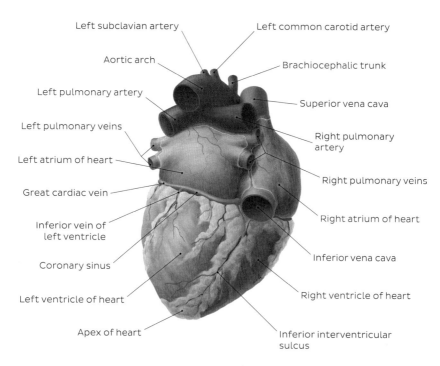

Left subclavian artery

Left common carotid artery

Aortic arch

Brachiocephalic trunk

Left pulmonary artery

Superior vena cava

Left pulmonary veins

Right pulmonary artery

Left atrium of heart

Right pulmonary veins

Great cardiac vein

Right atrium of heart

Inferior vein of left ventricle

Inferior vena cava

Coronary sinus

Left ventricle of heart

Right ventricle of heart

Apex of heart

Inferior interventricular sulcus

FIGURE 5.40. Posteroinferior view of the heart. The **inferior surface** is mostly made up of the left ventricle and part of the right ventricle and gently slopes anteroinferiorly from the base of the heart towards the apex. It is separated from the anatomical base (posterior surface) of the heart by the **posterior part of the coronary sulcus**. The inferior surface is also marked by the **inferior** (posterior) **interventricular sulcus**, which separates the ventricles and contains the inferior (posterior) interventricular artery and middle cardiac vein. The posterior surface is largely formed by the **left atrium** which is pierced by four pulmonary veins, as well a small portion of the right atrium which receives the superior and inferior venae cavae. The atria are separated by a shallow **interatrial sulcus**, which together with the coronary and inferior interventricular sulci, form the **crux of the heart**.

Key points about the surfaces of the heart		
Anterior (sternocostal) surface	**Components:** right atrium, ⅔ right ventricle, ⅓ left ventricle	
	Landmarks: right auricle of heart, coronary sulcus, anterior interventricular sulcus, cardiac apex	
	Vessels: right coronary artery, anterior interventricular artery/vein, anterior veins of right ventricle	
	Relations: sternum, sternocostal muscles, third to sixth costal cartilages	
Inferior (diaphragmatic) surface	**Components:** left ventricle, right ventricle	
	Landmarks: inferior (posterior) interventricular groove, atrioventricular groove, cardiac apex	
	Vessels: inferior (posterior) interventricular artery, middle cardiac vein, coronary sinus, inferior vein of right ventricle	
	Relations: sits mainly the central tendon of diaphragm, and a small portion of left muscular part of diaphragm	
Left (pulmonary) surface	**Components:** left ventricle, small part of left atrium and left auricle of heart	
	Landmarks: atrioventricular groove	
	Vessels: circumflex artery, great cardiac vein, left marginal vein	
	Relations: left pericardiacophrenic neurovascular bundle, left pleura/lung	

Key points about the surfaces of the heart	
Right (pulmonary) surface	**Components:** right atrium **Landmarks:** sulcus terminalis **Relations:** intrathoracic part of inferior vena cava, superior vena cava, right pleura/lung
Posterior surface (base)	**Components:** right atrium, left atrium **Vessels:** coronary sinus, left and right pulmonary veins, vena cavae **Relations:** principal bronchi, esophagus

 Heart

 Diagrams quizzes worksheets of the heart

RIGHT ATRIUM AND VENTRICLE

The **right atrium** occupies the upper right side of the heart. It is the first chamber of the heart to receive the **deoxygenated blood** from the body via 3 main sources: The superior vena cava, which drains blood from the upper parts of the body, the inferior vena cava, which collects blood from the lower parts, and the coronary sinus, which drains blood from the heart itself. One of the main features of the right atrium is the sinoatrial (SA) node that is placed within the wall of this chamber adjacent to the entrance of the superior vena cava. It is known as "**the human pacemaker**" that spontaneously generates electrical impulses and determines the normal heart rhythm.

The **right ventricle** takes up the majority of the anterior surface of the heart. It receives blood from the right atrium and pumps it via the pulmonary trunk into the lungs for blood oxygenation. The blood flow between these heart chambers is regulated by the **right atrioventricular (tricuspid) valve**, allowing only unidirectional flow from the right atrium to the right ventricle. Similarly, the **pulmonary valve** permits the blood to flow from the right ventricle to the pulmonary trunk without regurgitation.

Right auricle of heart

Crista terminalis

Superior vena cava

Pectinate muscles

Interatrial septum

Right pulmonary artery

Limbus of fossa ovalis

Right pulmonary veins

Right atrioventricular orifice

Fossa ovalis of right atrium

Right atrioventricular valve

Orifice of coronary sinus

Valve of inferior vena cava

Valve of coronary sinus

Inferior vena cava

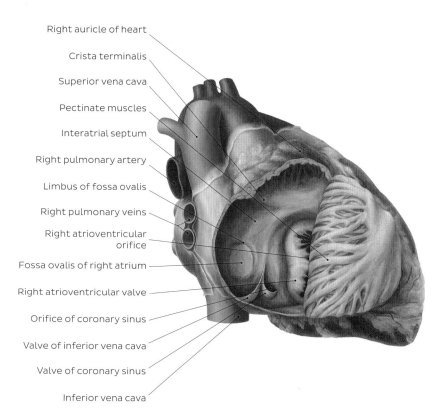

FIGURE 5.41. Overview of the right atrium. Interior of the right atrium with its anterior wall is reflected. The internal surface of the anterior wall has a roughened appearance due to the presence of the **pectinate muscles.** These are folds of muscle arranged in a comb-like fashion around the region of the right auricle which function to act as a volume reservoir, increasing the capacity of the right atrium during times of dilatation. The remaining walls of the right atrium are smooth and offer the appreciation of several anatomical landmarks: The fossa ovalis, valves of the inferior vena cava and coronary sinus, as well as the right atrioventricular orifice.

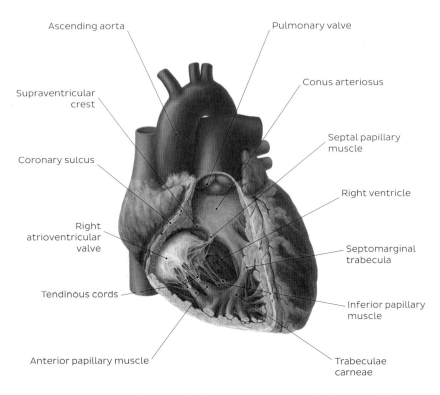

Ascending aorta

Pulmonary valve

Conus arteriosus

Supraventricular
crest

Septal papillary
muscle

Coronary sulcus

Right ventricle

Right
atrioventricular
valve

Septomarginal
trabecula

Tendinous cords

Inferior papillary
muscle

Anterior papillary muscle

Trabeculae
carneae

FIGURE 5.42. Overview of the right ventricle. Right ventricle, anterolateral wall removed. The structure of the right atrioventricular (tricuspid) valve with its three papillary muscles (anterior, inferior (a.k.a.posterior) and septal) and their tendinous cords (chordae tendineae) can be seen. The structure of the pulmonary valve is also illustrated as well, immediately superior to the conus arteriosus.

Key points about the right atrium	
Features	Receives deoxygenated blood from systemic circulation via the superior vena cava, inferior vena cava and coronary sinus
	Characteristics: thin wall; contains the sinoatrial and atrioventricular nodes; three internal surfaces (venous, vestibular, auricular)
	Landmarks: right auricle
	Function: reservoir for blood and an active pump that helps fill the ventricle
Right auricle of heart	Cone-shaped pouch which extends from the superoanterior part of right atrium
Pectinate muscles	Array of parallel muscular columns on the internal anterior wall of right atrium
Crista terminalis	Crescent-shaped muscular ridge on the internal aspect of right atrium that externally corresponds with the terminal sulcus
Sinus of venae cavae	Portion of right atrium that receives the superior and inferior venae cavae
Vestibule of right atrioventricular valve	Fibrous rings that support the leaflets of the right atrioventricular valve
Fossa ovalis	Oval depression on the interatrial septum (remnant of foramen ovale)

THORAX

Key points about the right atrium	
Sinoatrial (SA) node (natural pacemaker)	Collection of specialized nodal tissue that produces electrical impulses that travel through the electrical conduction system
Atrioventricular (AV) node	Part of electrical conduction system found near coronary sinus on the interatrial septum

Key points about the right ventricle	
Features	Receives deoxygenated blood from right atrium and pumps it to the lungs for oxygenation **Characteristics:** septomarginal trabecula (moderator band) **Landmarks:** three prominent papillary muscles **Function:** pumps blood into the pulmonary circulation
Supraventricular crest	Round accentuation of the internal muscular wall that separates the conus arteriosus from the rest of the ventricular cavity
Conus arteriosus	Conical pouch where the pulmonary trunk arises
Trabeculae carneae	Muscular elevations that course along mainly apical parts of ventricular wall
Papillary muscles, chordae tendineae	(Anterior/inferior/septal papillary muscles) Muscular projections attached to cusps of right atrioventricular valve via tendinous cords (chordae tendineae) preventing prolapse
Septomarginal trabecula	A muscular tissue that transmits the right branch of atrioventricular bundle from the interventricular septum to the anterior papillary muscle

 Atria of the heart

 Ventricles of the heart

 Heart

LEFT ATRIUM AND VENTRICLE

The **left atrium** occupies the **base** (posterior part) of the heart. It receives oxygenated blood from the lungs via four pulmonary veins and pumps it into the left ventricle via the left atrioventricular orifice. This orifice features the **left atrioventricular (mitral/bicuspid) valve** which functions to seal the atrioventricular opening during the ventricular contraction (systole). This prevents regurgitation of blood into the left atrium and redirects blood flow through the aortic orifice during ventricular systole.

The **left ventricle** is the largest of all heart chambers, mainly due to the thickness of its muscular walls. It occupies most of the left pulmonary and inferior surfaces of the heart, including its **apex**. Once filled with blood, the left ventricle contracts and strongly ejects most of its contents into the aorta. The left ventricle and aorta are separated by the aortic orifice, which features the **aortic (left semilunar) valve**. This valve is closed during ventricular diastole, preventing backflow of blood in the left ventricle, and open during systole to allow the blood to enter systemic circulation.

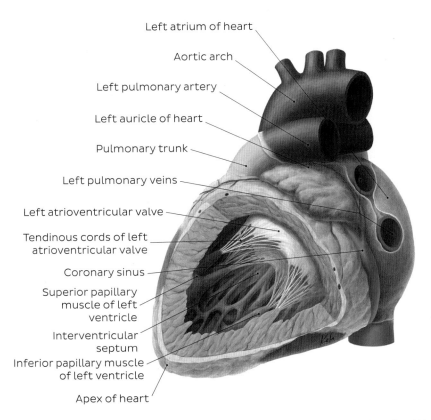

Left atrium of heart

Aortic arch

Left pulmonary artery

Left auricle of heart

Pulmonary trunk

Left pulmonary veins

Left atrioventricular valve

Tendinous cords of left atrioventricular valve

Coronary sinus

Superior papillary muscle of left ventricle

Interventricular septum

Inferior papillary muscle of left ventricle

Apex of heart

FIGURE 5.43. Interior of the left ventricle. The left ventricle has noticeably thicker muscular walls which facilitate the generation of sufficient force to overcome the higher blood systemic pressure of the aorta.

THORAX

Similar to its right counterpart, the internal structure of the ventricle features notable muscular ridges, known as the **trabeculae carneae**.

The **left atrioventricular** (mitral) **valve** has two leaflets, anterior and posterior. Each of these are connected to a corresponding superior (or anterior) and inferior (posterior) **papillary muscle** via tendinous cords, also known as **chordae tendineae**. A small conical projection of the left atrium, known as the left auricle (or atrial appendage) can be seen adjacent to the root of the pulmonary trunk. The posterior wall of the left atrium is also pierced by four pulmonary veins which carry oxygenated blood from the lungs.

Key points about the left atrium	
Features	Receives oxygenated blood from the lungs via the pulmonary veins (4 ostia)
	Characteristics: cuboidal chamber, thicker walls (compared to right atrium); has a small muscular pouch → left auricle of heart (contains pectinate muscles)
	Landmarks: T5 - T8 (supine), T6 - T9 (erect)
	Function: reservoir for blood and active pumps that help fill the ventricles
Sinus of pulmonary veins	Portion of posterior wall of left atrium that receives pulmonary veins
Vestibule of left atrioventricular valve	Contains fibrous ring that supports the leaflets of left AV valve

Key points about the left ventricle	
Features	Receives oxygenated blood from left atrium
	Characteristics: long conical shape, thicker walls (compared to right ventricle), smooth inflow/outflow tracts
	Function: pumps blood into systemic circulation
Aortic vestibule	Area immediately below aortic orifice, has fibrous walls that support leaflets of aortic valve
Trabeculae carneae	Muscular elevations that course along mainly apical parts of ventricular wall
Papillary muscles, chordae tendineae	(Superior/inferior papillary muscles)
	Muscular projections attached to cusps of left atrioventricular valve via tendinous cords (chordae tendineae) preventing prolapse
Apex of heart	Rounded anteroinferior extremity of heart formed by left ventricle;
	Located at left 5th intercostal space approximately 9 cm from median plane where apex beat (sounds of left AV valve closure) is maximal.

Atria of the heart

Ventricles of the heart

THORAX

HEART VALVES

There are four valves in the heart which can be divided into two groups: The atrioventricular valves and semilunar valves. The **atrioventricular valves** are located between the atria and ventricles; the **right atrioventricular valve (tricuspid valve)** is positioned between the right atrium and the right ventricle, while the **left atrioventricular valve (mitral or bicuspid valve)** lies between the left atrium and the left ventricle. On the other hand, the **semilunar valves** are the **pulmonary valve**, located between the right ventricle and the pulmonary trunk, and the **aortic valve**, between the left ventricle and aorta.

All the valves comprise a fibrous core covered by endocardial lining facing the chambers of the heart, and they promote unidirectional flow of blood through the heart.

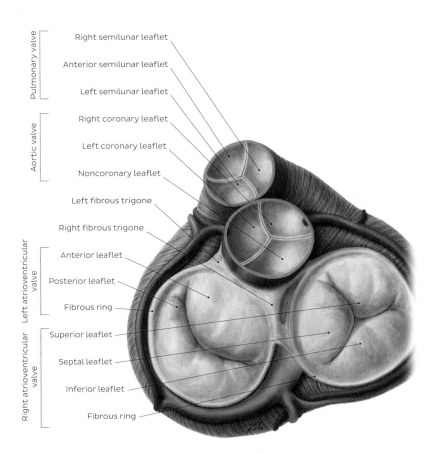

FIGURE 5.44. Overview of the valves of the heart (posterosuperior view). Posterosuperior view of the heart, with the atria removed to expose the heart valves and surrounding structures. All four heart valves have 3 **cusps** or leaflets each, except for the left atrioventricular (mitral valve), which only has 2 cusps (there may be small accessory cusps between the two major cusps of this valve).

The right, left and posterior semilunar cusps of the aortic valve are commonly referred to as the right coronary, left coronary and noncoronary leaflets in clinical practice. Other terminological variations include the anterior/posterior leaflets of the right atrioventricular valve which can more accurately be referred to as the superior/inferior leaflets, respectively. The heart valves are anchored by the fibrous skeleton of the heart, which can be seen as the fibrous rings of left and right atrioventricular valves (mitral and tricuspid valves).

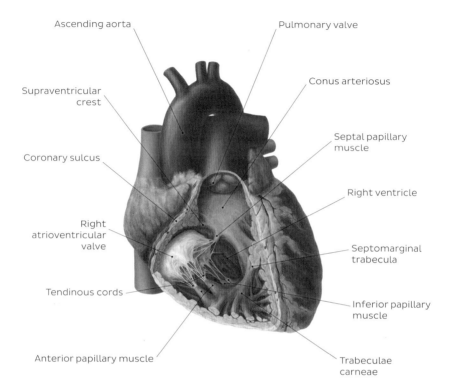

Ascending aorta

Pulmonary valve

Supraventricular crest

Conus arteriosus

Septal papillary muscle

Coronary sulcus

Right ventricle

Right atrioventricular valve

Septomarginal trabecula

Tendinous cords

Inferior papillary muscle

Anterior papillary muscle

Trabeculae carneae

THORAX

FIGURE 5.45. Right atrioventricular and semilunar valves. Overview of the right ventricle showing the valve apparatus which supports the right atrioventricular valve, a.k.a. tricuspid valve. This valve is attached to 3 sets of **papillary muscles** (anterior, medial (or septal), and inferior) via **tendinous cords** (chordae tendineae). These anchor the cusps and prevent them from prolapsing when closed and pressure inside the right ventricle increases. The pulmonary valve can also be seen, and together with the aortic valve they comprise the semilunar valves. These valves are smaller than the AV valves and do not have tendinous cords or papillary muscles supporting them.

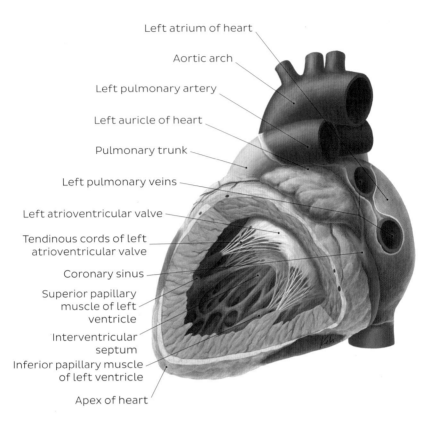

Left atrium of heart

Aortic arch

Left pulmonary artery

Left auricle of heart

Pulmonary trunk

Left pulmonary veins

Left atrioventricular valve

Tendinous cords of left atrioventricular valve

Coronary sinus

Superior papillary muscle of left ventricle

Interventricular septum

Inferior papillary muscle of left ventricle

Apex of heart

FIGURE 5.46. Left atrioventricular valve. Left view of the heart with a section of the left ventricular wall removed to reveal the interior of this chamber. The **left atrioventricular valve** (mitral or bicuspid valve) can be seen separating the left atrium and ventricle. The free edge of each leaflet receives multiple tendinous cords from both **papillary muscles** (superior/anterolateral and inferior/posterior).

The papillary muscles of the left ventricle are much larger than their right counterparts, most likely related to the fact that they must resist greater pressure in order to keep the left AV valve closed during ventricular systole. From the left ventricle blood flows to the root of the aorta via the aortic valve, not seen in this image.

Key points about the heart valves	
Right atrioventricular valve (tricuspid)	**Leaflets (cusps):** 3 – superior (anterior), inferior (posterior) and septal
	Papillary muscles: anterior, septal (medial) and inferior (posterior)
	Position: between right atrium and right ventricle
	Function: prevents backflow from right ventricle into right atrium
Left atrioventricular valve (mitral)	**Leaflets (cusps):** 2 – anterior (aortic) and posterior (mural)
	Papillary muscles: inferior (posterior) and superior (anterolateral)
	Position: between left atrium and left ventricle
	Function: prevents backflow from left ventricle into left atrium
Pulmonary valve	**Leaflets (cusps):** 3 – anterior (non-adjacent), right (right adjacent), and left (left adjacent)
	(No associated papillary muscles)
	Position: between right ventricle and root of pulmonary trunk
	Function: prevents backflow from pulmonary circulation into right ventricle

Key points about the heart valves		
Aortic valve	**Leaflets (cusps):** 3 – right coronary (right semilunar), left coronary (left semilunar), and non-coronary (posterior semilunar)	
	(No associated papillary muscles)	
	Position: between left ventricle and root of aorta	
	Function: prevents backflow from systemic circulation into left ventricle	

 Heart valves

 Heart

 Valvular heart disease

CORONARY ARTERIES AND CARDIAC VEINS

Coronary arteries and cardiac veins comprise the coronary circulation that is responsible for the blood supply and drainage of the heart muscle (myocardium). The two main coronary arteries are the **left** and **right coronary arteries**. The former is usually of a larger caliber and typically gives off two main branches that supply a larger area of the heart including most of the left atrium, the left ventricle and the interventricular septum. The smaller, right coronary artery supplies the right atrium, right ventricle, interatrial and interventricular septa, atrioventricular (AV) and sinuatrial (SA) nodes.

The **coronary veins** can be organized into two groups of veins: The greater and smaller cardiac venous system. The greater cardiac venous system comprises the coronary sinus and its tributaries, as well as the anterior cardiac veins, atrial veins, and the veins of the ventricular septum. The smaller cardiac venous system is composed of the 'smallest cardiac veins' (Thebesian veins) that drain blood directly into the heart chambers.

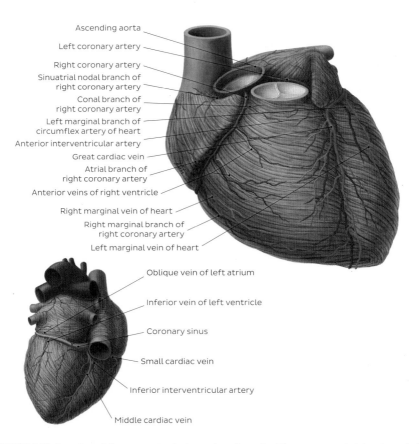

Ascending aorta
Left coronary artery
Right coronary artery
Sinuatrial nodal branch of right coronary artery
Conal branch of right coronary artery
Left marginal branch of circumflex artery of heart
Anterior interventricular artery
Great cardiac vein
Atrial branch of right coronary artery
Anterior veins of right ventricle
Right marginal vein of heart
Right marginal branch of right coronary artery
Left marginal vein of heart

Oblique vein of left atrium
Inferior vein of left ventricle
Coronary sinus
Small cardiac vein
Inferior interventricular artery
Middle cardiac vein

FIGURE 5.47. Overview of the coronary arteries and cardiac veins. The coronary arterial system starts with two main arteries which originate from the aortic sinuses of the root of the aorta. The **right coronary artery** wraps around the right side of the heart running in the coronary/atrioventricular sulcus. It gives rise to three groups of branches (anterior, marginal and inferior (formerly known as the posterior branch)) that vascularize the majority of structures located in the right aspect of the heart.

The **left coronary artery** courses towards the anterior interventricular groove where it bifurcates into its two terminal branches: The anterior interventricular artery and circumflex artery of the heart.

The largest vein of the heart is the **coronary sinus**. It runs in the coronary sulcus on the inferior aspect of the heart and drains blood from the majority of the heart into the right atrium. The coronary sinus has many tributaries including the great, middle and small cardiac veins, inferior vein of the left ventricle and the oblique vein of left atrium. The largest vein on the anterior aspect of the heart is the **great cardiac vein**. This vein receives blood from many venules of the ventricles and left atrium, left marginal vein and anterior interventricular vein.

Key points about the coronary arteries and cardiac veins	
Coronary arteries and their branches	**Left coronary artery:** anterior interventricular artery, circumflex artery of heart
	Right coronary artery: sinuatrial nodal branch, conal branch, atrial branches, ventricular branches, right marginal branch, inferior(/posterior) interventricular artery, atrioventricular nodal branch, right inferolateral branch
Main cardiac veins	Coronary sinus and its tributaries (great cardiac vein, middle cardiac vein, small cardiac vein, inferior vein of left ventricle); anterior cardiac veins, atrial and ventricular smallest cardiac veins (Thebesian veins)

Blood supply of the heart

Long ectopic left main coronary artery

THORAX

NERVES OF THE HEART

The heart receives intrinsic and extrinsic innervation, which allows it to continue to beat independently, even if its nerve supply is disrupted. The intrinsic **conducting system** initiates and controls the contractions of the heart. The contractions are regulated by an extrinsic regulatory system which consists of autonomic nerve fibers that originate from a network of nerves also known as the **cardiac plexus**.

The cardiac plexus is formed of both sympathetic and parasympathetic nerve fibers as well as visceral afferent fibers conveying reflexive and nociceptive fibers from the heart. It is located on the anterior surface of the trachea and along the posterior surface of the ascending aorta and pulmonary trunk. The sympathetic innervation to the heart comes from the sympathetic trunk, while the parasympathetic innervation originates from the **vagus nerve** (CN X). The cardiac plexus is responsible for influencing heart rate, cardiac output, and contraction force of the heart.

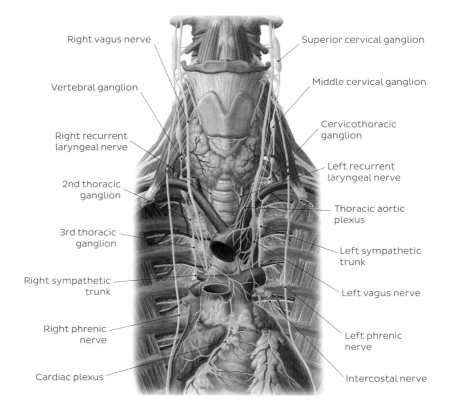

FIGURE 5.48. Overview of the innervation of the heart (anterior view). The heart is supplied mainly by the cardiac plexus, comprising fibers from both sympathetic and parasympathetic nervous systems. The **sympathetic supply** comes primarily from the presynaptic fibers that originate from the intermediolateral cell columns of the first four or five thoracic segments of the spinal cord. These fibers synapse in the

superior thoracic paravertebral sympathetic ganglia and cervical ganglia of the sympathetic trunks. Postganglionic fibers from these ganglia unite to form sympathetic **cardiac nerves**.

The **parasympathetic supply** comes from presynaptic fibers that arise from neurons either in the posterior nucleus of the vagus nerve or near the nucleus ambiguus, and run in cardiac branches of the vagus nerves. Postsynaptic parasympathetic cell bodies (intrinsic ganglia) are located in the atrial wall and interatrial septum near the SA and AV nodes and along the coronary arteries.

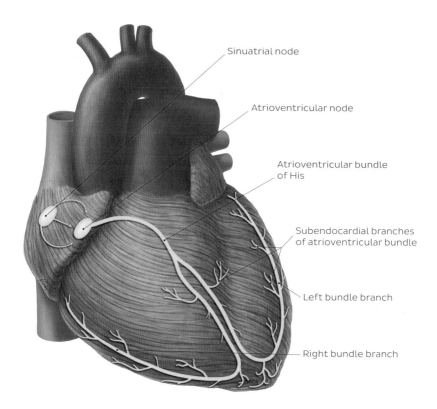

Sinuatrial node

Atrioventricular node

Atrioventricular bundle of His

Subendocardial branches of atrioventricular bundle

Left bundle branch

Right bundle branch

FIGURE 5.49. Conduction system of the heart. The conduction system of the heart is formed by the specialized cardiac muscle fibers that are responsible for the initiation and conduction of the cardiac impulse. The conduction system is composed of **five components**: The sinuatrial (SA) node, atrioventricular (AV) node, AV bundle, right and left branches of the atrioventricular bundles (of His) and the subendocardial fibers (Purkinje fibers). The **SA node** is the pacemaker of the heart and is located superior to the sulcus terminalis of the right atrium. The **AV node** is also located in the right atrium. It picks up and propagates action potentials produced by the sinuatrial node, however is also capable of producing its own action potentials. The **atrioventricular bundle (of His)** is made up of specialized cardiac muscle fibers that extend through the interatrial septum as far as the apex of the heart. These fibers then divide into **subendocardiac (Purkinje) fibers** that extend into the myocardium of the ventricles.

Key points about the nerves of the heart	
Parasympathetic efferent fibers	Cervical and thoracic cardiac branches of vagus nerves
	Function: decrease heart rate, decrease force of contraction of myocardium, vasoconstriction of coronary arteries
Sympathetic efferent fibers	Cardiac nerves from superior, middle and inferior cervical and upper thoracic ganglia
	Function: increase heart rate, increasing force of contraction of myocardium, increasing blood flow in coronary vessels

Key points about the nerves of the heart	
Afferent parasympathetic	Cervical and thoracic cardiac branches of vagus nerves
	Function: feedback on blood pressure
Afferent sympathetic fibers	Afferents to middle and inferior cervical and upper thoracic ganglia
	Function: feedback on blood pressure, pain sensation
Conduction system of the heart	Sinuatrial (SA) node
	Atrioventricular (AV) node
	AV bundle
	Right and left branches of atrioventricular bundles
	Subendocardial (Purkinje) fibers

 Innervation of the heart

 Conducting system of the heart

THORAX

LYMPHATICS OF THE HEART

Like the other organs in our body, the heart also needs to have interstitial fluid drained from its tissues. Small lymphatic vessels of the heart form three plexuses: The subendocardiac plexus, the myocardiac plexus and the subepicardiac plexus. The subendocardiac and myocardiac plexus drain into the subepicardiac plexus, which in turn gives rise to the **right** and **left coronary lymphatic trunks** (or cardiac collecting trunks) which drain the right and left sides of the heart, respectively.

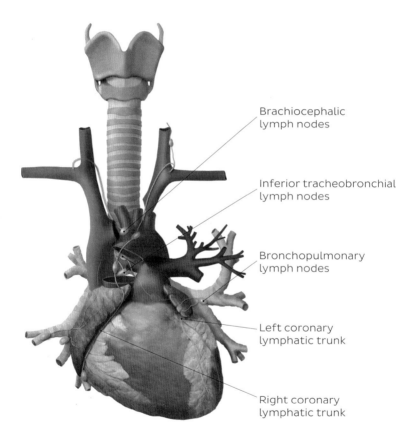

Brachiocephalic lymph nodes

Inferior tracheobronchial lymph nodes

Bronchopulmonary lymph nodes

Left coronary lymphatic trunk

Right coronary lymphatic trunk

FIGURE 5.50. Overview of the lymphatics of the heart. The **right coronary lymphatic trunk** travels within the coronary sulcus, courses anterior to the ascending aorta and ends in the brachiocephalic (anterior mediastinal) lymph nodes, usually on the left. Lymph drained from here is usually received by the **thoracic duct**.

The **left coronary trunk** travels superiorly within the anterior interventricular groove, passing between the pulmonary artery and left atrium before draining into the inferior tracheobronchial lymph nodes. Lymph is then drained to the **right lymphatic duct**.

Key points about the lymphatics of the heart	
Lymphatic plexuses of the heart	**Subendocardiac plexus:** drains into subepicardial plexus
	Myocardial plexus: drains into subepicardial plexus
	Subepicardiac plexus: efferents form the right and left coronary trunks
Right coronary trunk	**Drains:** right atrium, right border of heart and inferior (diaphragmatic) surface of right ventricle
	Empties into: brachiocephalic lymph nodes (usually on the left) → thoracic duct
Left coronary trunk	**Drains:** regions of right and left ventricles around anterior interventricular groove, as well as inferior (diaphragmatic) surface of left ventricle
	Empties into: inferior tracheobronchial lymph nodes → right lymphatic duct

 Heart

 Lymphatic system of the thoracic cavity and mediastinum

THORAX

ABDOMEN

6

REGIONS OF THE ABDOMEN

The abdomen is divided into several regions that allow precise communication about the location of anatomical structures within it, as well as any pathologies. There are two ways to map the abdomen: By nine regions or by four quadrants.

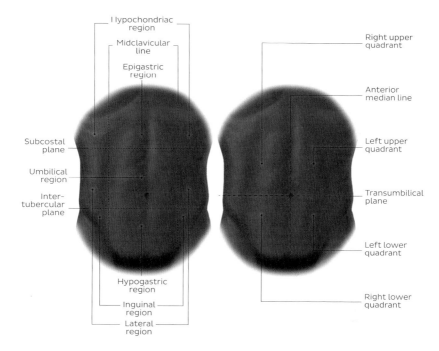

FIGURE 6.1. **Regions of the abdomen.** Two vertical and two horizontal planes divide the abdomen into **9 regions**: Right and left hypochondriac regions, epigastric region, umbilical region, right and left lateral regions of abdomen, hypogastric region, and right and left inguinal regions. The vertical planes are the left and right **midclavicular lines**. The first horizontal plane is the **subcostal plane** which runs at the level of the lower edge of the 10th costal cartilage. The second horizontal plane is the **intertubercular plane**, which passes through the tubercles of the iliac crest and the body of the fifth lumbar vertebra.

Another way to divide the abdomen is into **four quadrants** with one vertical and one horizontal line. The vertical line runs along the midline of the abdomen and the horizontal line along the abdomen at the level of the umbilicus. These divide the abdomen into the right upper quadrant, the left upper quadrant, the right lower quadrant and the left lower quadrant.

Key points about the regions of the abdomen	
Nine-region scheme	Right and left hypochondriac regions, epigastric region, umbilical region, right and left lateral regions, hypogastric region, right and left inguinal regions.
Four-quadrant scheme	Right upper quadrant, left upper quadrant, right lower quadrant, left lower quadrant.

Contents of the abdominal regions	
Left hypochondriac region	Left kidney, spleen, tail of pancreas; parts of stomach, left lobe of liver, small intestines, transverse colon, descending colon
Right hypochondriac region	Right lobe of liver, gallbladder, right colic flexure, upper half of right kidney and part of duodenum
Epigastric region	Abdominal part of esophagus, pylorus of stomach, spleen, pancreas, right and left suprarenal glands; parts of duodenum, liver, right and left kidneys, ureters
Umbilical region	Part of stomach, pancreas, lower part of duodenum, part of jejunum and ileum, cisterna chyli, transverse colon, part of kidneys, ureters
Left lateral region of abdomen	Lower part of left kidney, descending colon, parts of jejunum and ileum
Right lateral region of abdomen	Part of right lobe of liver, gallbladder, ascending colon, lower part of right kidney, parts of duodenum
Hypogastric region	Ileum, sigmoid colon, rectum, ureters, urinary bladder

Regions of the abdomen

Body regions learn with quizzes and labeled diagrams

MUSCLES OF THE ABDOMINAL WALL

The abdominal muscles are divided into the anterolateral and posterior groups.

- The **anterolateral abdominal muscles** compose the anterolateral abdominal wall. There are five muscles in this group (superficial to deep): Pyramidalis, external abdominal oblique, internal abdominal oblique and transversus abdominis muscles.
- The **posterior abdominal muscles** contribute to the posterior abdominal wall. This group consists of one true posterior wall muscle, the quadratus lumborum, as well as the iliopsoas muscle group which continues into the lower limb.

These muscles also support the abdominal viscera and participate in the formation of important anatomical passageways that allow structures from the abdomen and pelvis to reach the perineum and lower limb (e.g., inguinal canal)

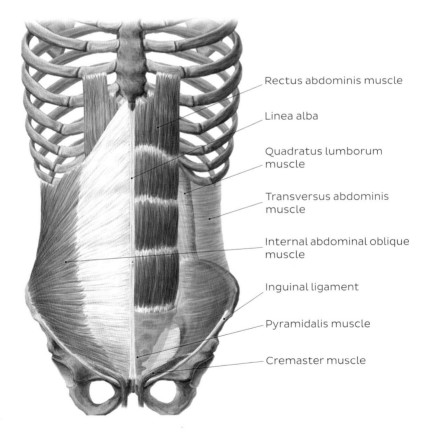

Rectus abdominis muscle

Linea alba

Quadratus lumborum muscle

Transversus abdominis muscle

Internal abdominal oblique muscle

Inguinal ligament

Pyramidalis muscle

Cremaster muscle

FIGURE 6.2. **Muscles of the anterior abdominal wall.** The external abdominal oblique muscle is removed to allow the appreciation of the internal abdominal oblique on the left side of the image. The right side of the image shows the muscles that lie deep to the internal oblique, namely the rectus abdominis,

ABDOMEN

pyramidalis and transversus abdominis muscle. The quadratus lumborum muscle is visible contributing to the posterior abdominal wall.

Muscles of abdominal wall	Origin	Insertion	Innervation	Function
External abdominal oblique	External surfaces of ribs 5-12	Linea alba, Pubic tubercle, Anterior half of iliac crest	Intercostal nerves (T7-T11), Subcostal nerve (T12), Iliohypogastric nerve (L1)	Bilateral contraction – Trunk flexion, Compresses abdominal viscera, Expiration Unilateral contraction – Trunk lateral flexion (ipsilateral), Trunk rotation (contralateral)
Internal abdominal oblique	Anterior two-thirds of iliac crest, Iliopectineal arch, Thoracolumbar fascia	Inferior borders of ribs 10-12, Linea alba, Pubic crest, Pecten pubis (via conjoint tendon)	Intercostal nerves (T7-T11), Subcostal nerve (T12), Iliohypogastric nerve (L1), Ilioinguinal nerve (L1)	Bilateral contraction – Trunk flexion, Compresses abdominal viscera, Expiration Unilateral contraction – Trunk lateral flexion (ipsilateral), Trunk rotation (ipsilateral)
Cremaster	Lateral part: lower edge of internal abdominal oblique and transversus abdominis muscles, Middle of inguinal ligament Medial part: pubic tubercle, Lateral part of pubic crest	Tunica vaginalis of testis	Genital branch of genitofemoral nerve (L1, L2)	Retraction of testis
Transversus abdominis	Internal surfaces of costal cartilages of ribs 7-12, Thoracolumbar fascia, Anterior two thirds of iliac crest, Iliopectineal arch	Linea alba, Aponeurosis of internal abdominal oblique muscle; Pubic crest, Pectineal line of pubis	Intercostal nerves (T7-T11), Subcostal nerve (T12), Iliohypogastric nerve (L1), Ilioinguinal nerve (L1)	Bilateral contraction – Compresses abdominal viscera, Expiration Unilateral contraction – Trunk rotation (ipsilateral)

ABDOMEN

Muscles of abdominal wall	Origin	Insertion	Innervation	Function
Rectus abdominis	Pubic symphysis, Pubic crest	Xiphoid process, Costal cartilages of ribs 5-7	Intercostal nerves (T7–T11), Subcostal nerve (T12)	Trunk flexion, Compresses abdominal viscera, Expiration
Pyramidalis	Pubic crest, Pubic symphysis	Linea alba	Subcostal nerve (T12)	Tenses linea alba
Quadratus lumborum	Iliac crest, Iliolumbar ligament	Inferior border of rib 12, Transverse processes of vertebrae L1-L4	Subcostal nerve (T12), Anterior rami of spinal nerves L1-L4	Bilateral contraction – Fixes Ribs 12 during inspiration, Trunk extension Unilateral contraction – Lateral flexion of trunk (ipsilateral)

 Anterior abdominal wall

 Anterior abdominal muscles

 Lateral abdominal muscles

ABDOMEN

ABDOMINAL SURFACE OF THE DIAPHRAGM

Two main arteries branch off the abdominal aorta and travel along the abdominal surface of the diaphragm, providing its arterial blood supply: The **left** and **right inferior phrenic arteries**. Another branch arising from the abdominal aorta is the **celiac trunk**, which in turn gives rise to three arteries that travel directly beneath the abdominal surface of the diaphragm: The common hepatic, left gastric and splenic arteries.

The diaphragm is closely related to components of the axial skeleton, including the ribs, sternum and lumbar vertebrae, as well as several muscles, such as the psoas major and quadratus lumborum muscles.

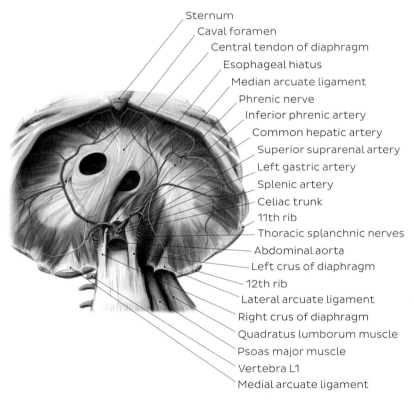

Sternum
Caval foramen
Central tendon of diaphragm
Esophageal hiatus
Median arcuate ligament
Phrenic nerve
Inferior phrenic artery
Common hepatic artery
Superior suprarenal artery
Left gastric artery
Splenic artery
Celiac trunk
11th rib
Thoracic splanchnic nerves
Abdominal aorta
Left crus of diaphragm
12th rib
Lateral arcuate ligament
Right crus of diaphragm
Quadratus lumborum muscle
Psoas major muscle
Vertebra L1
Medial arcuate ligament

FIGURE 6.3. **Abdominal surface of the diaphragm.** This inferior view (abdominal surface) of the diaphragm shows the muscular and tendinous components, as well as the three main openings of the diaphragm: The **aortic hiatus** (aorta, vena azygos and thoracic duct), **esophageal hiatus** (esophagus, branches of left gastric artery and vein and anterior vagal trunk) and **caval foramen** (inferior vena cava and branches of right phrenic nerve). These are formed with the help of tendinous structures, including the right and left crus of the diaphragm as well as the median arcuate ligament.

Two further ligaments, the **medial** and **lateral arcuate ligaments**, form openings posterior to the diaphragm, through which the psoas major and quadratus lumborum muscles pass. Also visible in this inferior view of the diaphragm are components of the axial skeleton, such as the ribs, sternum and the first three lumbar vertebrae. The major vessels supplying the diaphragm are also seen traveling along its abdominal surface: The phrenic nerves and inferior phrenic arteries.

Key points about the abdominal surface of the diaphragm	
Parts	Skeletal muscle (sternal, costal and lumbar parts), central tendon
Function	Main muscle responsible for respiration; increases abdominal pressure to expel feces, vomit and urine; applies pressure on the esophagus to prevent acid reflux
Openings (apertures)	Aortic hiatus: aorta, azygos vein, thoracic duct
	Esophageal hiatus: esophagus, branches of the left gastric artery and vein, anterior and posterior vagal trunks
	Caval foramen: inferior vena cava, branches of the right phrenic nerve
Blood supply	Left and right phrenic arteries (branches of the abdominal aorta)
Innervation	Left and right phrenic nerves (C3-C5)
Musculotendinous structures	Right and left crus of the diaphragm; median, medial and lateral arcuate ligaments

Diaphragm

Hiatal hernia

ABDOMEN

INGUINAL CANAL

The **inguinal canal** is an oblique tubular passage that connects the pelvis and perineum. It originates superolaterally at the **deep inguinal ring**, traverses the abdominal wall and terminates at the **superficial inguinal ring** near the pubic tubercle.

During fetal life, the inguinal canal in males allows for the physiological descension of the testes into the scrotum. In adult life, the inguinal canal serves as a conduit for the spermatic cord and ilioinguinal nerve in males. In females, the inguinal canal is less prominent due to the absence of the spermatic cord, however, it does provide the passage for the round ligament of uterus and ilioinguinal nerve.

The inguinal canal is the weakest point of the trunk wall and as such, an often site for herniations (inguinal hernia), especially so in males due to the descent of the testis.

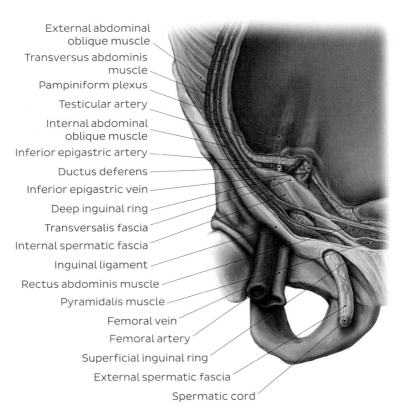

External abdominal oblique muscle
Transversus abdominis muscle
Pampiniform plexus
Testicular artery
Internal abdominal oblique muscle
Inferior epigastric artery
Ductus deferens
Inferior epigastric vein
Deep inguinal ring
Transversalis fascia
Internal spermatic fascia
Inguinal ligament
Rectus abdominis muscle
Pyramidalis muscle
Femoral vein
Femoral artery
Superficial inguinal ring
External spermatic fascia
Spermatic cord

FIGURE 6.4. Inguinal canal (male). The inguinal canal is shown originating at the deep inguinal ring, located at the midpoint between the anterior superior iliac spine and pubic tubercle. It continues between the anterior abdominal muscles and terminates at the superficial inguinal ring.

FIGURE 6.4. **(continued)**

The canal is bounded from four aspects:

The **roof** is formed by the internal oblique and transversus abdominis muscles. The **anterior wall** is derived from the aponeuroses of the internal and external abdominal oblique muscles. The **floor** is formed by the inguinal and lacunar ligaments (not shown). The **posterior wall** is formed by the transversalis fascia and conjoint tendon of the abdominal internal abdominal oblique muscles.

The image depicts the spermatic cord traversing the inguinal canal. The cord is enveloped by three fascial layers, derived from the musculofascial structures of the abdominal wall. From superficial to deep, they are: External spermatic fascia (derived from the aponeurosis of external abdominal oblique). Cremasteric muscle (derived from the internal abdominal oblique and its fascia). Internal spermatic fascia (derived from the transversalis fascia).

The cord itself transmits several structures to and from the testes: Testicular, cremasteric and artery of ductus deferens. Pampiniform venous plexus. Ilioinguinal nerve and genital branch of genitofemoral nerve. Ductus deferens.

Inguinal canal

NEUROVASCULATURE OF THE ABDOMINAL WALL

As the anterolateral abdominal wall is a particularly large region, formed by multiple layers of skin, connective tissue and muscles, it requires an abundant nervous and blood supply.

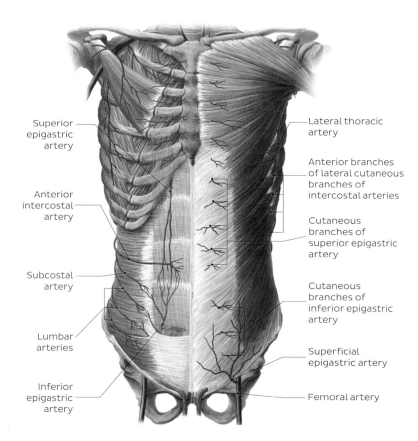

Superior epigastric artery

Anterior intercostal artery

Subcostal artery

Lumbar arteries

Inferior epigastric artery

Lateral thoracic artery

Anterior branches of lateral cutaneous branches of intercostal arteries

Cutaneous branches of superior epigastric artery

Cutaneous branches of inferior epigastric artery

Superficial epigastric artery

Femoral artery

FIGURE 6.5. Arteries of the anterolateral abdominal wall. Intercostal arteries 10-11, along with the **subcostal artery**, provide the anterior and lateral cutaneous branches that supply the skin and muscles of the upper lateral portion of the abdominal wall. The lower lateral portion is mainly supplied by the **lumbar arteries**, while the medial part is supplied by the branches of the **superior**, **inferior** and **superficial epigastric arteries**.

ABDOMEN

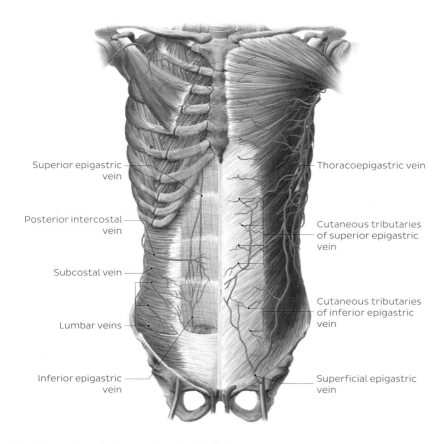

Superior epigastric vein

Thoracoepigastric vein

Posterior intercostal vein

Cutaneous tributaries of superior epigastric vein

Subcostal vein

Lumbar veins

Cutaneous tributaries of inferior epigastric vein

Inferior epigastric vein

Superficial epigastric vein

FIGURE 6.6. Veins of the anterolateral abdominal wall. The venous drainage of the anterolateral abdominal wall mainly mirrors the arterial supply. The posterior intercostal veins 10-11, as well as the subcostal vein, are tributaries of the hemiazygos vein. The superior epigastric vein drains into the internal thoracic vein, while the inferior epigastric vein drains into the external iliac vein. The lumbar veins drain directly into the inferior vena cava, while the superficial epigastric vein drains into the femoral vein.

Key points about the neurovasculature of the anterolateral abdominal wall	
Arteries	Internal thoracic artery and its branches (musculophrenic artery, superior epigastric artery), 10th and 11th posterior intercostal arteries, subcostal artery, inferior epigastric artery, deep circumflex iliac artery, superficial circumflex iliac artery, superficial epigastric artery
Veins	Superficial epigastric vein, superior epigastric vein, inferior epigastric vein, thoracoepigastric vein, subcostal vein
Nerves	Thoracoabdominal nerves, lateral cutaneous branches of intercostal nerves 7-11, subcostal nerve, iliohypogastric nerve, ilioinguinal nerve

ABDOMEN

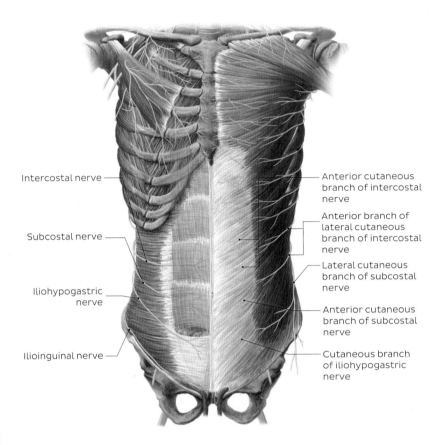

Intercostal nerve

Subcostal nerve

Iliohypogastric
nerve

Ilioinguinal nerve

Anterior cutaneous
branch of intercostal
nerve

Anterior branch of
lateral cutaneous
branch of intercostal
nerve

Lateral cutaneous
branch of subcostal
nerve

Anterior cutaneous
branch of subcostal
nerve

Cutaneous branch
of iliohypogastric
nerve

FIGURE 6.7. **Nerves of the anterolateral abdominal wall.** The anterolateral abdominal wall is innervated by four main sources:

- **Intercostal nerves 7-11** (the anterior rami of spinal nerves T7-T11)
- **Subcostal nerve** (anterior ramus of spinal nerve T12)
- **Iliohypogastric** and **ilioinguinal nerves** (branches of anterior ramus of spinal nerve L1)

The intercostal nerves 7-11 (sometimes referred to as thoracoabdominal nerves) and the subcostal nerve pass between the internal oblique and transversus abdominis muscles, giving off two cutaneous branches: Anterior and lateral. They supply the skin and muscles of the anterolateral abdominal wall.

The iliohypogastric and ilioinguinal nerves supply the skin and muscles of the inguinal and hypogastric regions.

Key points about the neurovasculature of the posterior abdominal wall	
Arteries	Abdominal aorta and its branches (subcostal artery, inferior phrenic artery, lumbar arteries, median sacral artery)
Veins	Inferior vena cava and its tributaries (inferior phrenic veins, lumbar veins, and common iliac veins)
Nerves	Aortic and periarterial nervous plexuses

ABDOMEN

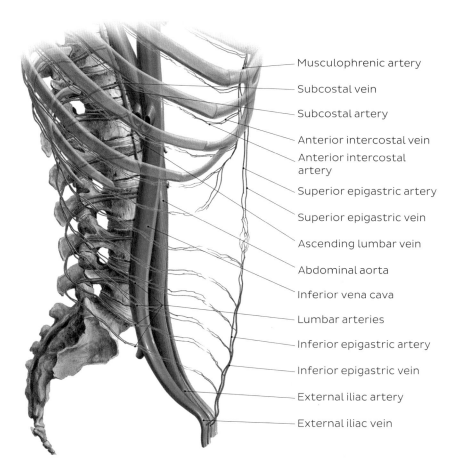

- Musculophrenic artery
- Subcostal vein
- Subcostal artery
- Anterior intercostal vein
- Anterior intercostal artery
- Superior epigastric artery
- Superior epigastric vein
- Ascending lumbar vein
- Abdominal aorta
- Inferior vena cava
- Lumbar arteries
- Inferior epigastric artery
- Inferior epigastric vein
- External iliac artery
- External iliac vein

FIGURE 6.8. Arteries and veins of the posterior abdominal wall (lateral view). The arteries that supply the posterior abdominal wall primarily stem from the **abdominal aorta**, often being referred to as the parietal branches of the aorta. The paired parietal branches are the subcostal, inferior phrenic and lumbar arteries. They respectively supply the regions at the levels of L2, T12 and L1-L4.

The veins of the posterior abdominal wall are predominantly the tributaries of the inferior vena cava. Namely, these are the inferior epigastric, lumbar and common iliac veins.

 Anterior abdominal wall

 Iliohypogastric nerve

 Lumbar plexus

PERITONEAL RELATIONS

The peritoneum is a double-layered serous membrane that envelopes the abdominal organs and lines the walls of the abdominal cavity. The two layers are the visceral and parietal peritoneum.

According to their position in relation to the peritoneum, the organs of the abdominopelvic region can be classified as:

- Intraperitoneal organs
- Extraperitoneal organs (retroperitoneal and infraperitoneal)

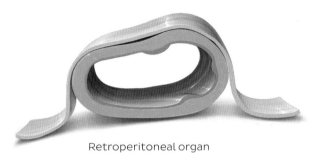

Retroperitoneal organ

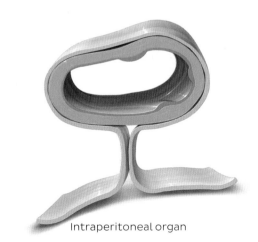

Intraperitoneal organ

FIGURE 6.9. Retroperitoneal vs. intraperitoneal organ. Organs which are completely surrounded by visceral peritoneum and connected by mesentery are called **intraperitoneal organs**. Most intraperitoneal structures are associated with the gastrointestinal tract as this organization allows for both support and movement.

In contrast, organs located behind the parietal peritoneum are referred to as the **retroperitoneal organs**. If they develop and remain outside the peritoneum, they are referred to as the **primary** retroperitoneal organs. **Secondary** retroperitoneal organs initially develop within the peritoneum and become retroperitoneal when their mesentery fuses with the posterior abdominal wall during embryonic development. **Infraperitoneal organs** are organs that lie inferior to the peritoneal cavity.

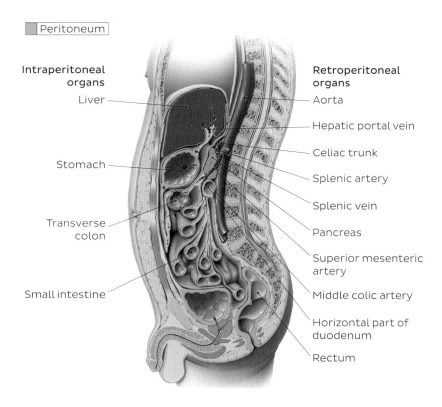

| Peritoneum |

Intraperitoneal organs
- Liver
- Stomach
- Transverse colon
- Small intestine

Retroperitoneal organs
- Aorta
- Hepatic portal vein
- Celiac trunk
- Splenic artery
- Splenic vein
- Pancreas
- Superior mesenteric artery
- Middle colic artery
- Horizontal part of duodenum
- Rectum

FIGURE 6.10. **Peritoneal relations.** Intraperitoneal organs are completely wrapped by visceral peritoneum. These organs are the liver, spleen, stomach, superior part of the duodenum, jejunum, ileum, transverse colon, sigmoid colon and superior part of the rectum. Retroperitoneal organs are found posterior to the peritoneum in the retroperitoneal space with only their anterior wall covered by the parietal peritoneum. If they develop and remain outside the peritoneum, they are primarily retroperitoneal organs: Kidney, adrenal glands and ureter. Other retroperitoneal organs develop inside the peritoneum, but then move posterior to it and fuse with the abdominal wall: Pancreas, distal duodenum, ascending and descending colons. Great blood vessels are also retroperitoneal.

Key points about the peritoneal relations	
Intraperitoneal structures	Stomach, superior part of the duodenum, jejunum, ileum, cecum/appendix, transverse colon, sigmoid colon, liver, gallbladder, spleen, pancreas (tail), female reproductive organs (ovaries, uterus and uterine tubes)
Primary retroperitoneal organs	Esophagus, anal canal, kidneys, suprarenal (adrenal) glands, ureters, aorta, inferior vena cava
Secondary retroperitoneal organs	Pancreas (head, neck and body), distal duodenum, ascending colon, descending colon, proximal one-third of rectum
Infraperitoneal organs	Inferior two thirds of rectum, urinary bladder
Recesses	Duodenal recesses, caecal recesses, intersigmoid recess

The peritoneum

Recesses of the peritoneal cavity

ABDOMEN

MESENTERY

The **mesentery** is an abdominal organ comprised of both layers of the perito-neum: Visceral and parietal. The main **function** of the mesentery is to attach/suspend the intraperitoneal organs (mainly the intestines) to the posterior abdominal wall and provide neurovascular communication between those organs and vessels/nerves of the posterior abdominal wall. Mesenteries include the:

- **Small intestine mesentery** (mesentery proper): Suspends the jejunum and the ileum
- **Mesoappendix:** Suspends the vermiform appendix and the cecum
- **Transverse mesocolon:** Suspends the transverse colon
- **Sigmoid mesocolon:** Suspends the sigmoid colon

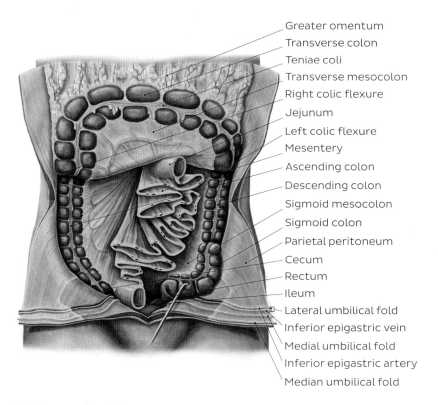

Greater omentum
Transverse colon
Teniae coli
Transverse mesocolon
Right colic flexure
Jejunum
Left colic flexure
Mesentery
Ascending colon
Descending colon
Sigmoid mesocolon
Sigmoid colon
Parietal peritoneum
Cecum
Rectum
Ileum
Lateral umbilical fold
Inferior epigastric vein
Medial umbilical fold
Inferior epigastric artery
Median umbilical fold

FIGURE 6.11. Overview of the mesentery. The **mesentery proper** is the largest mesentery that wraps around the jejunum and ileum, attaching them to the posterior abdominal wall. The **transverse mesocolon** supports the transverse colon, attaching it to the posterior abdominal wall. The **sigmoid mesocolon** provides support for the sigmoid colon. The **mesoappendix** is the mesentery of the appendix and the cecum.

Key points about the mesentery	
Definition	The mesentery is a peritoneal organ, composed of two layers of peritoneum, that wraps around the intestines and connects them to the posterior abdominal wall
Structure	Mesentery proper, transverse mesocolon, sigmoid mesocolon, mesoappendix
Function	Attaches intestines to the abdominal wall, supports digestion, stores fat, participates in immune functions, provides a pathway for the neurovascular structures that supply the intestines

Mesentery

GREATER OMENTUM

The **omenta** are fused peritoneal folds that connect the intraperitoneal organs to each other. The **greater omentum** is the largest, apron-like peritoneal fold which extends from the greater curvature of the stomach and duodenum to the posterior abdominal wall. The greater omentum is a site of fat deposition and functions to protect the abdominal organs by cushioning them and activating the immune response, as well as contributing to reparative processes.

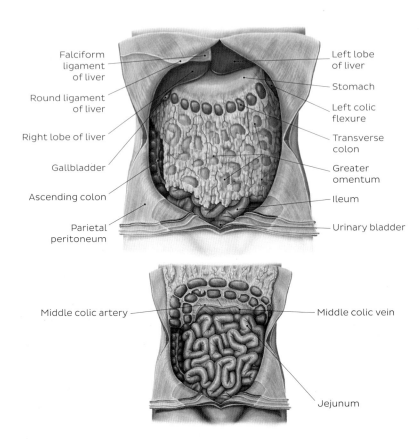

FIGURE 6.12. **Greater omentum.** The greater omentum is a four-layered peritoneal fold that hangs like an apron covering the abdominal organs. From left to right, the **upper margin** of the greater omentum is continuous with the gastrosplenic ligament, greater curvature of the stomach and the proximal part of the duodenum. It descends inferiorly over the transverse colon, jejunum and ileum. The omentum then turns posteriorly, passing anterior to the transverse colon and transverse mesocolon to attach to the posterior abdominal wall.

The **right margin** of the greater omentum is usually attached to the hepatic flexure and upper portion of the ascending colon. Its **left margin** is sometimes attached to the anterior surface of the descending colon. The greater omentum is vascularized by the **gastroomental arteries**, and the blood is drained by **gastroomental veins**, which run between its layers.

Key points about the greater omentum	
Definition	The greater omentum is the largest peritoneal fold located in the abdominal cavity.
Blood supply	Right gastroomental artery, left gastroomental artery
Venous drainage	Right gastroomental vein, left gastroomental vein
Related organs	Stomach, duodenum, colon, jejunum, ileum
Function	Site of fat deposition, protection, reparation

Greater and lesser omentum

The peritoneum

OMENTAL BURSA

The **omental bursa** is a large peritoneal recess located in the abdomen formed by a double-layered fold of visceral peritoneum. It is situated posterior to the stomach and the lesser omentum, inferior to the liver and anterior to the pancreas. The omental bursa is also known as the **lesser sac**, in contrast to the larger part of the peritoneal cavity which is referred to as the **greater sac**. These two cavities are connected by the **epiploic foramen (of Winslow)**. The size of the omental bursa varies greatly, mainly due to the volume of the organs that make up its walls.

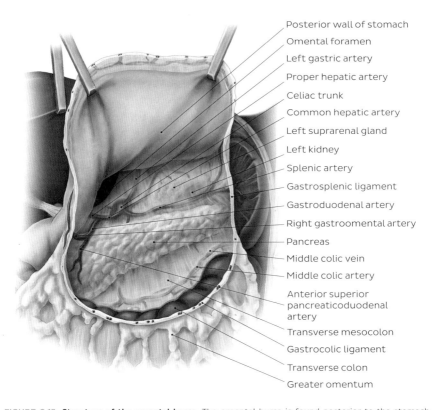

Posterior wall of stomach
Omental foramen
Left gastric artery
Proper hepatic artery
Celiac trunk
Common hepatic artery
Left suprarenal gland
Left kidney
Splenic artery
Gastrosplenic ligament
Gastroduodenal artery
Right gastroomental artery
Pancreas
Middle colic vein
Middle colic artery
Anterior superior pancreaticoduodenal artery
Transverse mesocolon
Gastrocolic ligament
Transverse colon
Greater omentum

FIGURE 6.13. Structure of the omental bursa. The omental bursa is found posterior to the stomach, inferior to the liver and anterior to the pancreas and duodenum. It has an irregular shape with one superior and one inferior recess. The superior recess is bordered by the diaphragm and the coronary ligament of the liver, while the inferior recess is found between the folding layers of the greater omentum.

The omental bursa communicates with the greater sac via the epiploic foramen (omental foramen) found posterior to the free edge of the lesser omentum. This foramen has clear borders:

- Anterior – hepatoduodenal ligament
- Posterior – inferior vena cava and the right crus of the diaphragm
- Superior – caudate lobe of the liver
- Inferior – superior part of the duodenum

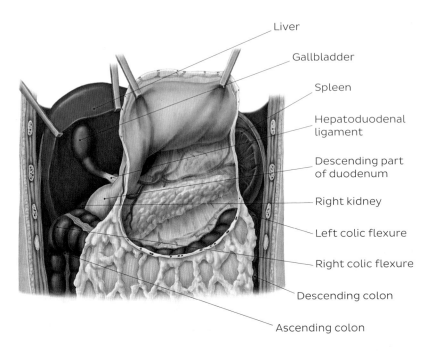

Liver

Gallbladder

Spleen

Hepatoduodenal ligament

Descending part of duodenum

Right kidney

Left colic flexure

Right colic flexure

Descending colon

Ascending colon

FIGURE 6.14. **Posterior relations of the omental bursa.** The omental bursa is a potential space whose function is to provide space for unhindered movements of the stomach. It is filled with peritoneal fluid and provides a cushion between the posterior surface of the stomach and several other structures: Celiac trunk and its branches, pancreas, left kidney and left suprarenal glands. The omental bursa allows normal peristalsis of the stomach without friction against the above mentioned structures.

Key points about the omental bursa	
Definition	Omental bursa (lesser sac) is a hollow space formed by the greater and lesser omentum and its adjacent organs.
Walls	**Anterior:** hepatogastric ligament, posterior surface of stomach, posterior layers of the lesser and greater omenta
	Posterior: transverse colon, transverse mesocolon, pancreas, left adrenal gland, and the upper end of the left kidney, abdominal aorta, coeliac trunk, diaphragm
Borders	**Superior:** extends between esophagus and ligamentum venosum
	Inferior: from gastrosplenic ligament to duodenum
	Left: gastrosplenic ligament, spleen, phrenicosplenic ligament
	Right: epiploic foramen, lesser omentum, greater sac
Recesses	Superior omental recess
	Inferior omental recess
	Splenic recess

Omental bursa

ABDOMEN

RETROPERITONEUM

The **retroperitoneum** is a potential anatomical space located posterior to the peritoneal cavity and anterior to the posterior abdominal wall. It contains several organs which, due to their location behind the parietal peritoneum, are referred to as the **retroperitoneal organs**. The retroperitoneum is divided into three individual spaces:

- Anterior pararenal space
- Posterior pararenal space
- Perirenal space

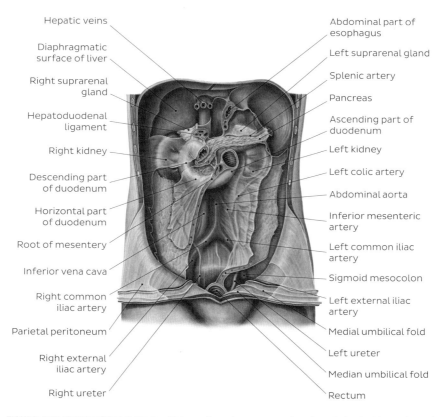

Hepatic veins	Abdominal part of esophagus
Diaphragmatic surface of liver	Left suprarenal gland
Right suprarenal gland	Splenic artery
Hepatoduodenal ligament	Pancreas
Right kidney	Ascending part of duodenum
Descending part of duodenum	Left kidney
Horizontal part of duodenum	Left colic artery
Root of mesentery	Abdominal aorta
Inferior vena cava	Inferior mesenteric artery
Right common iliac artery	Left common iliac artery
Parietal peritoneum	Sigmoid mesocolon
Right external iliac artery	Left external iliac artery
Right ureter	Medial umbilical fold
	Left ureter
	Median umbilical fold
	Rectum

FIGURE 6.15. Retroperitoneal organs. Retroperitoneal organs are found posterior to the peritoneal cavity in the **retroperitoneal space** with only their anterior wall covered by the parietal peritoneum. If they develop and remain outside the peritoneum, they are referred to as the **primary retroperitoneal organs**. These are the kidneys, suprarenal glands, ureters, aorta/inferior vena cava and rectum. **Secondary retroperitoneal organs** initially develop within the peritoneum, however, they become retroperitoneal as they lose their mesentery during embryonic development. These include the pancreas, distal duodenum, ascending and descending colons.

Key points about the retroperitoneum	
Definition	The retroperitoneum is a potential anatomical space located posterior to the parietal peritoneum.
Primary retroperitoneal organs	Kidneys, suprarenal (adrenal) glands, ureter, aorta/inferior vena cava
Secondary retroperitoneal organs	Pancreas, distal duodenum, ascending colon, descending colon
Spaces	Anterior pararenal space, posterior pararenal space, perirenal space

The peritoneum

Recesses of the peritoneal cavity

ABDOMEN

STOMACH *IN SITU*

The **stomach** is a hollow muscular organ and the most dilated portion of the gastrointestinal tract. It is located on the left upper quadrant of the abdomen between the esophagus and duodenum. The stomach consists of four main **parts**: The cardia, fundus, body, and pyloric part.

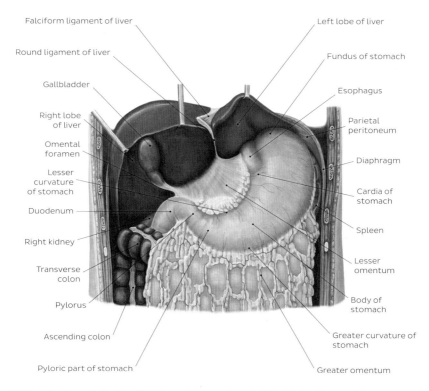

Falciform ligament of liver

Round ligament of liver

Gallbladder

Right lobe of liver

Omental foramen

Lesser curvature of stomach

Duodenum

Right kidney

Transverse colon

Pylorus

Ascending colon

Pyloric part of stomach

Left lobe of liver

Fundus of stomach

Esophagus

Parietal peritoneum

Diaphragm

Cardia of stomach

Spleen

Lesser omentum

Body of stomach

Greater curvature of stomach

Greater omentum

FIGURE 6.16. **Stomach in situ.** The stomach has a characteristic 'J-shape' created by two unequal **curvatures**: The longer, convex greater curvature (located on the left side) and the shorter, concave lesser curvature (on the right). Between the curvatures, the four main parts of the stomach are visible: Cardia, fundus, body and the pyloric part. Anterior relations of the stomach are not fully visible in the illustration however they include the diaphragm, left lobe of the liver (retracted), and the anterior abdominal wall.

Key points about the stomach and its relations	
Definition	The stomach is a hollow muscular organ of the digestive system, specialized in the mechanical and chemical digestion of food.
Main parts	Cardia, fundus, body, pyloric part
Relations	**Anterior:** diaphragm, left lobe of liver, and anterior abdominal wall
	Posterior: omental bursa (lesser sac), pancreas, left kidney and adrenal gland, splenic artery and spleen
	Superior: esophagus and diaphragm
	Inferior: transverse colon/mesocolon, greater omentum
Functions	Mechanical and chemical digestion (of proteins and fats especially), absorption, hormone secretion

ABDOMEN

STRUCTURE OF THE STOMACH

The wall of the stomach consists of **four histological layers**: Mucosa, sub-mucosa, muscular coat (muscularis externa) and serosa. The muscular coat is further divided into three separate layers: The oblique, circular and longitudi-nalmuscle fibers. The main function of the stomach involves the mechanical and chemical digestion of ingested food.

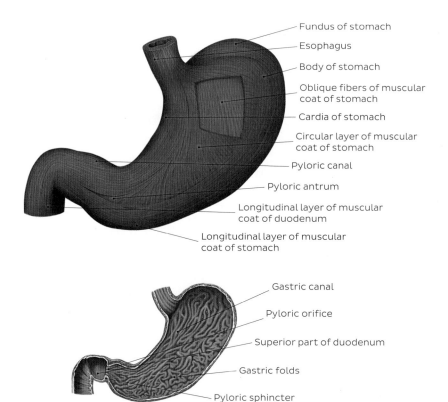

FIGURE 6.17. **Musculature and mucosa of the stomach.** Outer and inner surfaces of the stomach. The upper image shows the external features of the stomach and its three muscular layers. The outermost layer is the **longitudinal muscle layer**. Its fibers are mostly situated on the greater and lesser curvatures. The middle layer is the **circular muscle layer** composed of circular muscle fibers. This layer comprises the pyloric sphincter which serves to regulate the passage of digested food into the duodenum. When these two layers are removed, the innermost layer, the **oblique muscle fibers** become visible. This layer is responsible for the peristaltic movement that churns and breaks down food in the stomach.

In the lower image, the anterior wall of the stomach has been removed to reveal its internal features. The most prominent features seen on the mucosa of the stomach are the **gastric folds** (gastric rugae). The **gastric canal** runs along the lesser curvature of the stomach and is formed by the longitudinal muscle fibers of the stomach. The **pylorus** represents the terminal part of the stomach. It is divided into two parts, the **pyloric antrum**, which connects to the body of the stomach, and the **pyloric canal**, which connects to the duodenum by the pyloric orifice.

Key points about the structure of the stomach	
Definition	The stomach is a hollow muscular organ of the digestive system, specialized in the accumulation and digestion of food.
Main parts	Cardia, fundus, body, pyloric part
Layers of the gastric wall	Mucosa, submucosa, muscular layer, serosa
Muscular layers	Longitudinal layer, circular layer, oblique fibers
Function	Mechanical and chemical digestion, absorption, hormone secretion

The stomach

Stomach histology

STRUCTURE OF THE SPLEEN

The **spleen** is a soft, delicate, fist-sized, intraperitoneal organ covered by a fibroelastic capsule. It is located in the left upper quadrant of the abdomen (left hypochondrium), at the level of the ninth to eleventh ribs, posterior to the stomach and anterior to the left hemidiaphragm and costodiaphragmatic recess. It plays an important role in the immune system, by participating both in the humoral and the cell-mediated responses.

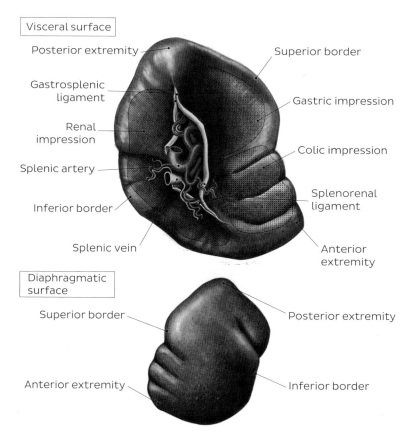

Visceral surface
Posterior extremity
Gastrosplenic ligament
Renal impression
Splenic artery
Inferior border
Splenic vein
Superior border
Gastric impression
Colic impression
Splenorenal ligament
Anterior extremity

Diaphragmatic surface
Superior border
Anterior extremity
Posterior extremity
Inferior border

FIGURE 6.18. **Surfaces of the spleen.** The spleen has two surfaces: Visceral and diaphragmatic. The convex **diaphragmatic surface** faces the diaphragm and is shown on the lower half of the image, while the upper image on represents the visceral surface of the spleen.

The **hilum** is located centrally on the visceral surface with the splenic vessels (splenic artery and vein) surrounded by the gastrosplenic and splenorenal ligaments. The visceral surface also bears three impressions, named by the structures directly in contact with them: These are the **gastric, colic** and **renal impressions**.

ABDOMEN

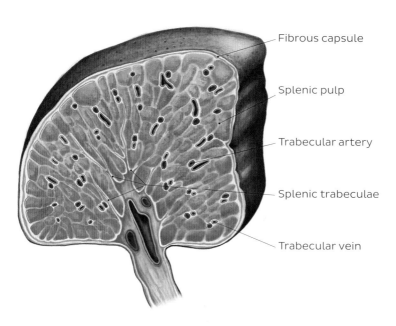

Fibrous capsule

Splenic pulp

Trabecular artery

Splenic trabeculae

Trabecular vein

FIGURE 6.19. **Transverse section of the spleen.** Transverse section through the hilum shows the parenchyma/splenic pulp being divided into small sections by numerous septa called trabeculae.

Key points about the spleen	
Definition	Intraperitoneal lymphatic organ found on the left side of the abdomen, inferior to the diaphragm
Relations of spleen	**Superolateral:** diaphragm
	Anteromedial: stomach
	Posteroinferior: left kidney (and superior pole of the left suprarenal gland)
	Inferior pole: left flexure of the colon
Neurovascular supply	**Arterial supply:** splenic artery
	Venous drainage: splenic vein
	Lymphatic drainage: celiac node
	Innervation: celiac plexus

Spleen

Histology of the spleen

Splenic artery rupture

ABDOMEN

OVERVIEW OF THE LIVER

The **liver** is a large accessory organ of the gastrointestinal tract with metabolic, endocrine and exocrine functions. It is located mainly in the right hypochondrium and epigastrium, with a small portion extending into the left hypochondrium. The liver is divided into the right, left, quadrate and caudate lobes. It is covered in visceral peritoneum, except for the **bare area**, where it is in contact with the diaphragm and therefore has diaphragmatic and visceral surfaces. Its location gives it numerous relations to other organs and structures of the body:

- Superior: Diaphragm
- Anterior: Ribs (7-11th), anterior abdominal wall
- Posteroinferior: Esophagus, right kidney and adrenal gland, right colic flexure, lesser omentum, duodenum, gallbladder, stomach

The **position of the liver** is secured with the following ligaments: Coronary, left and right triangular, falciform, round ligaments, ligamentum venosum and lesser omentum.

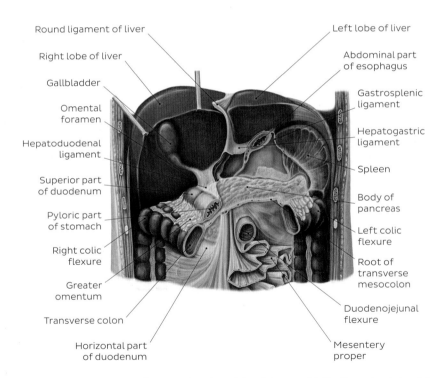

Round ligament of liver
Right lobe of liver
Gallbladder
Omental foramen
Hepatoduodenal ligament
Superior part of duodenum
Pyloric part of stomach
Right colic flexure
Greater omentum
Transverse colon
Horizontal part of duodenum

Left lobe of liver
Abdominal part of esophagus
Gastrosplenic ligament
Hepatogastric ligament
Spleen
Body of pancreas
Left colic flexure
Root of transverse mesocolon
Duodenojejunal flexure
Mesentery proper

FIGURE 6.20. **Relations of the liver.** Anterior view of the abdomen with the liver retracted and the stomach removed to expose the underlying structures. **Right** and **left lobes** of the liver can be seen, with the **gallbladder** on the posterior surface of the right lobe and with the blood vessels and the bile duct enclosed in the **hepatoduodenal ligament** (part of the lesser omentum).

The rest of the lesser omentum is formed by the **hepatogastric ligament**. It extends between the liver and the stomach, but only a small part of it is visible around the cardiac orifice of the esophagus. The **falciform ligament** is located between the right and left lobes and is continuous inferiorly with the round ligament

ABDOMEN

of the liver, which is exposed due to the reflected liver. The **round ligament** extends posteroinferiorly to join the ligamentum venosum. A section of the greater omentum, the superior part of the duodenum and the transverse colon are all shown and form the posteroinferior anatomical relations of the liver. Not shown in the image are the posterior relations of the liver to the right kidney and the adrenal gland.

Key points about the liver	
Location	Right hypochondriac and epigastric regions
Anatomy	**Lobes:** right, left, caudate, quadrate **Surfaces:** diaphragmatic, visceral **Fissures:** main portal fissure, right portal fissure, left portal fissure, umbilical fissure (fissure for ligamentum teres, fissure for ligamentum venosum) **Ligaments:** coronary, left triangular, right triangular, falciform, round, ligamentum venosum, hepatogastric, hepatoduodenal
Function	Metabolic, endocrine and exocrine functions (xenobiotic biotransformation, protein synthesis, nutrient storage, bile production)
Relations	**Superior:** diaphragm **Anterior:** ribs 7–11, anterior abdominal wall **Posteroinferior:** esophagus, stomach, gallbladder, duodenum, right kidney, right adrenal gland, right colic flexure, lesser omentum

 Liver

 Functional division of the liver

 Liver ligaments

ABDOMEN

SURFACES OF THE LIVER

The liver has two surfaces which are separated by a narrow inferior border:

- The **diaphragmatic surface**, lying just below the diaphragm
- The **visceral surface**, which faces the abdominal organs

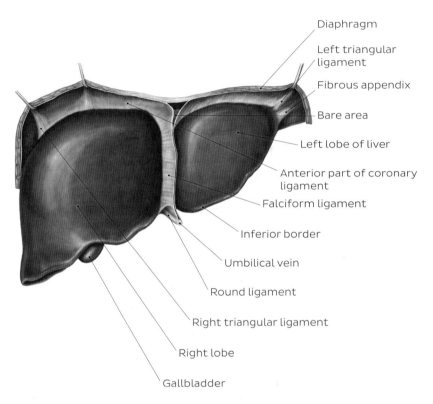

Diaphragm

Left triangular ligament

Fibrous appendix

Bare area

Left lobe of liver

Anterior part of coronary ligament

Falciform ligament

Inferior border

Umbilical vein

Round ligament

Right triangular ligament

Right lobe

Gallbladder

FIGURE 6.21. Anterior view of the liver. Observing the liver from an anterior perspective allows the appreciation of its superior, anterior and right **surfaces**, which are collectively dome-shaped due to their contact with the overlying diaphragm. All are covered mainly with **peritoneum** which is reflected superiorly as **the anterior part of the coronary ligament**, forming the **bare area** of the liver posterior to it. The peritoneum covering the anterior surface meets its posterior counterpart at the upper right and left corners of the liver, forming the **right** and **left triangular ligaments**. The left and right lobes of the liver are separated by the **falciform ligament**, whose inferior margin encloses the **round ligament**.

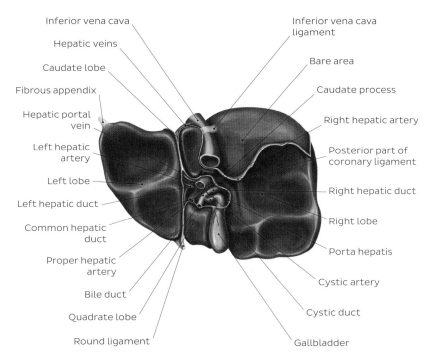

Inferior vena cava

Hepatic veins

Caudate lobe

Fibrous appendix

Hepatic portal vein

Left hepatic artery

Left lobe

Left hepatic duct

Common hepatic duct

Proper hepatic artery

Bile duct

Quadrate lobe

Round ligament

Inferior vena cava ligament

Bare area

Caudate process

Right hepatic artery

Posterior part of coronary ligament

Right hepatic duct

Right lobe

Porta hepatis

Cystic artery

Cystic duct

Gallbladder

FIGURE 6.22. Inferior view of the liver. Several vascular and ligamentous structures, together with the gallbladder, form the shape of the letter "H" on the posteroinferior aspect of the liver. The horizontal limb is represented by the **hilum of the liver (porta hepatis)**, which gives passage to the hepatic portal vein, proper hepatic artery and biliary ducts. The right limb of the H is formed by the **groove for inferior vena cava** and **gallbladder** below it. The left limb, which separates the left lobe from the caudate and quadrate lobes, is defined by the fissures for **ligamentum venosum** and **round ligament**.

Between the porta hepatis and inferior vena cava is the **posterior part of the coronary ligament** that extends to the right, marking the inferior boundary of the bare area of the liver. Below it on the right lobe are **impressions** of the suprarenal gland, kidney and hepatic flexure of the colon. The posteroinferior aspect of the left lobe presents a well defined impression of the stomach, while the quadrate lobe is adjacent to the first part of the duodenum.

ABDOMEN

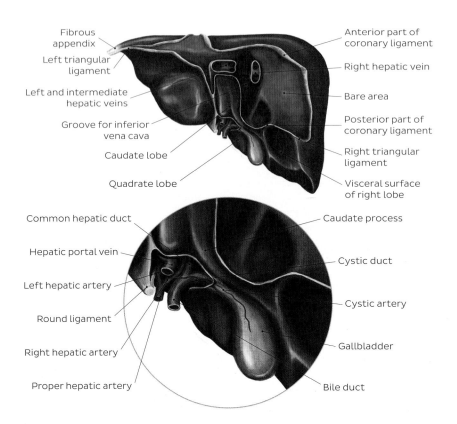

FIGURE 6.23. Posterior view of the liver. The posterior surface of the liver is attached to the diaphragm at the **bare area**. This area is bounded by the anterior and posterior parts of the coronary ligament which merge to the left and right as the triangular ligaments of the liver. In the center of the bare area are the **right**, **middle** and **left hepatic veins**.

The **caudate lobe** is limited by the posterior part of coronary ligament, fissure for ligamentum venosum and porta hepatis. The **left lobe** carries an impression of the stomach, while to the right of the gallbladder are additional impressions of the suprarenal gland and kidney.

Key points about the surfaces of the liver	
Lobes of the liver	**Right lobe:** largest lobe of the liver
	Left lobe: separated anteriorly from right lobe by falciform ligament
	Quadrate lobe: visceral surface, between gallbladder and left lobe
	Caudate lobe: visceral surface, between inferior vena cava and left lobe
Diaphragmatic surface	**Surfaces:** superior, anterior, right, posterior
	Landmarks: cardiac impression, bare area, groove for inferior vena cava, hepatic veins
Visceral surface	Also known as inferior surface;
	Landmarks: porta hepatis, fossa for gallbladder, omental tuberosity,
	Fissures: main portal fissure, right portal fissure, left portal fissure, umbilical fissure (fissure for ligamentum teres, fissure for ligamentum venosum)
	Impressions: esophageal, gastric, duodenal, colic, renal, suprarenal
Ligaments of liver	Coronary (anterior and posterior parts), left triangular, right triangular, falciform, round, ligamentum venosum, hepatogastric, hepatoduodenal

GALLBLADDER

The **gallbladder** is a small intraperitoneal organ, located below the liver, to which it is functionally connected through the extrahepatic duct system. While the liver produces bile, the gallbladder's main function is to **store bile** that it receives from the liver and **concentrate** it by removing water and electrolytes.

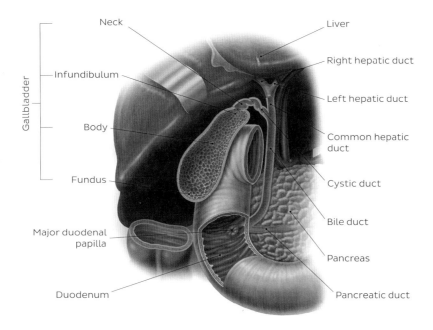

FIGURE 6.24. **Overview of the gallbladder.** The gallbladder is a small pear-shaped sac, which is divided into four anatomical **parts**: Fundus, body, infundibulum and neck. It is located on the inferior aspect of the right lobe of the liver. The gallbladder empties its contents via the **cystic duct**, which joins with the **common hepatic duct** from the liver to form the bile duct. The **bile duct** extends into the pancreas, where it joins the main pancreatic duct to form the **hepatopancreatic ampulla** (ampulla of Vater). This short duct then empties into the duodenum via the **major duodenal papilla**.

Key points about the gallbladder	
Definition	Gastrointestinal, intraperitoneal sac-like organ, located on the inferior aspect of the liver
Parts	Fundus, body, infundibulum, neck
Function	Storage, concentration and release of bile
Extrahepatic duct system	Left and right hepatic ducts, common hepatic duct, cystic duct, bile duct, pancreatic duct, hepatopancreatic ampulla, major duodenal papilla
Neurovascular supply	**Arterial supply:** cystic artery
	Venous drainage: small tributaries of the segmental portal veins
	Lymph: intrahepatic lymph vessels, cystic node
	Innervation: hepatic plexus

PANCREAS *IN SITU*

The **pancreas** is an accessory retroperitoneal organ of the digestive system that has both exocrine and endocrine functions. It helps digestion by producing pancreatic juices which are secreted into the duodenum. These juices consist of enzymes that break down sugars, lipids, and starches. The pancreas also produces important hormones (insulin, glucagon, and somatostatin) that regulate blood glucose levels.

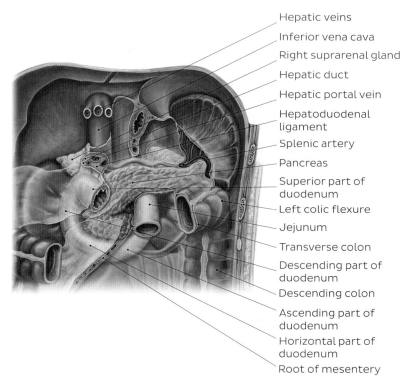

Hepatic veins
Inferior vena cava
Right suprarenal gland
Hepatic duct
Hepatic portal vein
Hepatoduodenal ligament
Splenic artery
Pancreas
Superior part of duodenum
Left colic flexure
Jejunum
Transverse colon
Descending part of duodenum
Descending colon
Ascending part of duodenum
Horizontal part of duodenum
Root of mesentery

FIGURE 6.25. Pancreas in situ. The pancreas is an elongated organ which lies mainly **retroperitoneally** across the posterior abdominal wall. It is divided into five anatomical parts: Head, neck, body, tail and uncinate process. The descending and horizontal parts of the C-shaped **duodenum** wrap around the pancreatic head. The aorta, superior mesenteric artery, left renal vessels, left kidney, and left suprarenal gland are situated posterior to the pancreatic body. The tail is the last part of the pancreas and lies intraperitoneally. It is situated in close proximity to the hilum of the spleen and runs with the splenic vessels in the splenorenal ligament.

Key points about the pancreas	
Definition	Accessory gland of the digestive system with endocrine and exocrine functions
Location	Retroperitoneal, behind the stomach
Relations	**Anterior:** stomach, transverse mesocolon
	Posterior: common bile duct, aorta, inferior vena cava, hepatic portal vein, left kidney, left suprarenal gland
	Superior: splenic artery
	Lateral-right: duodenum
	Lateral-left: spleen
Parts	Head, uncinate process, neck, body, tail
Function	**Exocrine:** secretes enzymatic fluids that break down nutrients
	Endocrine: secretes hormones that regulate metabolism (insulin, glucagon, somatostatin)
Neurovascular supply	**Arterial supply:** superior and inferior pancreaticoduodenal arteries splenic artery, gastroduodenal artery, superior mesenteric artery
	Venous drainage: pancreaticoduodenal veins, superior mesenteric vein, hepatic portal vein, pancreatic veins, splenic vein
	Innervation: vagus nerve (parasympathetic), greater and lesser splanchnic nerves (sympathetic)

Pancreas

Pancreas histology

ABDOMEN

PANCREATIC DUCT SYSTEM

The **pancreatic duct system** is a system of excretory ducts within the pancre-atic tissue which convey the pancreatic digestive enzymes (pancreatic juices) and bile into the duodenum.

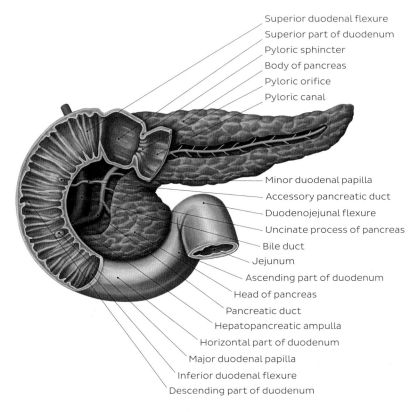

Superior duodenal flexure
Superior part of duodenum
Pyloric sphincter
Body of pancreas
Pyloric orifice
Pyloric canal

Minor duodenal papilla
Accessory pancreatic duct
Duodenojejunal flexure
Uncinate process of pancreas
Bile duct
Jejunum
Ascending part of duodenum
Head of pancreas
Hepatopancreatic ampulla
Horizontal part of duodenum
Major duodenal papilla
Inferior duodenal flexure
Descending part of duodenum

FIGURE 6.26. **Pancreatic duct system.** The **pancreatic duct** (of Wirsung) originates in the pancreatic tail and courses through the entire length of the body of pancreas, from which it receives the contents of the smaller interlobular ducts. At the head of the pancreas, it converges with the bile duct to form the **hepatopancreatic ampulla** (of Vater). The bile and pancreatic juices are then passed into the duodenum through the **major duodenal papilla**. The **hepatopancreatic sphincter** (of Oddi) surrounds the hepatopancreatic ampulla to allow for a controlled flow of pancreatic juices and bile. The smaller **accessory pancreatic duct**, when present, drains the head of the pancreas and empties into the duodenum at the **minor duodenal papilla**.

Key points about the pancreatic duct system	
Main pancreatic duct (of Wirsung)	Extends from tail to head of pancreas
	Joins bile duct to form hepatopancreatic ampulla
	Drains into duodenum at major duodenal papilla
Accessory pancreatic duct (of Santorini)	Arises at head of pancreas
	Communicates with main pancreatic duct
	Empties into duodenum at minor duodenal papilla
Function	Drains pancreatic digestive enzymes and bile into the duodenum where further digestion of food takes place

ABDOMEN

DUODENUM

The **duodenum** is the first segment of the small intestine, extending from the pyloric sphincter of the stomach to the jejunum. It is divided into the superior, descending, horizontal and ascending parts. Only the **proximal section** of the superior part is **intraperitoneal**, and thus the most mobile, while the rest of the duodenum is retroperitoneal.

Its **functions** are to dilute and neutralize digestive juices, digest and process chyme passed on from the stomach, receive pancreatic enzymes and bile, as well as absorb various nutrients.

The wall of the duodenum consists of three main layers: An inner **mucosa** with defined circular folds (of Kerckring), an underlying **submucosa** and a double-layered **muscular coat**.

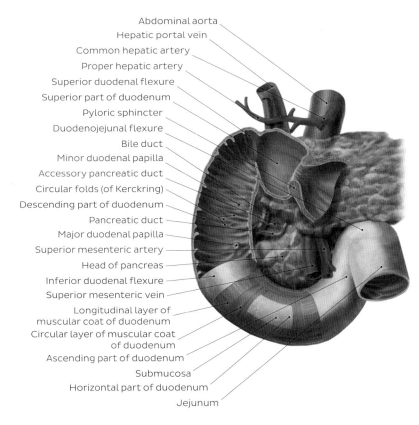

Abdominal aorta
Hepatic portal vein
Common hepatic artery
Proper hepatic artery
Superior duodenal flexure
Superior part of duodenum
Pyloric sphincter
Duodenojejunal flexure
Bile duct
Minor duodenal papilla
Accessory pancreatic duct
Circular folds (of Kerckring)
Descending part of duodenum
Pancreatic duct
Major duodenal papilla
Superior mesenteric artery
Head of pancreas
Inferior duodenal flexure
Superior mesenteric vein
Longitudinal layer of muscular coat of duodenum
Circular layer of muscular coat of duodenum
Ascending part of duodenum
Submucosa
Horizontal part of duodenum
Jejunum

FIGURE 6.27. **Overview of the duodenum with related structures.** The anterior wall of the superior and descending parts of the duodenum is removed to reveal its internal structure. **Circular folds (of Kerckring)** define the mucosa from the descending part onwards. Two small openings are seen amongst them in the descending part of the duodenum. The **major duodenal papilla** allows pancreatic enzymes and bile to enter the duodenum from the union of the pancreatic duct and bile duct, known as the hepatopancreatic ampulla. The **minor duodenal papilla** is an opening for pancreatic enzymes from the accessory pancreatic duct.

ABDOMEN

The different layers of the duodenum are exposed on its horizontal part. The head of the pancreas sits within the curve of the duodenum. The abdominal aorta, hepatic portal vein (pictured) inferior vena cava, pancreaticoduodenal arteries, bile duct, right kidney, ureter and psoas major, gonadal vessels and L3 vertebra (not pictured) are located posterior to the duodenum. The superior mesenteric artery and vein (pictured), right lobe of the liver and the gallbladder (not pictured) extend over the anterior surface of the duodenum.

Key points about the duodenum	
Parts	**Superior:** from pyloric sphincter to superior duodenal flexure
	Descending: from superior duodenal flexure to inferior duodenal flexure
	Horizontal: from inferior duodenal flexure to ascending part
	Ascending: from horizontal part to the duodenojejunal flexure
Internal structure	Mucosa (with circular folds [of Kerckring])
	Submucosa
	Muscular coat (outer longitudinal, inner circular layers)
Openings	Major duodenal papilla: from hepatopancreatic ampulla
	Minor duodenal papilla: from accessory pancreatic duct
Ligaments	Hepatoduodenal ligament (part of lesser omentum)
	Suspensory muscle of duodenum (ligament of Treitz)
Relations	In curve of duodenum – head of pancreas
	Posterior – abdominal aorta, hepatic portal vein, inferior vena cava, gastroduodenal artery, bile duct, right kidney, ureter and psoas major, L3 vertebra, right gonadal vessels
	Anterior – superior mesenteric artery/vein, gallbladder, right lobe of liver

Duodenum

Small intestine

ABDOMEN

JEJUNUM AND ILEUM

The **jejunum** and **ileum** are the middle and terminal parts of the small intestine, extending from the duodenojejunal flexure to the ileocecal junction. Together, they measure around five meters on average, with the jejunum comprising the proximal two-fifths and the ileum the distal three-fifths. They occupy much of the mid-to-lower abdominal cavity where they are largely enclosed by the large intestine. In the supine position, the jejunum is generally situated within the left lateral and umbilical regions of the abdomen, while the ileum is characteristically found within the hypogastric and right inguinal/iliac regions.

The main **function** of the jejunum and ileum is to absorb nutrients from food (chyme). The jejunum absorbs most of the sugars, fatty and amino acids as well as other nutrients. The ileum absorbs remaining nutrients after passage through the jejunum and is specifically responsible for the absorption of vitamin B$_{12}$ and reabsorption of conjugated bile salts.

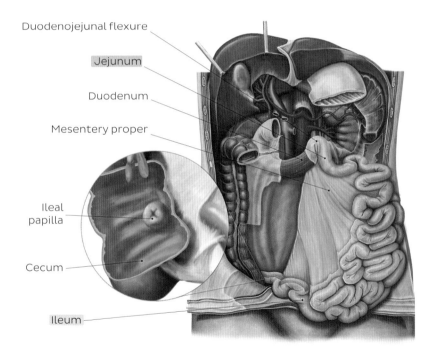

Duodenojejunal flexure

Jejunum

Duodenum

Mesentery proper

Ileal papilla

Cecum

Ileum

FIGURE 6.28. **Jejunum and ileum reflected (anterior view).** The **jejunum** begins at the **duodenojejunal flexure**, an abrupt bend after which the small intestine becomes intraperitoneal again. From this point, both the jejunum and ileum are suspended from the posterior abdominal wall by the mesentery *proper*, which gives them a great degree of mobility within the abdominal cavity. The walls of both the jejunum and ileum are enveloped by visceral peritoneum except along their mesenteric borders where the peritoneum is reflected onto the mesentery behind.

There is no clear demarcation between the jejunum and ileum, but rather a gradual transition in their internal morphology from one part to the next. At a gross level, the jejunum has a somewhat 'redder' appearance due its more profuse blood supply compared with the ileum. The distal 30cm of the ileum is referred to as the terminal ileum (due to specialized morphology and functions of this part). It terminates at the ileocecal junction, featuring the **ileal papilla**, through which the contents of the small intestine pass from the ileum to the cecum of the large intestine.

Key points about the jejunum and ileum		
	Jejunum	**Ileum**
Definition/ location	Middle part of small intestine, located in umbilical and left lateral regions	Terminal part of small intestine, located in hypogastric and right inguinal/iliac regions
Length	Proximal ⅖ of small intestine (after duodenojejunal flexure)	Distal ⅗ of small intestine
Structure	• Mucosa (with circular folds [of Kerckring]) • Submucosa • Muscular coat (outer longitudinal, inner circular layers) • Visceral peritoneum	
Internal anatomy	Thicker wall with more numerous and pronounced circular folds, more profuse blood supply	Thinner walls with fewer, less defined circular folds, contains high amounts of MALT (mucosa associated lymphoid tissue)
Functions	Absorbs digested sugars, amino and fatty acids, nutrients etc.	Absorbs remaining nutrients after jejunum, (specifically responsible for absorption vitamin B_{12} and conjugated bile salts)

Jejunum

Ileum

ARTERIES AND VEINS OF THE SMALL INTESTINE

The small intestine comprises three separate segments: The duodenum, jejunum and ileum, each of which with different vasculature. The proximal half of the duodenum, which is part of the foregut, is mainly supplied by branches of the **gastroduodenal artery** (a terminal branch of the common hepatic artery). Tributaries draining this part of the duodenum mostly empty directly into the **portal vein**.

The rest of the small intestine, which belongs to the midgut, receives its arterial supply and venous drainage from the main vessels associated with the midgut: The **superior mesenteric artery (SMA)** and **vein**. It is important to note that both the arterial supply and the venous drainage of the small intestine is highly variable.

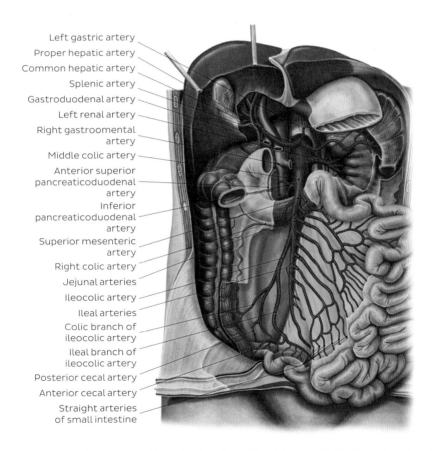

Left gastric artery
Proper hepatic artery
Common hepatic artery
Splenic artery
Gastroduodenal artery
Left renal artery
Right gastroomental artery
Middle colic artery
Anterior superior pancreaticoduodenal artery
Inferior pancreaticoduodenal artery
Superior mesenteric artery
Right colic artery
Jejunal arteries
Ileocolic artery
Ileal arteries
Colic branch of ileocolic artery
Ileal branch of ileocolic artery
Posterior cecal artery
Anterior cecal artery
Straight arteries of small intestine

FIGURE 6.29. Arteries of the small intestine. Overview of the abdomen with the liver reflected, and parts of the stomach, pancreas and large intestine removed. The proximal part of the duodenum (as far as the major duodenal papilla), is primarily supplied by **superior pancreaticoduodenal branches** of the gastroduodenal artery (which also provides supply via the supraduodenal, retroduodenal and right gastroomental arteries). There are also small contributions to the duodenum from the **right gastric artery**, a branch of the proper hepatic artery. The **superior mesenteric artery** supplies the remainder of the duodenum via the inferior pancreaticoduodenal and first jejunal arteries.

ABDOMEN

The jejunal and ileal branches of the superior mesenteric artery form loops known as **arterial arcades**. They give off branches known as **straight arteries** or vasa recta which supply the jejunum and the ileum. The terminal part of the ileum receives its supply from branches of the **ileocolic artery**.

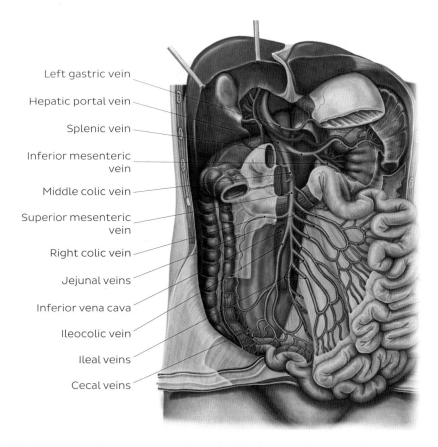

Left gastric vein
Hepatic portal vein
Splenic vein
Inferior mesenteric vein
Middle colic vein
Superior mesenteric vein
Right colic vein
Jejunal veins
Inferior vena cava
Ileocolic vein
Ileal veins
Cecal veins

FIGURE 6.30. **Veins of the small intestine.** Overview of the abdomen with the liver reflected and parts of the stomach, pancreas and large intestine removed. The venous drainage of the small intestine is more variable, but tends to generally follow the same pattern as the arteries. The **superior mesenteric vein**, however, drains into the hepatic portal vein rather than the inferior vena cava. The blood then goes through the portal venous system to the liver, where nutrients and toxins are removed, before being emptied into the inferior vena cava.

Key points about the vascular supply of the small intestine	
Duodenum arterial supply (proximal part)	**Main arteries:** anterior superior pancreaticoduodenal artery, posterior superior pancreaticoduodenal artery (from gastroduodenal artery)
	Minor contributions: right gastric (from proper hepatic artery), supraduodenal, retroduodenal and right gastroomental arteries (from gastroduodenal artery)
Duodenum arterial supply (distal part)	**Main arteries:** anterior inferior pancreaticoduodenal artery, posterior inferior pancreaticoduodenal artery (from SMA)
	Minor contributions: first jejunal artery (from SMA)
Duodenum venous drainage	**Proximal part:** superior pancreaticoduodenal vein (drains into right gastroepiploic vein and hepatic portal vein)
	Distal part: inferior pancreaticoduodenal vein (drains into superior mesenteric vein)

Key points about the vascular supply of the small intestine	
Jejunum vascular supply	**Arteries:** jejunal arteries (arterial arcades) to straight arteries (from SMA)
	Veins: jejunal veins (drain to superior mesenteric vein)
Ileum vascular supply	**Arteries:** ileal arteries (arterial arcades) to straight arteries, Ileal branch of ileocolic artery (from SMA)
	Veins: ileal veins, Ileocolic vein (drain to superior mesenteric vein)

Blood supply and innervation of the small intestine

Superior mesenteric artery

INNERVATION OF THE SMALL INTESTINE

The small intestine has an extrinsic and intrinsic innervation. The **extrinsic innervation** is provided by the sympathetic and parasympathetic divisions of the autonomic nervous system, while the **intrinsic innervation** comes from the enteric nervous system.

Preganglionic sympathetic fibers from the thoracolumbar spinal cord travel as the **greater** and **lesser thoracic splanchnic nerves** to the celiac, aorticorenal and superior mesenteric ganglia. From there, postganglionic fibers are distributed via the **celiac/superior mesenteric plexus** to the duodenum, jejunum and ileum to inhibit digestion. Both the anterior and posterior vagal **trunks of the vagus nerve** send parasympathetic contributions via the celiac ganglia which then follow the same pathway as the sympathetic fibers to stimulate digestion. Postganglionic parasympathetic fibers are located in the target organ wall.

The **enteric nervous system** regulates muscle tone and contractions, nutrient absorption and enzyme secretion via the myenteric plexus (plexus of Auerbach) and the submucosal plexus (Meissner's plexus).

ABDOMEN

Anterior vagal trunk

Hepatic branch of
anterior vagal trunk

Hepatic plexus

Celiac branch of
anterior vagal trunk

Celiac branches of
posterior vagal trunk

Pyloric branch of
anterior vagal trunk

Right greater thoracic
splanchnic nerve

Left greater thoracic
splanchnic nerve

Celiac ganglia

Left lesser thoracic
splanchnic nerve

Aorticorenal ganglia

Superior mesenteric
ganglion

Pancreatic plexus

Superior mesenteric
plexus

Periarterial plexus

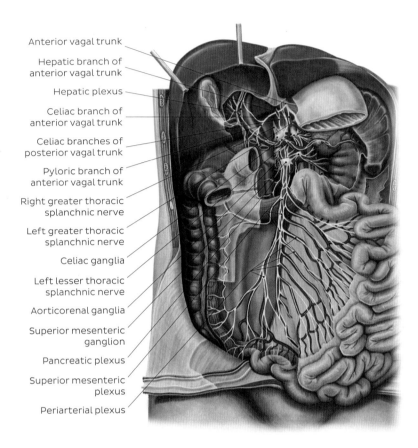

FIGURE 6.31. **Nerves of the small intestine.** Overview of the abdomen with the liver reflected, and parts of the stomach, pancreas and large intestine removed. The **greater** and **lesser splanchnic nerves** transmit sympathetic innervation from the thoracolumbar spinal cord to the celiac, aorticorenal and superior mesenteric ganglia on both sides of the celiac trunk. Parasympathetic information is provided by the **anterior** and **posterior vagal trunks**, following the same periarterial pathways and passing through the sympathetic ganglia. From here, sympathetic and parasympathetic nerve fibers are distributed via periarterial plexuses to the duodenum, jejunum and ileum.

Key points about the innervation of the small intestine	
Sympathetic Innervation	**Preganglionic:** greater and lesser splanchnic nerves from thoracolumbar spinal cord to celiac, aorticorenal and superior mesenteric ganglia
	Postganglionic: fibers from celiac and superior mesenteric ganglia to small intestine
	Function: inhibits digestion
Parasympathetic innervation	**Preganglionic:** anterior and posterior vagal trunks to celiac and superior mesenteric plexus
	Postganglionic: fibers from celiac and superior mesenteric ganglia to small intestine
	Function: stimulates digestion
Intrinsic innervation	**Myenteric plexus (of Auerbach):** regulates smooth muscle tone and contractions
	Submucosal plexus (Meissner's Plexus): regulates intestinal enzyme secretion, food absorption and (sub)mucosal muscle movement

ABDOMEN

Blood supply and innervation of the small intestine

 Celiac plexus

LYMPHATICS OF THE SMALL INTESTINE

The lymph nodes of the duodenum include the superior and inferior pancreaticoduodenal lymph nodes, superior mesenteric lymph nodes, celiac lymph nodes and again drain into the cisterna chyli.

The distal part of the ileum is drained by the **ileocolic lymph nodes**. Lymph drained from the proximal ileum and the jejunum is carried to the **juxtaintestinal lymph nodes** which are located within the mesentery in close proximity to the small intestine. From here, lymph continues to the **superior mesenteric lymph nodes** via the intermediate mesenteric lymph nodes, ultimately reaching the **cisterna chyli** via the intestinal lymph trunk.

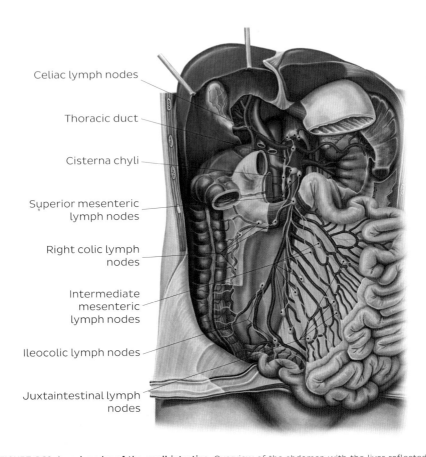

Celiac lymph nodes

Thoracic duct

Cisterna chyli

Superior mesenteric
lymph nodes

Right colic lymph
nodes

Intermediate
mesenteric
lymph nodes

Ileocolic lymph nodes

Juxtaintestinal lymph
nodes

FIGURE 6.32. Lymph nodes of the small intestine. Overview of the abdomen with the liver reflected and the stomach, pancreas and parts of the large intestine removed. The lymph nodes of the small intestine compose one the largest groups in the body, consisting of 100–150 nodes dispersed throughout the mesentery. The **juxtaintestinal lymph nodes** are located peripherally close to the ileal and jejunal wall. From here, lymph is transported towards the **superior mesenteric lymph nodes** via intermediate mesenteric nodes located alongside the jejunal and ileal arteries. **Pancreaticoduodenal lymph nodes drain most of the duodenum**. Lymph is then transported to the celiac and superior mesenteric nodes before reaching the **cisterna chyli** and continuing into the **thoracic duct**.

Key points about the lymph nodes of the small intestine	
Ileum	**Distal:** ileocolic lymph nodes
	Proximal: juxtaintestinal lymph nodes → superior mesenteric lymph nodes via intermediate mesenteric lymph nodes
Jejunum	Juxtaintestinal lymph nodes → superior mesenteric lymph nodes via intermediate mesenteric lymph nodes
Duodenum	Mainly drained by superior and inferior pancreaticoduodenal lymph nodes (in addition to pyloric and inferior pancreatic nodes) → celiac & superior mesenteric lymph nodes

Lymphatics of
abdomen and pelvis

Lymphatic system

LARGE INTESTINE

The **large intestine** is the penultimate part of the gastrointestinal tract. It is responsible for the absorption of water and electrolytes and converting indigestible matter to feces, which is stored temporarily until defecation. The large intestine begins at the **ileocaecal junction** and it consists of the cecum, vermiform appendix, colon, rectum and anal canal. The colon is the longest part of the large intestine, subdivided into four main segments: The ascending, transverse, descending and sigmoid colon. All parts of the large intestine are located **retroperitoneally**, with the exception of the transverse and sigmoid colon, which are **intraperitoneal** organs.

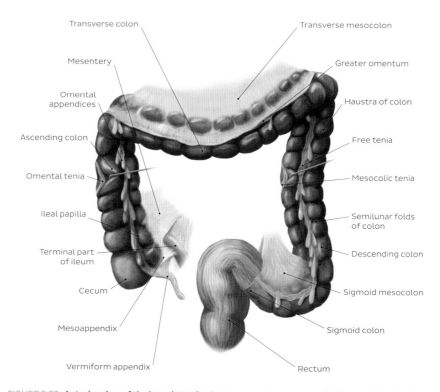

Transverse colon

Transverse mesocolon

Mesentery

Greater omentum

Omental appendices

Haustra of colon

Ascending colon

Free tenia

Omental tenia

Mesocolic tenia

Ileal papilla

Semilunar folds of colon

Terminal part of ileum

Descending colon

Cecum

Sigmoid mesocolon

Mesoappendix

Sigmoid colon

Vermiform appendix

Rectum

FIGURE 6.33. Anterior view of the large intestine (greater omentum removed). The large intestine begins at the **cecum**, which continues on from the terminal part of the ileum. Protruding from the cecum is the **vermiform appendix**, which usually lies intraperitoneally and is held in position by its mesentery, the **mesoappendix**.

Continuing on from the cecum is the **colon**, divided into ascending, transverse, descending and sigmoid colon. Of these, the transverse and sigmoid colon are located intraperitoneally and suspended by the transverse and sigmoid mesocolon, respectively. The large intestine ends with the **rectum** and **anal canal**.

Important features unique to the large intestine are the **epiploic appendages**, which are small pouches of the peritoneum filled with adipose tissue, the longitudinal bands of smooth muscle called taenia coli, as well as the pouch-like sacculations called haustra coli.

Key points about the large intestine	Location	Blood supply	Innervation	Lymphatic drainage	Mesentery
Cecum	Intraperitoneal	Ileocolic artery	Superior mesenteric plexus	Ileocolic lymph nodes	/
Vermiform appendix	Intraperitoneal (or in the pelvic cavity)	Appendicular arteries	Superior mesenteric plexus (sympathetic), vagus nerve (parasympathetic)		Mesoappendix
Ascending colon	Retroperitoneal	Ileocolic and right colic arteries	Superior mesenteric plexus	Epicolic and paracolic lymph nodes	/
Transverse colon	Intraperitoneal	Right, middle and left colic arteries	Superior and inferior mesenteric plexuses	Middle colic lymph nodes	Transverse mesocolon
Descending colon	Retroperitoneal	Left colic and superior sigmoid arteries	Superior hypogastric plexus (sympathetic), pelvic splanchnic nerves (parasympathetic)	Paracolic and epicolic lymph nodes	/
Sigmoid colon	Intraperitoneal				Sigmoid mesocolon
Rectum	Intraperitoneal (superior segment), retroperitoneal (inferior segment)	[Ano]rectal arteries	Superior and inferior hypogastric plexuses	Pararectal and epirectal lymph nodes	/
Anal canal	Pelvic cavity (extraperitoneal)				

Neurovascular supply of the large intestine

Colon

ABDOMEN

RECTUM AND ANAL CANAL

The rectum and anal canal are located in the pelvic cavity and are the **terminal structures of the gastrointestinal tract**. The rectum is a direct continuation of the sigmoid colon and is followed by the anal canal, which opens itself to the external environment through the anus. The main functions of these structures is to absorb water and electrolytes, and store feces prior to defecation.

The rectum and anal canal lie posteriorly against the sacrum and coccyx, the anococcygeal ligament and the median sacral vessels. In males, the urinary bladder, distal parts of the ureters, ductus deferens, seminal glands, and prostate are found anterior to the rectum and anal canal, whereas in females the vagina occupies this position.

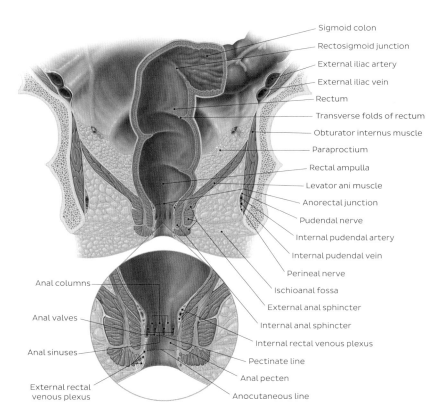

Sigmoid colon
Rectosigmoid junction
External iliac artery
External iliac vein
Rectum
Transverse folds of rectum
Obturator internus muscle
Paraproctium
Rectal ampulla
Levator ani muscle
Anorectal junction
Pudendal nerve
Internal pudendal artery
Internal pudendal vein
Perineal nerve
Ischioanal fossa
External anal sphincter
Internal anal sphincter
Internal rectal venous plexus
Pectinate line
Anal pecten
Anocutaneous line

Anal columns
Anal valves
Anal sinuses
External rectal venous plexus

FIGURE 6.34. Rectum and anal canal (coronal view). The rectum extends from the **rectosigmoid junction** superiorly to the **anorectal junction** inferiorly. Four transverse folds create the three lateral flexures of the rectum (superior, intermediate, and inferior). The anal canal houses the **anal columns**, which are connected to each other distally end by folds known as **anal valves**. Found between the anal columns are **anal sinuses**, into which the excretory ducts of the anal glands open. The anal valves form an irregular line called the **pectinate line**, which is an important anatomic landmark.

The anal canal extends down to the **anocutaneous line**, which represents its transition into the anus and perianal skin. The region between the pectinate line and anocutaneous line is termed as the **anal pecten**. The internal anal sphincter can be seen surrounding the upper two thirds of the anal canal, whereas the external anal sphincter is observed external to the lower two thirds of the anal canal. The levator ani

ABDOMEN

muscle can be seen extending inferiorly, where its puboanalis part (puboanalis, a.k.a. puborectalis muscle) slings around the anorectal junction. The region constituted by adipose tissue that is interposed in between the anal canal and the ischium is termed **ischioanal fossa**.

Key points about the rectum and anal canal	
Location	**Superior third of rectum:** intraperitoneal
	Middle third of rectum: retroperitoneal
	Inferior third of rectum and anal canal: infraperitoneal
Function	**Rectum:** absorption of water and electrolytes and feces storage
	Anal canal: absorption of water and electrolytes and defecation
Major landmarks of rectum	**Vertical flexures:** sacral flexure (dorsal bend) and anorectal flexures (ventral bend)
	Lateral flexures: superior flexure (convexes to the right), intermediate flexure (convexes to the left) and inferior lateral flexure (convexes to the right)
Major landmarks of anal canal	**Columnar zone:** contains anal columns, valves and sinuses
	Intermediate zone: separated from the columnar zone by the pectinate (dentate) line
	Cutaneous zone: made of perianal skin and progresses to the anus

Rectum

Anal canal

ARTERIES OF THE LARGE INTESTINE

The blood supply of the large intestine complies with the pattern of its embryological development. The proximal half of the large intestine is a midgut derivative, while the rest of it belongs to the hindgut.

- The **midgut** derived part, from ileocecal junction to the proximal two-thirds of the transverse colon, is supplied by the branches of the **superior mesenteric artery**.
- The **hindgut** derived part, from the final third of transverse colon to the termination of anal canal, is supplied by the branches of the **inferior mesenteric artery** and **internal iliac artery**.

These terminal branches of the superior and inferior mesenteric arteries anastomose to form the **marginal artery of colon** (of Drummond), which contributes to the supply of the entire large intestine.

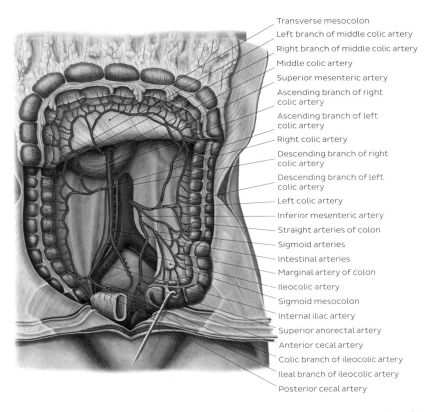

Transverse mesocolon
Left branch of middle colic artery
Right branch of middle colic artery
Middle colic artery
Superior mesenteric artery
Ascending branch of right colic artery
Ascending branch of left colic artery
Right colic artery
Descending branch of right colic artery
Descending branch of left colic artery
Left colic artery
Inferior mesenteric artery
Straight arteries of colon
Sigmoid arteries
Intestinal arteries
Marginal artery of colon
Ileocolic artery
Sigmoid mesocolon
Internal iliac artery
Superior anorectal artery
Anterior cecal artery
Colic branch of ileocolic artery
Ileal branch of ileocolic artery
Posterior cecal artery

FIGURE 6.35. Arteries of the large intestine. The large intestine is supplied mainly by branches of the superior mesenteric, inferior mesenteric and internal iliac arteries. The **superior mesenteric artery** supplies the cecum, ascending colon and a part of the transverse colon. The **inferior mesenteric artery** supplies the terminal part of the transverse colon, the descending colon and the proximal part of the rectum. Finally, the **internal iliac artery** supplies the distal part of rectum. The branches of these arteries anastomose close to the large intestine, forming the marginal artery of colon.

Key points about the arteries of the large intestine	
Superior mesenteric artery	Supplies the derivatives of the midgut:
	Cecum: anterior cecal artery, posterior cecal artery (branches of ileocolic artery)
	Appendix: appendicular artery (branch of ileocolic artery)
	Ascending colon: colic branch (of ileocolic artery), right colic artery
	Proximal ⅔ of transverse colon: middle colic artery
Inferior mesenteric artery	Supplies a part of the hindgut derivatives:
	Distal ⅓ of transverse colon: left colic artery
	Descending colon: left colic artery
	Sigmoid colon: sigmoid arteries
	Superior part of rectum: superior anorectal artery
Internal iliac artery	Supplies the rest of the hindgut derivatives:
	Middle and inferior parts of rectum: middle anorectal artery, inferior anorectal artery

ABDOMEN

INNERVATION OF THE LARGE INTESTINE

Similar to the small intestine, the large intestine receives both intrinsic and extrinsic innervation. Intrinsic innervation is facilitated by the enteric nervous system (ENS). The **myenteric** and **submucosal plexuses** are constituents of the ENS and are responsible for regulating peristaltic contractions of the large intestine as well as mucosal secretions and blood flow. Although the ENS is capable of autonomously driving various motor patterns in the large intestine, its functions are modulated by sympathetic, parasympathetic and visceral afferent pathways.

Extrinsic innervation is largely dependent on the embryological origin of the large intestine:

- Midgut-derived structures (i.e. cecum → proximal two-thirds of transverse colon) receive parasympathetic fibers from the **vagus nerve/vagal trunks** (i.e. cranial origin), and sympathetic fibers which originate from the **thoracic splanchnic nerves (T5–T12)**.
- Hindgut-derived structures (distal third of transverse colon → rectum) receive their parasympathetic innervation from the **pelvic splanchnic nerves (S2–S4)** (i.e. sacral origin), and sympathetic innervation via the **lumbar splanchnic nerves (L1–L2)**

Functionally, parasympathetic fibers are responsible for increasing secretomotor activity along this segment of the digestive tract, while sympathetic fibers play an inhibitory role in the activity of the large intestine.

Besides the regulation of secretomotor activity via efferent innervation, the large intestine equally sends visceral afferent signals to the brainstem and thalamus. Pain sensation is carried via sympathetic fibers to the thoracolumbar spinal sensory ganglia, while reflex information reaches the vagal sensory ganglia through parasympathetic pathways.

ABDOMEN

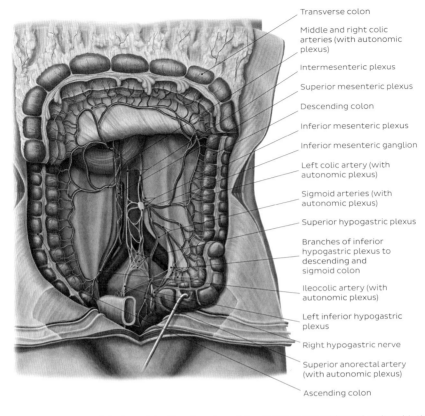

Transverse colon

Middle and right colic arteries (with autonomic plexus)

Intermesenteric plexus

Superior mesenteric plexus

Descending colon

Inferior mesenteric plexus

Inferior mesenteric ganglion

Left colic artery (with autonomic plexus)

Sigmoid arteries (with autonomic plexus)

Superior hypogastric plexus

Branches of inferior hypogastric plexus to descending and sigmoid colon

Ileocolic artery (with autonomic plexus)

Left inferior hypogastric plexus

Right hypogastric nerve

Superior anorectal artery (with autonomic plexus)

Ascending colon

FIGURE 6.36. **Nerves of the large intestine.** Overview of the abdomen and peritoneal cavity with the greater and lesser omenta reflected and small intestine removed. The colon can be seen along with its arterial supply.

Preganglionic parasympathetic fibers from the anterior and posterior vagal trunks, destined to supply the derivatives of the midgut (i.e. cecum → proximal two-thirds of transverse colon), pass through the **superior mesenteric plexus** (without synapsing) and continue their course to synapse with cell bodies of postganglionic neurons in the enteric plexuses. The hindgut receives its parasympathetic innervation via preganglionic parasympathetic fibers **(pelvic splanchnic nerves (S2–4))** which enter the **inferior hypogastric plexus**, in which some synapse. From here, most fibers ascend via retroperitoneal tissues, independent of the periarterial plexuses, to supply this part of the colon (some fibers may ascend via the hypogastric nerve/superior hypogastric plexus to pass through the **inferior mesenteric plexus** to reach the hindgut). Most preganglionic parasympathetic fibers synapse in intramural plexuses.

Preganglionic sympathetic fibers to the **midgut** originate from **spinal nerves T5–T12** which form the greater and lesser thoracic splanchnic nerves. These course via the superior mesenteric plexuses, where they synapse. Postganglionic fibers reach the midgut via periarterial plexuses found along the superior mesenteric artery and its branches. Sympathetic innervation to the hindgut originates from spinal nerves L1–L2 (lumbar splanchnic nerves). Preganglionic fibers synapse in the aortic and inferior mesenteric plexuses and emerge as postganglionic sympathetic neurons to supply the hindgut via periarterial plexuses of the inferior mesenteric artery and its branches.

Key points about the innervation of the small intestine	
Sympathetic innervation	**Midgut-derived structures** • *Preganglionic*: greater and lesser thoracic splanchnic nerves (T5–T12) → superior mesenteric plexuses • *Postganglionic*: fibers from celiac and superior mesenteric ganglia → large intestine via periarterial plexuses along superior mesenteric artery and branches **Hindgut-derived structures** • *Preganglionic*: lumbar splanchnic nerves (L1–L2) to aortic, inferior mesenteric plexuses • *Postganglionic*: fibers from aortic, inferior mesenteric, hypogastric plexuses to large intestine (hindgut-derived structures) **Function:** inhibits digestion
Parasympathetic innervation	**Midgut-derived structures** • *Preganglionic*: anterior and posterior vagal trunks → celiac and superior mesenteric plexuses (no synapse) → synapse in myenteric and submucosal plexuses • *Postganglionic*: fibers extend from enteric plexuses to innervate glands (secreto-motor) and muscle (motor) of the large intestine. **Hindgut-derived structures** • *Preganglionic*: pelvic splanchnic nerves (S2–S4) → inferior hypogastric plexus (some synapse here) → most synapse in myenteric and submucosal plexuses • *Postganglionic*: fibers from inferior hypogastric plexus to parasympathetic ganglia of large intestine (hindgut-derived structures) **Function:** stimulates digestion
Intrinsic innervation	**Myenteric plexus** (Auerbach's plexus): regulates smooth muscle tone and contractions **Submucosal plexus** (Meissner's plexus): regulates intestinal enzyme secretion, food absorption and (sub)mucosal muscle movement

Neurovascular supply
of the large intestine

NEUROVASCULATURE OF THE RECTUM AND ANAL CANAL

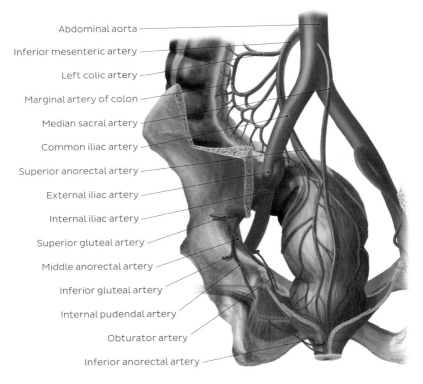

Abdominal aorta
Inferior mesenteric artery
Left colic artery
Marginal artery of colon
Median sacral artery
Common iliac artery
Superior anorectal artery
External iliac artery
Internal iliac artery
Superior gluteal artery
Middle anorectal artery
Inferior gluteal artery
Internal pudendal artery
Obturator artery
Inferior anorectal artery

FIGURE 6.37. **Arteries of the rectum and anal canal (posterior view, sacrum removed).** The rectum and anal canal are supplied by the three **anorectal arteries**: Superior, middle and inferior, previously known as the 'rectal' arteries. From superior to inferior, these arteries branch from the inferior mesenteric, internal iliac and internal pudendal arteries, respectively.

Key points about the blood vessels of the rectum and anal canal	
Superior anorectal artery	**Origin:** inferior mesenteric artery
	Supply: upper two thirds of the rectum
Middle anorectal artery	**Origin:** internal iliac artery
	Supply: middle and lower parts of the rectum
Inferior anorectal artery	**Origin:** internal pudendal artery (branch of the internal iliac artery)
	Supply: anal canal, internal and external anal sphincter, perianal skin
Anorectal veins	**Superior anorectal veins** → Superior mesenteric vein
	Middle anorectal veins → Internal iliac vein
	Inferior anorectal veins → Internal pudendal vein (drains into the internal iliac vein)

ABDOMEN

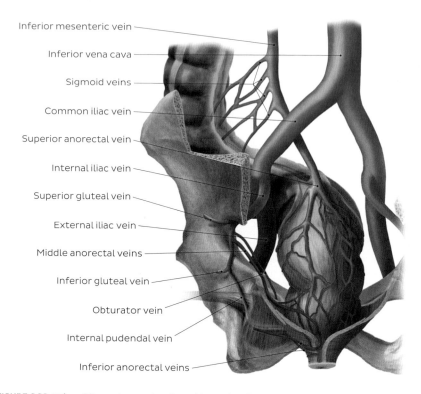

Inferior mesenteric vein

Inferior vena cava

Sigmoid veins

Common iliac vein

Superior anorectal vein

Internal iliac vein

Superior gluteal vein

External iliac vein

Middle anorectal veins

Inferior gluteal vein

Obturator vein

Internal pudendal vein

Inferior anorectal veins

FIGURE 6.38. **Veins of the rectum and anal canal (posterior view sacrum removed).** The three anorectal veins follow the same path as arteries, draining into the corresponding vessels: Inferior mesenteric, internal iliac and internal pudendal veins. The anorectal veins form a **hemorrhoidal venous plexus** which has a special clinical significance, as it can swell and present as different types of hemorrhoids.

Key points about the innervation of the rectum and anal canal	
Intrinsic innervation of rectum and anal canal	**Enteric nervous system** • Submucosal plexus (of Meissner) • Enteric plexus (of Auerbach) Control peristaltic contractions and mucous secretions.
Extrinsic innervation of rectum and upper half of anal canal (above pectinate line)	**Autonomic nervous system** • Sympathetic input: sacral splanchnic nerves • Parasympathetic input: pelvic splanchnic nerves Splanchnic nerves synapse within the superior and inferior hypogastric plexuses and give the superior anal (rectal) nerves.
Extrinsic innervation of lower half of anal canal (below pectinate line)	**Somatic nervous system** • Pudendal nerve: inferior anal (rectal) nerve • Provides voluntary control over external anal sphincter and defecation

KIDNEYS

The **kidneys** are a pair of bilateral, retroperitoneal abdominal organs of the urinary system which are located on either side of the vertebral column. They are surrounded by a **fibrous capsule** and **adipose tissue** that protect them from injury. Functionally, the main parts of the kidney are the cortex, medulla and hilum. The main **function** of the kidneys is to regulate the amount of fluid and electrolytes in the body. They also excrete metabolic waste products and produce hormones that facilitate several metabolic processes.

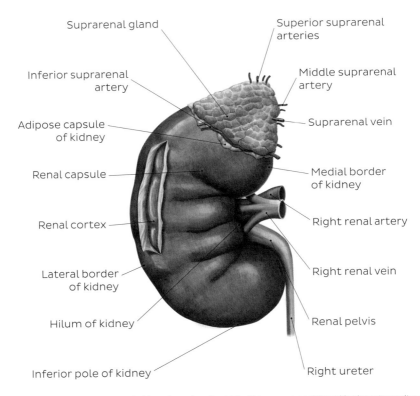

FIGURE 6.39. Gross anatomy of kidney (anterior view). The kidneys are positioned in the retroperitoneal space at the level of vertebrae **T12–L3**. They are bean-shaped and feature two **poles** (superior and inferior) and two **borders** (medial and lateral).

Located at the superior pole is the **suprarenal gland**. The medial border of the kidney is defined by the **hilum** of the kidney, which is the entry and exit point for the neurovascular structures of the kidney (renal artery and vein, renal plexus) and the ureter. The most superior vessel is the renal vein which exits the kidney, just below which is the renal artery that enters in, with the ureter located most inferiorly of the three. The anterior to posterior orientation follows the same pattern: Renal vein, renal artery and ureter.

ABDOMEN

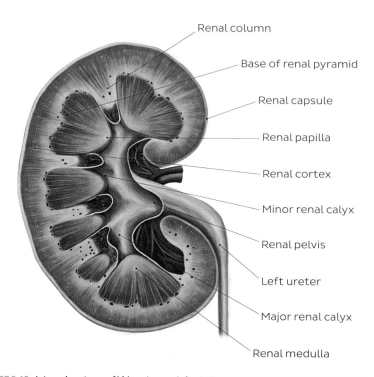

FIGURE 6.40. **Internal anatomy of kidney (coronal view).** The internal structure (parenchyma) of the kidney consists of the outer **renal cortex** and inner **renal medulla** which is characterized by renal pyramids. The **pyramids** are separated by extensions of the cortex known as **renal columns**. The apices of the pyramids project medially toward the renal sinus where they each open into a **minor calyx** that unite to form a **major calyx**. Usually, there are two to three major calyces in the kidney (superior, middle, and inferior), which further unite to form the **renal pelvis**. The renal pelvis gives off a single **ureter** that leaves the kidney via the hilum.

Key points about the kidneys	
Definition	Paired retroperitoneal organs of the urinary system.
Main external features	2 poles (superior and inferior)
	2 borders (lateral and medial)
	Fibrous capsule, hilum
Main internal features	Renal cortex, renal medulla, renal pelvis
Neurovascular structures	Renal artery (branch of the abdominal aorta)
	Renal vein (drains to the inferior vena cava)
	Renal plexus (derived from celiac plexus, intermesenteric plexus, aorticorenal ganglia and lumbar splanchnic nerves)
Functions	Elimination of toxic metabolites through urine, regulation of blood homeostasis and blood pressure, production of some hormones

Kidneys

Coronal section of the kidney

RENAL ARTERIES

The **renal arteries** arise from the abdominal aorta just inferior to the superior mesenteric artery in the retroperitoneum. Each courses posterior to the ipsilateral renal vein and nerves towards the renal hilum, through which they enter their respective kidney. The right renal artery originates slightly inferior to its left counterpart and is also longer, traveling posterior to the inferior vena cava.

The renal arteries supply oxygenated blood to the kidney parenchyma and simultaneously deliver the blood to be filtered by the kidneys.

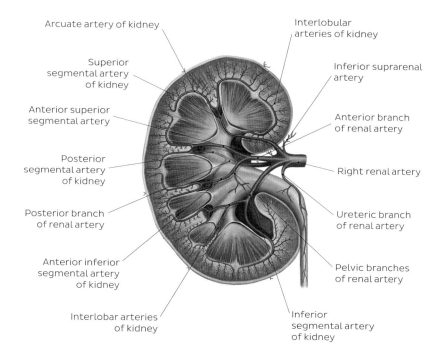

Arcuate artery of kidney

Interlobular arteries of kidney

Superior segmental artery of kidney

Inferior suprarenal artery

Anterior superior segmental artery

Anterior branch of renal artery

Posterior segmental artery of kidney

Right renal artery

Posterior branch of renal artery

Ureteric branch of renal artery

Anterior inferior segmental artery of kidney

Pelvic branches of renal artery

Interlobar arteries of kidney

Inferior segmental artery of kidney

FIGURE 6.41. **Renal arteries (coronal section of the kidney).** Overview of a coronal section of the right kidney, exposing the right renal artery and its branches. Upon traversing the renal hilum, the renal artery divides into an anterior branch and a posterior branch. The **anterior branch** further divides into four segmental arteries: The superior or apical, anterior superior, anterior inferior and inferior segmental arteries. The **posterior branch** divides into the posterior segmental arteries to supply the posterior segment of the kidney.

The **segmental arteries** of both branches then divide into the **interlobar arteries** which are located in between the renal lobes. At the base of the medullary pyramids of the lobe these arteries receive the name of **arcuate arteries**, and they give origin to the **interlobular arteries**. These then enter the nephrons as **afferent glomerular arterioles** to bring blood to the glomerulus to be filtered. The inferior suprarenal artery is a branch to the renal pelvis. The ureteric branch of the renal artery supplies the suprarenal gland, renal pelvis and ureter, respectively.

ABDOMEN

Key points about the renal arteries	
Origin	Abdominal aorta, at the level of the IV disc between the L1 and L2 vertebrae, inferior to the origin of the superior mesenteric artery
Branches	**Anterior branch:** superior (apical), anterior superior, anterior inferior and inferior segmental arteries
	Posterior branch: posterior segmental arteries
	Inferior suprarenal artery
	Branch to renal pelvis
	Ureteric branch
Functions	Supply kidney parenchyma with oxygenated blood
	Deliver blood to be filtered by the kidney
Supply	Kidneys, suprarenal glands, ureters

Renal artery

Neurovascular supply of the kidney

URETERS

The **ureters** are a pair of muscular, tubular structures that are responsible for transporting urine from the kidneys to the urinary bladder by peristalsis for temporary storage, until urination. Each ureter arises as a continuation of the funnel-shaped renal pelvis at the hilum of the kidney in the posterior abdomen and runs distally into the pelvic cavity to enter the base of the urinary bladder. The ureters are closely related to several structures along their course, including psoas major muscle, parts of the intestines, several blood vessels in the abdominopelvic cavity, ductus deferens in males and the uterine cervix in females.

The **blood supply** of the ureters comes from the abdominal aorta through multiple direct and indirect branches along its length. The ureters receive both sympathetic and parasympathetic **innervation** through several plexuses in the abdomen and pelvis.

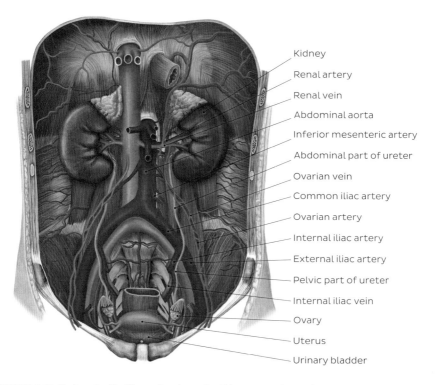

Kidney
Renal artery
Renal vein
Abdominal aorta
Inferior mesenteric artery
Abdominal part of ureter
Ovarian vein
Common iliac artery
Ovarian artery
Internal iliac artery
External iliac artery
Pelvic part of ureter
Internal iliac vein
Ovary
Uterus
Urinary bladder

FIGURE 6.42. **Ureters** *in situ.* The ureters leave the kidneys posterior to the renal vessels and course distally on the anterior surface of the psoas major muscle, posterior to the ovarian vessels (or testicular vessels in males). They cross the bifurcation of the common iliac arteries at the pelvic brim to enter the pelvic cavity, where they run below the ductus deferens in males and below the uterine arteries in females, to enter the base of the urinary bladder.

Key points about the ureters	
Parts	Abdominal, pelvic
Function	Transport of urine from the kidneys to urinary bladder
Major relations	**Right ureter:** psoas major muscle, genitofemoral nerve, duodenum (descending part), branches of the superior mesenteric vessels, gonadal vessels, common iliac artery, uterine artery, urinary bladder
	Left ureter: psoas major, genitofemoral nerve, branches of the inferior mesenteric vessels, gonadal vessels, common iliac artery, uterine artery urinary bladder
Blood supply	Ureteric branches of renal artery, ovarian/testicular artery, ureteric branches of the abdominal aorta and common iliac arteries, ureteric branches of the superior and inferior vesical and uterine arteries
Innervation	Renal plexus and ganglia, aortic plexus, ureteric branches of intermesenteric plexus, pelvic splanchnic nerves, superior and inferior hypogastric plexuses
Lymphatic drainage	Internal iliac, external iliac nodes, common iliac, and lumbar lymph nodes

Ureters

 Urinary system

 Kidneys ureters and suprarenal glands

ABDOMEN

LUMBAR PLEXUS

The **lumbar plexus** is a collection of spinal nerves located deep in the lumbopelvic region, close to the psoas major muscle. Formed from the **anterior rami of spinal nerves L1–L4**, the plexus provides innervation to the muscles, joints and skin of the anterolateral aspects of the pelvis and thigh.

The lumbar plexus has six major terminal branches. According to their anatomical position, the branches are grouped into anterior and posterior divisions. The **anterior division** innervates the pelvis, while the **posterior division** supplies branches to the thigh. Fibers from spinal nerve L4 join with fibers from L5 to form the lumbosacral trunk. This large nerve links the lumbar plexus with the sacral plexus, thus these nerve complexes are often given the combined name of **lumbosacral plexus**. Together these two plexuses supply all innervation to the pelvis and lower limb.

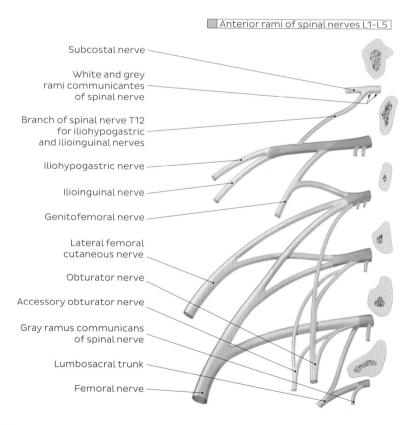

Anterior rami of spinal nerves L1–L5

- Subcostal nerve
- White and grey rami communicantes of spinal nerve
- Branch of spinal nerve T12 for iliohypogastric and ilioinguinal nerves
- Iliohypogastric nerve
- Ilioinguinal nerve
- Genitofemoral nerve
- Lateral femoral cutaneous nerve
- Obturator nerve
- Accessory obturator nerve
- Gray ramus communicans of spinal nerve
- Lumbosacral trunk
- Femoral nerve

FIGURE 6.43. **Lumbar plexus.** The lumbar plexus is formed by the anterior rami of spinal nerves L1–L4. These six **terminal branches** arise from the plexus: The iliohypogastric nerve, ilioinguinal nerve genitofemoral nerve, obturator nerve, lateral femoral cutaneous nerve and femoral nerve. Occasionally, in approximately 29% of the people, an **accessory obturator nerve** can be present. The **iliohypogastric** and **ilioinguinal nerves** arise from the anterior ramus of spinal nerve L1. **Genitofemoral** (L2-L3) and **obturator nerves** (L2-L4) are anterior divisions of anterior rami of spinal nerves and they supply the anterolateral hip region. The **lateral femoral cutaneous** (L2-L3) and **femoral nerves** (L2-L4) are posterior divisions of anterior rami of spinal nerves and they supply innervation to the anterolateral thigh.

ABDOMEN

Key points about the lumbar plexus	
Roots	L1, L2, L3, L4
Structural organization	Branches from spinal nerve L1 Branches from anterior division of spinal nerves L2–L4 Branches from posterior division of spinal nerves L2–L4
Terminal branches	Iliohypogastric nerve, ilioinguinal nerve, genitofemoral nerve, obturator nerve, lateral femoral cutaneous nerve and femoral nerve.
Function	Sensory and motor innervation of the lower abdomen, pelvis, anterolateral hip and thigh regions

 Lumbar plexus

 Femoral nerve

ARTERIES OF THE STOMACH, LIVER AND GALLBLADDER

The stomach, liver and gallbladder (foregut derivatives) are supplied by the three branches of the **celiac trunk:** Left gastric, common hepatic and splenic arteries.

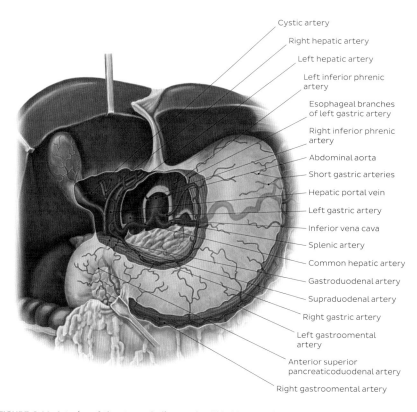

Cystic artery

Right hepatic artery

Left hepatic artery

Left inferior phrenic artery

Esophageal branches of left gastric artery

Right inferior phrenic artery

Abdominal aorta

Short gastric arteries

Hepatic portal vein

Left gastric artery

Inferior vena cava

Splenic artery

Common hepatic artery

Gastroduodenal artery

Supraduodenal artery

Right gastric artery

Left gastroomental artery

Anterior superior pancreaticoduodenal artery

Right gastroomental artery

FIGURE 6.44. Arteries of the stomach, liver and gallbladder. Arterial supply of the stomach, liver and gallbladder with the liver retracted.

The blood supply of the stomach originates from the **celiac trunk** and is provided from two anastomotic systems along the curvatures and several direct branches. The **anastomosis along the lesser curvature** is created by the union of the right and left gastric arteries which originate from the common hepatic artery and celiac trunk, respectively. The **greater curvature anastomosis** is formed by the union of the right and left gastroomental arteries (gastroepiploic), which originate from the gastroduodenal and splenic arteries, respectively. **Short** and **posterior gastric arteries**, which arise from the splenic artery supply the fundus and posterior wall.

The liver is supplied by the **proper hepatic artery** which is a continuation of the common hepatic artery and courses alongside the hepatic portal vein and common bile duct (porta hepatis). The right hepatic artery gives off the **cystic artery** which supplies the gallbladder.

Key points about the arteries of the stomach	
Right gastric artery	Arises from proper hepatic artery, forms anastomosis with left gastric artery; supplies lesser curvature, anterior and posterior sides of the stomach
Left gastric artery	Arises from common hepatic artery, forms anastomosis with right gastric artery; supplies lesser curvature, cardia, right upper and posterior walls
Right gastroomental (gastroepiploic) artery	Arises from gastroduodenal artery; forms anastomosis with left gastroomental artery and supplies inferior part of greater curvature
Left gastroomental (gastroepiploic) artery	Arises from splenic artery; forms anastomosis with right gastroomental artery and supplies superior part of greater curvature
Short and posterior gastric arteries	Arise from splenic artery; supply fundus and posterior wall of stomach
Gastroduodenal artery	Arises from common hepatic artery; supplies pyloric part

Key points about the arteries of the liver	
Common hepatic artery	Originates from the celiac trunk, supplies liver (via proper hepatic artery → right/left hepatic arteries)

Key points about the arteries of the gallbladder	
Cystic artery	Arises from right hepatic artery, supplies the gallbladder, common hepatic duct, cystic duct and the proximal part of the common bile duct

 Blood vessels of abdomen and pelvis

 Celiac trunk

ARTERIES OF THE PANCREAS, DUODENUM AND SPLEEN

The pancreas, duodenum and spleen are supplied with oxygenated blood by arteries that stem from the **celiac trunk** and **superior mesenteric artery**, both of which originate from the abdominal aorta.

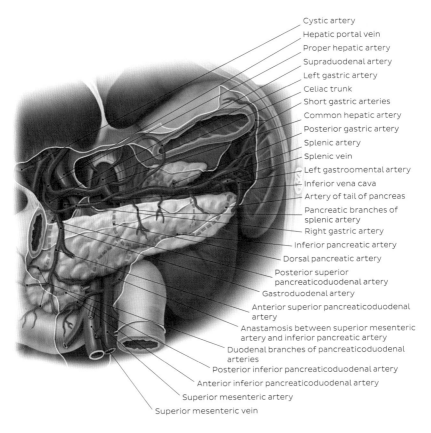

Cystic artery
Hepatic portal vein
Proper hepatic artery
Supraduodenal artery
Left gastric artery
Celiac trunk
Short gastric arteries
Common hepatic artery
Posterior gastric artery
Splenic artery
Splenic vein
Left gastroomental artery
Inferior vena cava
Artery of tail of pancreas
Pancreatic branches of splenic artery
Right gastric artery
Inferior pancreatic artery
Dorsal pancreatic artery
Posterior superior pancreaticoduodenal artery
Gastroduodenal artery
Anterior superior pancreaticoduodenal artery
Anastamosis between superior mesenteric artery and inferior pancreatic artery
Duodenal branches of pancreaticoduodenal arteries
Posterior inferior pancreaticoduodenal artery
Anterior inferior pancreaticoduodenal artery
Superior mesenteric artery
Superior mesenteric vein

FIGURE 6.45. **Arterial supply of the pancreas, duodenum and spleen.** Anterior view with the liver retracted and stomach removed. The **posterior superior pancreaticoduodenal artery** arises as a proximal branch of the gastroduodenal artery, while its anterior counterpart arises as the smaller terminal branch of the same vessel. The **anterior** and **posterior inferior pancreaticoduodenal arteries** arise from a common branch of the superior mesenteric artery. The pancreaticoduodenal arteries project around the pancreatic neck where they form arterial arcades to supply the head, neck and uncinate process of the pancreas.

The duodenum is also supplied by these arteries, and additionally by the **supraduodenal artery**. The **splenic artery** is the longest branch of the celiac trunk and runs horizontally towards the spleen. It courses along the superior border of the pancreas and supplies its body and tail with numerous branches (dorsal pancreatic artery, great pancreatic artery, artery of tail of pancreas). Upon reaching the splenic hilum, it divides into 2-3 terminal branches supplying the spleen.

Key points about the arteries of the pancreas	
Superior pancreaticoduodenal arteries	Branches of gastroduodenal artery, form pancreaticoduodenal arcades which run anteriorly and posteriorly with inferior pancreaticoduodenal arteries; supply head and neck of pancreas
Inferior pancreaticoduodenal arteries	Branches of superior mesenteric artery, form pancreaticoduodenal arcades which run anteriorly and posteriorly with superior pancreaticoduodenal arteries; supply head and uncinate process of pancreas
Splenic artery	Direct branch of celiac trunk; supplies body and tail of pancreas (via dorsal and great pancreatic arteries and artery of tail of pancreas)

Key points about the arteries of the duodenum	
Superior pancreaticoduodenal arteries	Branches of gastroduodenal artery; form pancreaticoduodenal arcades with inferior pancreaticoduodenal arteries, supply superior and descending part of duodenum
Inferior pancreaticoduodenal arteries	Branches of the superior mesenteric artery, form pancreaticoduodenal arcades with superior pancreaticoduodenal arteries; supply horizontal and ascending part of duodenum
Supraduodenal and retroduodenal arteries	Branches of gastroduodenal artery (or common hepatic artery); mainly supplies superior/posterior part of duodenum

Key points about the arteries of the spleen	
Splenic artery	Direct branch of celiac trunk; divides into 2 or 3 splenic branches

Blood vessels of abdomen and pelvis

Celiac trunk

HEPATIC PORTAL SYSTEM

The **hepatic portal system** is a venous system that drains the spleen, pancreas, gallbladder and upper parts of the gastrointestinal tract.

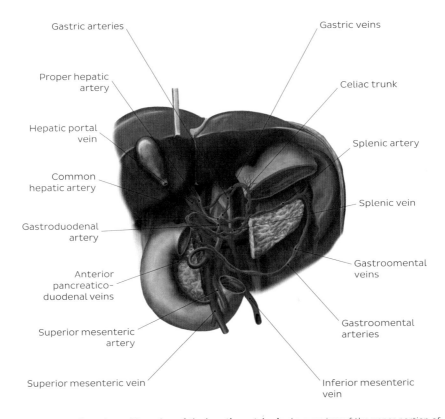

Gastric arteries

Gastric veins

Proper hepatic artery

Celiac trunk

Hepatic portal vein

Splenic artery

Common hepatic artery

Splenic vein

Gastroduodenal artery

Gastroomental veins

Anterior pancreatico-duodenal veins

Gastroomental arteries

Superior mesenteric artery

Inferior mesenteric vein

Superior mesenteric vein

FIGURE 6.46. Tributaries and branches of the hepatic portal vein. An overview of the upper portion of the abdomen with the liver reflected and parts of the stomach, pancreas and small intestine removed. The hepatic portal vein is formed by the union of the **superior mesenteric** and **splenic veins** just posterior to the neck of the pancreas. The **superior mesenteric vein** receives venous blood from the small intestine, cecum, ascending colon and transverse colon through its tributaries. The **splenic vein** can be found along the posterior length of the pancreas and receives several tributaries which drain the spleen, parts of the stomach and pancreas. The **hepatic portal vein** ascends obliquely alongside the proper hepatic artery within the hepatoduodenal ligament to reach the liver before bifurcating into left and right branches.

Key points about hepatic portal system	
Hepatic portal vein	**Branches:** anterior and posterior right branches of hepatic portal vein, transverse and umbilical parts of left branch of hepatic portal vein
	Tributaries: superior mesenteric, splenic, posterior superior pancreaticoduodenal, cystic, paraumbilical and gastric veins
	Course: hepatoduodenal ligament → porta hepatis
Superior mesenteric vein	**Tributaries:** jejunal, ileal, ileocolic, right and middle colic, right gastro-omental, and pancreaticoduodenal veins
Splenic vein	**Tributaries:** short gastric, left gastro-omental, inferior mesenteric and pancreatic veins

ABDOMEN

LYMPHATICS OF THE PANCREAS, DUODENUM AND SPLEEN

The lymphatic drainage of the pancreas, duodenum and spleen is closely related to their venous drainage. For example, as in the case of the arterial supply of the pancreas, the lymphatic drainage of the head of the pancreas is different than of the body and tail. Similarly, the lymphatic drainage of the superior part of the duodenum is different from its inferior part.

Lymphatic capillaries within the pancreas, duodenum and spleen collect lymph from these tissues and transport it into adjacent lymph nodes. The lymph is then passed along a series of lymph nodes to reach the terminal lymph nodes, which in this case, are known as the **preaortic lymph nodes**. The preaortic lymph nodes consist of three groups of nodes: The celiac, superior mesenteric and inferior mesenteric lymph nodes out of which the former two drain the pancreas, duodenum and spleen.

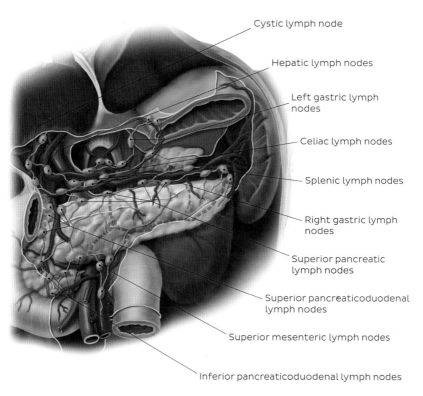

Cystic lymph node

Hepatic lymph nodes

Left gastric lymph nodes

Celiac lymph nodes

Splenic lymph nodes

Right gastric lymph nodes

Superior pancreatic lymph nodes

Superior pancreaticoduodenal lymph nodes

Superior mesenteric lymph nodes

Inferior pancreaticoduodenal lymph nodes

FIGURE 6.47. **Lymphatic drainage of the pancreas, duodenum and spleen.** An overview of the upper portion of the abdomen with the liver retracted and the stomach removed to provide a clear view of the pancreas, duodenum and spleen. The body and tail of the pancreas are drained by the **superior and inferior pancreatic lymph nodes**. The head of the pancreas is drained by the **superior and inferior pancreaticoduodenal lymph nodes**, which also drain the majority of the duodenum. The exception is the

ABDOMEN

superior part of the duodenum, which is drained by the **pyloric lymph nodes** and the ascending part of the duodenum, drained by the **inferior pancreatic** and **superior mesenteric lymph nodes**.

The spleen is drained by the **splenic lymph nodes**, which may also drain the tail of the pancreas and therefore can also be known as the **pancreaticosplenic lymph nodes**. The majority of these lymph nodes eventually drain into the **celiac lymph nodes**, which ultimately drain into the **cisterna chyli**.

Key points about the lymphatics of the pancreas	
Head	Superior pancreaticoduodenal lymph nodes → hepatic lymph nodes → celiac lymph nodes → cisterna chyli
	Inferior pancreaticoduodenal lymph nodes → superior mesenteric lymph nodes → celiac lymph nodes → cisterna chyli
Body	Superior and inferior pancreatic lymph nodes → celiac lymph nodes → cisterna chyli
Tail	Superior and inferior pancreatic lymph nodes → celiac lymph nodes → cisterna chyli
	Splenic lymph nodes → celiac lymph nodes → cisterna chyli

Key points about the lymphatics of the duodenum	
Superior part	Pyloric lymph nodes → hepatic lymph nodes → celiac lymph nodes → cisterna chyli
Ascending part	Inferior pancreatic lymph nodes → celiac lymph nodes → cisterna chyli
	Superior mesenteric lymph nodes → cisterna chyli
Descending and horizontal parts	Superior pancreaticoduodenal lymph nodes → hepatic lymph nodes → celiac lymph nodes → cisterna chyli
	Inferior pancreaticoduodenal lymph nodes → superior mesenteric lymph nodes → celiac lymph nodes → cisterna chyli

Key points about the lymphatics of the spleen	
Spleen	Splenic nodes → celiac lymph nodes → cisterna chyli

Lymphatics of the
retroperitoneal space

Lymphatics of
abdomen and pelvis

ABDOMEN

LYMPHATICS OF THE STOMACH, LIVER AND GALLBLADDER

The lymphatic drainage of the stomach is somewhat variable between individuals however several major lymph nodes are generally involved. These are the:

- **Juxtacardial nodes**, located in the region of the cardia of the stomach,
- **Right/left gastric nodes**, short gastric nodes, right/left gastroomental (a.k.a. gastroepiploic) nodes (all of which are related to the arteries of the same names),
- **Pyloric nodes** (made up of the supra-, sub- and retropyloric groups), related to the pylorus of the stomach.

The lymphatic drainage of the liver is elaborate and can generally be split into superficial and deep pathways:

- The **superficial pathway** transports lymph via channels in the subserosal areolar tissue which envelopes the liver. The anterior and inferior surfaces largely drain to hepatic nodes, while lymph from other surfaces is mainly received by various node groups of the inferior mediastinum or the celiac/superior mesenteric nodes.
- The **deep pathway** consists of hepatic lymph vessels which follow branches of the hepatic arteries and portal vein and flow towards the hepatic nodes at the hilum of the liver. Other lymphatic vessels course along the hepatic veins which exit via the bare area of the liver; these are received by the right lumbar (a.k.a. caval) nodes or inferior diaphragmatic nodes.

Lymph drained from the gallbladder is mainly received either directly by hepatic nodes or first via a cystic lymph node.

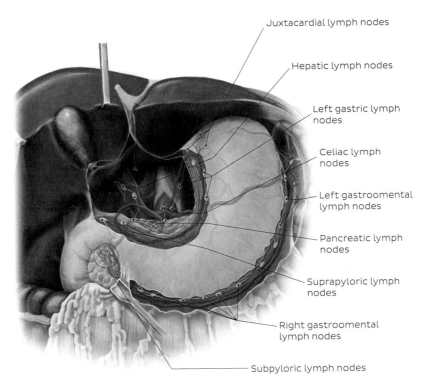

Juxtacardial lymph nodes

Hepatic lymph nodes

Left gastric lymph nodes

Celiac lymph nodes

Left gastroomental lymph nodes

Pancreatic lymph nodes

Suprapyloric lymph nodes

Right gastroomental lymph nodes

Subpyloric lymph nodes

FIGURE 6.48. Lymphatics of the stomach, liver and gallbladder (anterior view). Anterior view with the liver retracted showing a section of the lymphatic system of the upper abdomen. The nodes draining the stomach are labeled. The **right** and **left gastric nodes** follow the arteries of the same name along the lesser curvature of the stomach while the **right** and **left gastroomental nodes** follow their homonymous arteries on the greater curvature of the stomach. Lymph drained from these nodes is largely received by the **celiac nodes** which in turn drain into the **cisterna chyli** via the left lumbar nodes (paraaortic nodes) or intestinal lymphatic trunk.

ABDOMEN

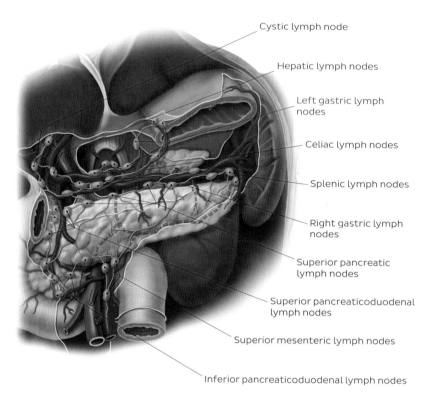

Cystic lymph node

Hepatic lymph nodes

Left gastric lymph nodes

Celiac lymph nodes

Splenic lymph nodes

Right gastric lymph nodes

Superior pancreatic lymph nodes

Superior pancreaticoduodenal lymph nodes

Superior mesenteric lymph nodes

Inferior pancreaticoduodenal lymph nodes

FIGURE 6.49. Lymphatics of the stomach, liver and gallbladder (retrogastric view). Anterior view of abdomen with the stomach removed to show the lymphatic pathways of the upper abdomen. The **hepatic lymph nodes** can be identified around the porta hepatis, as well as a **cystic lymph node** which drains the gallbladder. The hepatic nodes largely drain to the **celiac nodes** via lymphatic vessels which course along the common and proper hepatic arteries. The **right** and **left gastric nodes** can also be clearly observed along their related arteries.

Key points about the lymphatics of the stomach	
Cardia	Juxtacardial nodes
Fundus	Short gastric nodes
Lesser curvature	Right/left gastric nodes
Greater curvature	Right/left gastroomental nodes
Pyloric part	Pyloric nodes (suprapyloric, retropyloric, subpyloric nodes)
Drainage path	Celiac nodes → intestinal lymphatic trunk → cisterna chyli → thoracic duct

Key points about the lymphatics of the liver		
Superficial pathway	Anterior surface	Hepatic nodes
	Inferior surface	Hepatic nodes (or directly to lumbar nodes)
	Superior surface	Hepatic nodes/parasternal/pericardiac nodes
	Posterior surface	Celiac/superior mesenteric or posterior mediastinal nodes

ABDOMEN

Key points about the lymphatics of the liver	
Deep pathway	Hepatic nodes → celiac nodes
	Posterior mediastinal/ right lumbar nodes

Key points about the lymphatics of the gallbladder	
Superior aspect	Cystic node or directly to hepatic nodes
Inferior aspect	Cystic node, posterior pancreaticoduodenal nodes or preaortic nodes

Lymphatics of
abdomen and pelvis

Lymphatics of the
retroperitoneal space

LYMPHATICS OF THE POSTERIOR ABDOMINAL AND PELVIC WALL

There are several groups of lymph nodes present in the posterior abdominal and pelvic walls. Most of those groups are named according to their anatomical relation to the aorta/inferior vena cava and their branches/tributaries.

The main lymph node groups of this region are the **lumbar lymph nodes**, composed of the right lumbar (caval), intermediate lumbar and left lumbar (aortic) nodes. They receive lymph from abdominal organs and also from the common, internal and external iliac lymph nodes, which drain the pelvic organs.

The lymph is then drained by lymph trunks:

- **Left lumbar lymph trunk**: Drains left lumbar lymph nodes
- **Right lumbar lymph trunk**: Drains right lumbar and intermediate lumbar lymph nodes.
- **Intestinal lymph trunk**: Drains celiac, superior mesenteric and phrenic lymph nodes.
- **Cisterna chyli**: Receives the lymph from the trunks mentioned above (directly or indirectly) and ultimately drains all the lymph from the posterior abdomen and pelvis.

ABDOMEN

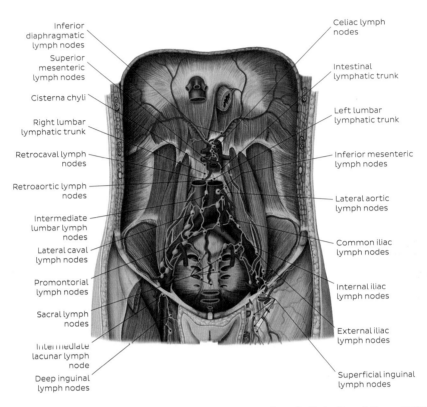

Inferior diaphragmatic lymph nodes

Superior mesenteric lymph nodes

Cisterna chyli

Right lumbar lymphatic trunk

Retrocaval lymph nodes

Retroaortic lymph nodes

Intermediate lumbar lymph nodes

Lateral caval lymph nodes

Promontorial lymph nodes

Sacral lymph nodes

Intermediate lacunar lymph node

Deep inguinal lymph nodes

Celiac lymph nodes

Intestinal lymphatic trunk

Left lumbar lymphatic trunk

Inferior mesenteric lymph nodes

Lateral aortic lymph nodes

Common iliac lymph nodes

Internal iliac lymph nodes

External iliac lymph nodes

Superficial inguinal lymph nodes

FIGURE 6.50. **Lymphatics of the posterior abdominal and pelvic wall.** Illustration of the posterior abdominal wall and pelvic cavity, with the organs and other structures removed to reveal the lymph nodes and neighboring vessels. In the center of the figure, adjacent to the abdominal aorta, is the **cisterna chyli**, the main drainage pathway of the posterior abdominal wall. Two trunks converge to form the cisterna chyli: The **right lumbar lymph trunk** and **left lumbar lymph trunk** (which usually receives the intestinal lymph trunk). These structures receive the lymph mainly from the **lumbar lymph nodes** (which are composed of the left lumbar nodes, also known as aortic lymph nodes and the right lumbar nodes, also called caval lymph nodes) as well as the **celiac** and **superior/inferior mesenteric nodes** which drain the gastrointestinal tract.

Pelvic organs drain to the **common**, **internal** and **external iliac lymph nodes**, which in turn drain to **lumbar lymph nodes**.

Key points about the lymphatics of the posterior abdominal wall	
Main trunks	**Cisterna chyli:** ultimately drains most of the lymph from the posterior abdominal wall, pelvis and lower limbs
	Intestinal lymph trunk: drains phrenic, celiac, superior mesenteric, and some inferior mesenteric lymph nodes
	Left lumbar lymph trunk: drains left lumbar lymph nodes (may receive intestinal lymph trunk)
	Right lumbar lymph trunk: drains right lumbar and intermediate lymph nodes

Key points about the lymphatics of the posterior abdominal wall	
Main abdominal lymph node groups	**Phrenic nodes:** drain inferior surface of diaphragm, abdominal part of esophagus, and suprarenal glands
	Celiac nodes: drain stomach, duodenum, pancreas, liver, spleen, and greater omentum
	Superior mesenteric nodes: drain jejunum, ileum, cecum, vermiform appendix, ascending, and transverse colons
	Inferior mesenteric nodes: drain regions irrigated by the inferior mesenteric artery
	Left/right lumbar nodes: directly drain kidneys, superior abdominal part of ureters, gonads, also receives efferents from GIT
Main pelvic lymph node groups	Common, internal and external iliac lymph nodes: drain the pelvis and the lower limbs

Lymphatics of abdomen and pelvis

Lymphatics of the retroperitoneal space

ABDOMEN

PELVIS AND PERINEUM

7

BONY PELVIS

The bony pelvis is a complex, basin-shaped structure that comprises the skeletal framework of the pelvic region and houses the pelvic organs. It consists of the right and left hip bones and the sacrum, which are connected via the sacroiliac joints.

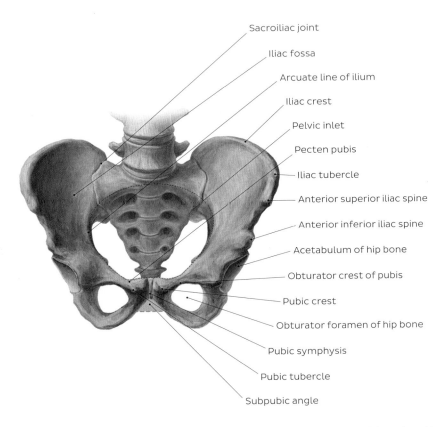

Sacroiliac joint
Iliac fossa
Arcuate line of ilium
Iliac crest
Pelvic inlet
Pecten pubis
Iliac tubercle
Anterior superior iliac spine
Anterior inferior iliac spine
Acetabulum of hip bone
Obturator crest of pubis
Pubic crest
Obturator foramen of hip bone
Pubic symphysis
Pubic tubercle
Subpubic angle

FIGURE 7.1a. Bony pelvis (anterior and posterior views). The bilateral ischiopubic rami form the pubic arch, the vertex of which is known as the subpubic angle. In fig 7.1a of a female pelvis, the subpubic angle measures around 90° (approximating to the angle between the widely extended thumb and index finger); in a male pelvis (fig 7.1b), it measures closer to 60° (approximate angle between abducted index and middle fingers).

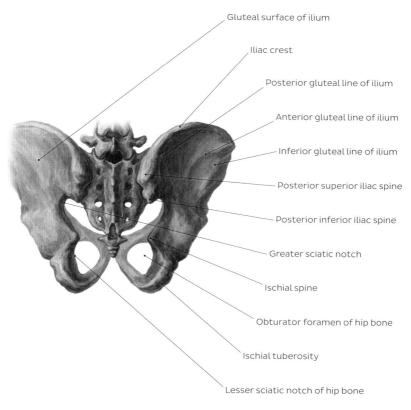

Gluteal surface of ilium

Iliac crest

Posterior gluteal line of ilium

Anterior gluteal line of ilium

Inferior gluteal line of ilium

Posterior superior iliac spine

Posterior inferior iliac spine

Greater sciatic notch

Ischial spine

Obturator foramen of hip bone

Ischial tuberosity

Lesser sciatic notch of hip bone

FIGURE 7.1b. **Bony pelvis (anterior and posterior views).** (Continued)

PELVIS AND
PERINEUM

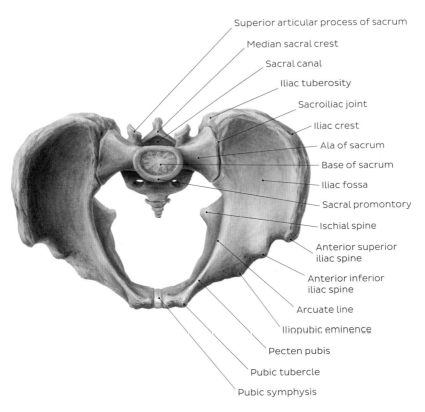

Superior articular process of sacrum
Median sacral crest
Sacral canal
Iliac tuberosity
Sacroiliac joint
Iliac crest
Ala of sacrum
Base of sacrum
Iliac fossa
Sacral promontory
Ischial spine
Anterior superior iliac spine
Anterior inferior iliac spine
Arcuate line
Iliopubic eminence
Pecten pubis
Pubic tubercle
Pubic symphysis

FIGURE 7.2. **Bony pelvis (superior view).** The bony pelvis is divided into the greater and lesser pelvis by the **pelvic inlet** (superior pelvic aperture). Posteriorly, the pelvic inlet is bounded by the sacral promontory and alae of the sacrum. The anterolateral borders are defined by a right and left linea terminalis, which are formed by the arcuate line of the ilium and pectin pubis/pubic crest of the pubis.

The **greater** (a.k.a false) **pelvis** is found superior to the pelvic inlet and contains the inferior parts of the abdominal organs. The **lesser** (a.k.a. true) **pelvis** is located between the pelvic inlet and pelvic outlet, and it includes the intrapelvic urinary organs, internal reproductive organs and the perineum.

PELVIS AND
PERINEUM

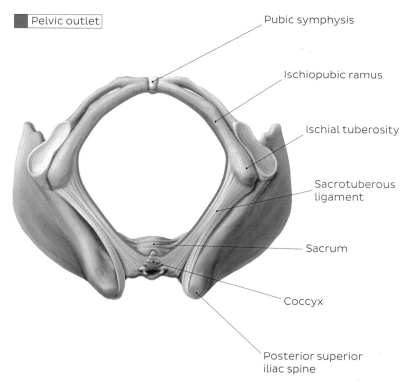

Pelvic outlet

Pubic symphysis

Ischiopubic ramus

Ischial tuberosity

Sacrotuberous ligament

Sacrum

Coccyx

Posterior superior iliac spine

FIGURE 7.3. **Bony pelvis (inferior view).** The pelvic outlet (a.k.a. inferior pelvic aperture) is the inferior opening of the true pelvis. It is formed anteriorly by the pubic arch, ischiopubic rami and ischial tuberosities, and posteriorly by inferior borders of the sacrotuberous ligaments and apex of the coccyx. Since the latter structures are both slightly yielding, this results in a less rigid posterior half of the pelvic outlet.

Key points about the bony pelvis	
Bones	Hip bone: ilium, ischium, pubis
	Sacrum
	Coccyx
Hip bone	Acetabulum, ischiopubic ramus, obturator foramen, greater sciatic notch, greater sciatic foramen
Ilium	Body of ilium, ala, gluteal surface, sacropelvic surface
Ischium	Body of ischium, ramus of ischium, ischial spine, lesser sciatic notch, lesser sciatic foramen, ischial tuberosity
Pubis	Body of pubis, superior pubic ramus, inferior pubic ramus
Sacrum	Base of sacrum, apex of sacrum, lateral part, pelvic surface, dorsal surface
Coccyx	Base of coccyx, coccygeal horn, apex of coccyx
Joints	Sacroiliac joint, pubic symphysis, lumbosacral joint, sacrococcygeal symphysis, hip joint

PELVIS AND
PERINEUM

The pelvis

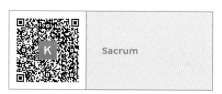

Sacrum

LIGAMENTS OF THE PELVIS

The robust structure of the pelvic girdle is held together by important mechanical stabilizers, the **ligaments of the pelvis**, which provide structural support in and around the pelvis. Pelvic ligaments can be categorized according to their associated joints and are therefore divided into the ligaments of the: Lumbosacral, sacroiliac, sacrococcygeal, and pubic symphyseal joints of the pelvis.

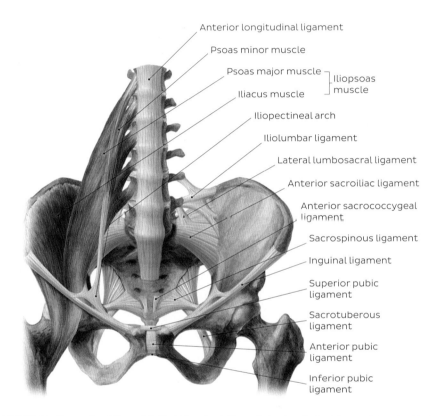

Anterior longitudinal ligament

Psoas minor muscle

Psoas major muscle ⎤ Iliopsoas
                     ⎦ muscle
Iliacus muscle

Iliopectineal arch

Iliolumbar ligament

Lateral lumbosacral ligament

Anterior sacroiliac ligament

Anterior sacrococcygeal ligament

Sacrospinous ligament

Inguinal ligament

Superior pubic ligament

Sacrotuberous ligament

Anterior pubic ligament

Inferior pubic ligament

FIGURE 7.4. Ligaments of the pelvis (Anterior view). The anterior longitudinal ligament travels along the entire length of the vertebral column. It extends from the basilar part of the occipital bone to the anterior surface of the sacrum, passing over the lumbosacral joint in doing so. It functions to prevent hyperextension of the vertebral column and reinforces the anterior aspect of the sacrum.

Ligaments of the lumbosacral joint limit the range of movement at this junction and include the **iliolumbar** and **lateral lumbosacral ligaments**. The former is made up of two bands (superior and inferior) originating from the transverse processes of vertebra L5. The superior band extends over the sacroiliac joint and across the iliac crest to blend with the thoracolumbar fascia, while the inferior band crosses the anterior sacroiliac ligament to insert in the posterior region of the iliac fossa. Continuous with the lower border of the iliolumbar ligament is the **lateral lumbosacral ligament** which arises from the lower margin of the transverse process of L5 vertebra and passes inferolaterally to attach to the ala of the sacrum.

The sacroiliac joint is strengthened by three ligaments, of which only the **anterior sacroiliac ligament** is seen in this view. It comprises the anteroinferior thickening of the joint capsule and connects the preauricular surface of the ilium to the third sacral segment.

On the anterior aspect of the bony pelvis, the pubic symphysis is strengthened by the **superior**, **anterior** and **inferior pubic ligaments**. Two ligaments crossing the pubic bone can equally be seen: The **iliopectineal arch**, a thickened band of iliopsoas fascia, running from the anterior superior iliac spine (ASIS) to the iliopectineal eminence of the pubic bone as well as the **inguinal ligament** extending from the ASIS to the pubic tubercle. Anterior stabilization of the sacrococcygeal joint is achieved by the **anterior sacrococcygeal ligament**, which is a continuation of the anterior longitudinal ligament.

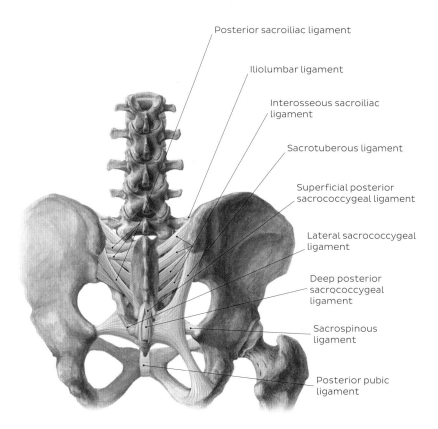

Posterior sacroiliac ligament

Iliolumbar ligament

Interosseous sacroiliac ligament

Sacrotuberous ligament

Superficial posterior sacrococcygeal ligament

Lateral sacrococcygeal ligament

Deep posterior sacrococcygeal ligament

Sacrospinous ligament

Posterior pubic ligament

FIGURE 7.5. **Ligaments of the pelvis (Posterior view).** The sacroiliac joint is strengthened by three ligaments, namely the **anterior** (see previous image), **interosseous** and **posterior sacroiliac ligaments**. The **interosseous sacroiliac ligament** constitutes the major bond between the ilium and sacrum, filling the gaps between these two bones at the posterosuperior aspect of the joint. The **posterior sacroiliac ligament** lies superficial to the interosseous sacroiliac ligament and consists of several fibers connecting the posterior superior iliac spine (PSIS), iliac crest as well as the lateral and intermediate sacral crests. The two bones of the pelvic spine (sacrum and coccyx) are strengthened by the **anterior** (see previous image) and **posterior sacrococcygeal ligaments**.

The **superficial posterior sacrococcygeal ligament** arises from the margin of the sacral hiatus and attaches to the dorsum of the coccyx. The **deep posterior sacrococcygeal ligament** extends from the dorsal surface of the fifth sacral vertebral body to the dorsal surface of the coccyx. Bilaterally, the **lateral posterior sacrococcygeal ligament** spans from the inferolateral angles of the sacrum to the transverse processes of the coccyx. Two major ligaments situated on the posterior aspect of the bony pelvis are the **sacrospinous** and **sacrotuberous ligaments**. These transform the lesser and greater sciatic notches into the lesser and greater sciatic foramina. The former extends from the margins of the coccyx and sacrum to the spine of the ischium, while the latter has several attachments to the posterior superior iliac spine, the posterior sacroiliac ligaments, lateral sacral crest as well as the lateral margins of the lower sacrum and upper coccyx.

Lastly, the **posterior pubic ligament**, blending with the periosteum of both pubic bodies posteriorly, can be seen in this view.

Key points about the ligaments of the pelvis	
Lumbosacral joint	Iliolumbar ligament, lateral lumbosacral ligament
Sacroiliac joint	Anterior sacroiliac ligament, interosseous sacroiliac ligament, posterior sacroiliac ligament
Sacrococcygeal joint	Anterior sacrococcygeal ligament, superficial posterior sacrococcygeal ligament, deep posterior sacrococcygeal ligament, lateral sacrococcygeal ligament
Pubic symphysis	Superior pubic ligament, anterior pubic ligament, inferior pubic ligament, posterior pubic ligament
Nonarticular ligaments	Anterior longitudinal ligament, sacrospinous ligament, sacrotuberous ligament, iliopectineal arch, inguinal ligament
Function	Mechanical stabilizers of the pelvic girdle

MUSCLES OF THE PELVIC FLOOR AND PERINEUM

The **pelvic floor** is formed by the bowl- or funnel-shaped pelvic diaphragm, consisting of the levator ani and coccygeus muscles and their investing fascia. **Structurally**, the pelvic floor separates the pelvic cavity from the perineum. **Functionally**, these pelvic floor muscles support the pelvic organs, keeping them in place and preventing prolapse upon straining. It also aids in maintaining both urinary and fecal continence until one can conveniently void.

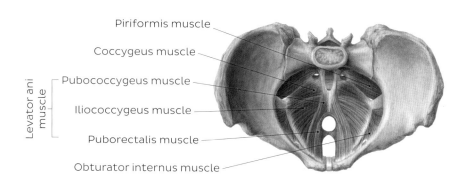

Piriformis muscle
Coccygeus muscle
Levator ani muscle
— Pubococcygeus muscle
Iliococcygeus muscle
Puborectalis muscle
Obturator internus muscle

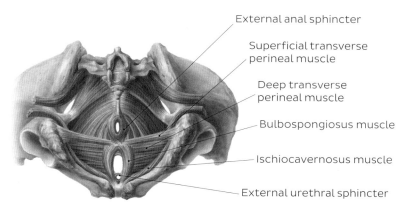

External anal sphincter
Superficial transverse perineal muscle
Deep transverse perineal muscle
Bulbospongiosus muscle
Ischiocavernosus muscle
External urethral sphincter

FIGURE 7.6. **Muscles of the pelvic floor and perineum.** The upper image shows the superior view of the pelvic floor, while the lower image demonstrates the inferior view. From the superior view, the **levator ani muscle** and its three components are visible: The puborectalis (puboanalis), pubococcygeus and iliococcygeus muscles. Extending between the ischial spines and coccyx is the **coccygeus muscle**. Moving posterosuperiorly, the **piriformis muscle** forms the posterolateral wall of the pelvic cavity, while the **obturator internus muscle** forms part of the anterolateral wall of the pelvic cavity.

From the inferior view, the muscles of the perineum can be identified. Beginning in the deep perineal space/pouch, there is the **deep transverse perineal muscle** and **external urethral sphincter**. Moving inferiorly to the superficial perineal space/pouch, the **superficial transverse perineal muscle, bulbospongiosus**, and paired **ischiocavernosus muscles** are found. Finally, heading posteriorly to the anal triangle of the perineum, the **external anal sphincter** is depicted.

Pelvic diaphragm		Origin	Insertion	Innervation	Function
Levator ani	Puborectalis	Posterior surface of bodies of pubic bones	None (forms 'puborectal sling' posterior to rectum)	Nerve to levator ani (S4) (pubococcygeus also receives branches via inferior rectal/perineal branches of pudendal nerve (S2–S4))	Supports pelvic viscera, Increases intraabdominal pressure, Assists with fecal and urinary continence
	Pubococcygeus	Posterior surface of bodies of pubic bones (lateral to puborectalis)	Anococcygeal ligament, Coccyx, Perineal body and musculature of prostate/vagina		
	Iliococcygeus	Tendinous arch of internal obturator fascia, Ischial spine	Anococcygeal ligament, Coccyx		
Coccygeus		Ischial spine	Inferior end of sacrum, Coccyx	Anterior rami of spinal nerves S4 & S5	Supports pelvic viscera, Flexes coccyx
Obturator internus		Ischiopubic ramus, Posterior surface of obturator membrane	Greater trochanter of femur	Nerve to obturator internus (L5–S2)	Hip joint: thigh external rotation, thigh abduction (from flexed hip); stabilizes head of femur in acetabulum
Piriformis		Anterior surface of S2-S4 segments of sacrum, Superior margin of greater sciatic notch, Sacrotuberous ligament	Greater trochanter of femur	Nerve to piriformis (S1, S2)	

Muscles of the pelvic floor

Perineal region

INTRODUCTION TO THE FEMALE PELVIC CAVITY

The **female pelvic cavity** contains several organs from the digestive, reproductive and urinary systems, some of which pass into the perineum. These include the:

- Terminal part of the sigmoid colon, which continues distally as the rectum
- Ovaries, uterine tubes and uterus
- Pelvic part of the ureters and urinary bladder

The female pelvic organs are surrounded by **pelvic visceral fascia**. Additionally, the parietal peritoneum of the abdominal cavity reflects onto the superior surfaces of some of these organs, forming pouches/spaces between adjacent organs. The **pelvic floor** is formed by a musculofascial pelvic diaphragm composed of the levator ani and coccygeus muscles, that separates the pelvic cavity above from the perineum below.

The female pelvic cavity is supplied by various branches of the internal iliac artery, the superior [ano]rectal artery and the median sacral artery, with the ovary receiving the ovarian artery from the abdominal aorta. Various visceral plexuses carry both sympathetic and parasympathetic fibers that provide innervation to the organs as well as visceral afferent fibers which mostly carry pain sensation to the central nervous system.

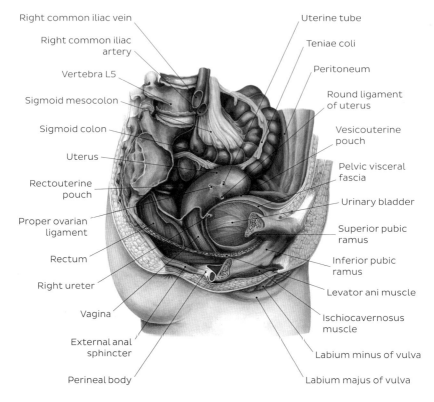

Right common iliac vein

Right common iliac artery

Vertebra L5

Sigmoid mesocolon

Sigmoid colon

Uterus

Rectouterine pouch

Proper ovarian ligament

Rectum

Right ureter

Vagina

External anal sphincter

Perineal body

Uterine tube

Teniae coli

Peritoneum

Round ligament of uterus

Vesicouterine pouch

Pelvic visceral fascia

Urinary bladder

Superior pubic ramus

Inferior pubic ramus

Levator ani muscle

Ischiocavernosus muscle

Labium minus of vulva

Labium majus of vulva

FIGURE 7.7. Female pelvis and perineum (parasagittal section). Parasagittal section of the female pelvis and perineum (right view) with parts of the right pelvic wall, fascia, ovary and other structures removed to show the relations of the female pelvic organs. The **urinary bladder** (full of urine) is located anteriorly, just posterior to the pubic bone, with the distal part of the right pelvic **ureter** at its base.

The **uterus** sits between the urinary bladder and the rectum and shows pieces of the right proper ovarian ligament, uterine tube and round ligament of the uterus. The **vagina** extends inferiorly from the cervical region of the uterus and opens into the perineum at the vaginal orifice (opening). The terminal part of the **sigmoid colon** continues distally as the **rectum**, both of which are located in the posterior aspect of the pelvic cavity, anterior to the sacrum and coccyx.

Key points about the female pelvic cavity		
Walls and floors	**Bones**: hip bone (Ilium, ischium, pubis), sacrum, coccyx	
	Ligaments: sacroiliac, sacrospinous, and sacrotuberous	
	Muscles: levator ani, coccygeus, piriformis, obturator internus	
Digestive organs	**Organs**: sigmoid colon, rectum	
	Functions: absorption of minerals, vitamins, water and electrolytes, temporary storage of fecal matter and elimination during defecation	
Reproductive organs	**Organs**: ovary, uterine tube, uterus, vagina	
	Functions: formation and development of ova, production of estrogen and progesterone, implantation of embryo, fetal development	
Urinary organs	**Organs**: pelvic part of ureter, urinary bladder	
	Functions: transport and elimination of urine from from the body	

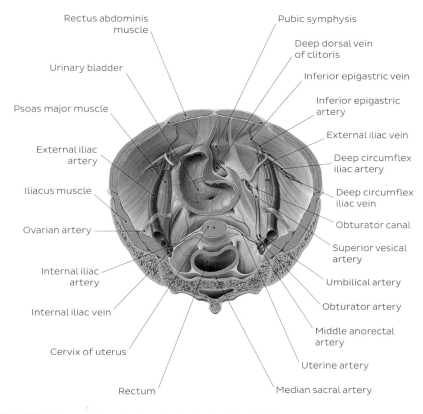

FIGURE 7.8. Organs and vessels (superior view). The **urinary bladder** (opened and retracted) is situated posterior the anterior pelvic wall. Immediately posterior to it is the **uterus** (body removed, with only the cervix remaining). Finally, in the posterior part of the pelvic cavity is the **rectum**.

This superior view also allows the appreciation of the distribution of the vessels in the pelvic cavity. The arteries of this area stem mainly from the internal and external iliac arteries, which are shown bifurcating from the common iliac artery. The **internal iliac artery** supplies the pelvic walls and organs, as well as the gluteal and medial thigh regions of the lower limb. The **external iliac artery** provides arterial supply to the lower abdominal wall (via the inferior epigastric and deep circumflex iliac arteries); it passes beneath the inguinal ligament, where it becomes the femoral artery (main artery of the lower limb).

Key points about the female pelvic cavity	
Peritoneal pouches/ depressions	Vesicouterine pouch (between urinary bladder and uterus)
	Rectouterine pouch (between uterus and rectum)
	Pararectal fossae (lateral to the recum)
Blood supply	**Internal iliac artery**: superior vesical arteries, inferior vesical artery, internal pudendal artery, middle [ano]rectal artery
	Superior [ano]rectal artery (from inferior mesenteric artery)
	Median sacral artery (from aortic bifurcation)
	Ovarian artery (from abdominal aorta)
Innervation	**Sympathetic**: lumbar splanchnic nerves, hypogastric and pelvic plexuses
	Parasympathetic: pelvic splanchnic nerves, left and right inferior hypogastric plexuses, and rectal (pelvic) plexus

PELVIS AND PERINEUM

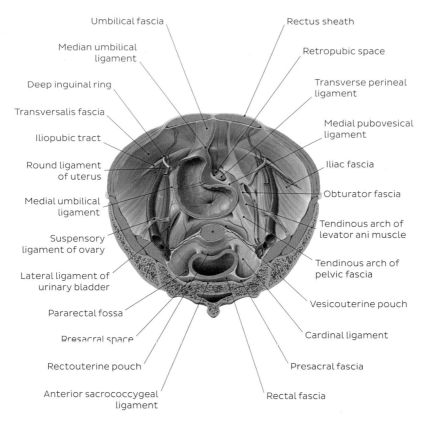

Umbilical fascia

Median umbilical ligament

Deep inguinal ring

Transversalis fascia

Iliopubic tract

Round ligament of uterus

Medial umbilical ligament

Suspensory ligament of ovary

Lateral ligament of urinary bladder

Pararectal fossa

Presacral space

Rectouterine pouch

Anterior sacrococcygeal ligament

Rectus sheath

Retropubic space

Transverse perineal ligament

Medial pubovesical ligament

Iliac fascia

Obturator fascia

Tendinous arch of levator ani muscle

Tendinous arch of pelvic fascia

Vesicouterine pouch

Cardinal ligament

Presacral fascia

Rectal fascia

FIGURE 7.9. Fasciae/ligaments and anatomical spaces (superior view). The peritoneum covers the pelvic wall as well as parts of the viscera. Consequently, a number of spaces and pouches are created. The most significant ones are the vesicouterine pouch, rectouterine pouch (of Douglas, lowest part of the female peritoneal cavity), pararectal fossae and presacral space.

Female reproductive organs

Anatomical spaces of the pelvic cavity

UTERUS, UTERINE TUBES AND OVARIES

The vagina, uterus, uterine tubes and ovaries represent the **internal organs** of the female reproductive system (female internal genitalia).

The **uterus**, commonly known as the womb, is a pear-shaped muscular organ situated in the pelvis anterior to the rectum and posterior to the urinary bladder. It is about 8 cm long and is divided into 4 parts: The cervix, isthmus, corpus, and fundus. The uterus has many functions, such as providing vaginal and uterine secretions, hosting the fetus during pregnancy, and allowing sperm to pass to the uterine tubes in order to fertilize an egg (ovum). During childbirth, the uterus contracts to move the fetus through the pelvis/birth canal.

The **ovaries** are paired disc-shaped endocrine glands, responsible for the production of eggs (ova) and the secretion of the hormones progesterone and estrogen. An **ovum** is released every 3 to 4 weeks into the uterine tube, which is a paired, 10 cm long muscular tube. The **uterine tube** extends laterally from each side of the uterus, serving as a passageway between the ovaries and the uterus.

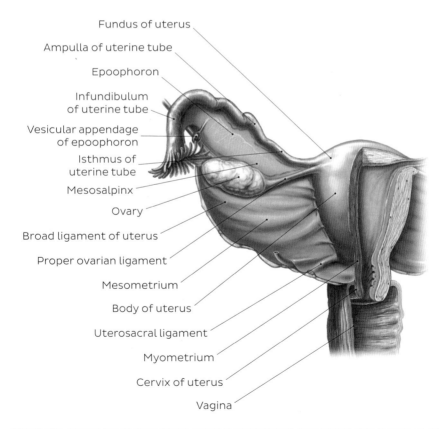

Fundus of uterus

Ampulla of uterine tube

Epoophoron

Infundibulum of uterine tube

Vesicular appendage of epoophoron

Isthmus of uterine tube

Mesosalpinx

Ovary

Broad ligament of uterus

Proper ovarian ligament

Mesometrium

Body of uterus

Uterosacral ligament

Myometrium

Cervix of uterus

Vagina

FIGURE 7.10. **Internal female reproductive organs (posterior view).** Each **uterine tube** is made up of 4 parts: The infundibulum, ampulla (where eggs are usually fertilized), isthmus and the intramural part. The **uterus** has 3 layers: The endometrium, myometrium, and the perimetrium. The uterus, uterine tubes and ovaries are supported by various **ligaments**, including the uterosacral ligament inferiorly, the ovarian ligament laterally, the suspensory ligament and the broad ligament of uterus. The most prominent of them is the broad ligament of uterus, which is subdivided into 3 components: The **mesometrium, mesosalpinx** and **mesovarium**.

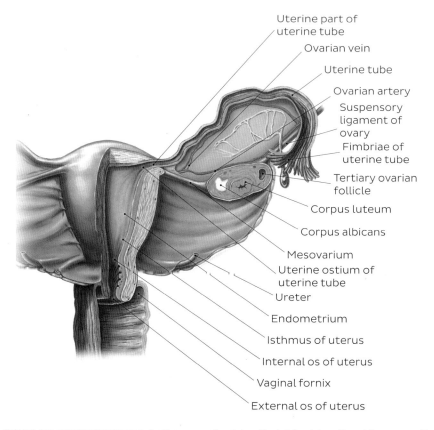

Uterine part of uterine tube
Ovarian vein
Uterine tube
Ovarian artery
Suspensory ligament of ovary
Fimbriae of uterine tube
Tertiary ovarian follicle
Corpus luteum
Corpus albicans
Mesovarium
Uterine ostium of uterine tube
Ureter
Endometrium
Isthmus of uterus
Internal os of uterus
Vaginal fornix
External os of uterus

FIGURE 7.11. Internal female reproductive organs (frontal section). A frontal-section of the ovary, with the **ovarian follicles** in different stages of maturation. When a follicle has matured, it undergoes **ovulation** and releases an egg (ovum) into the peritoneal cavity and ultimately into the uterine tube.

Key points about the uterus	
Definition	Pear-shaped muscular organ, 8 cm long
Parts	Cervix, isthmus, corpus, and fundus
Layers	Endometrium (innermost mucous membrane layer) Myometrium (smooth muscle layer) Perimetrium (serosa or outer serosal layer)
Ligaments	Uterosacral ligament, broad ligament of uterus (mesometrium, mesosalpinx, mesovarium)
Relations	Vagina (inferior), urinary bladder (anterior), rectum (posterior), uterine tubes (left and right), ovaries (left and right)
Function	Provide vaginal and uterine secretions, host the fetus during pregnancy, allow sperm to pass through the uterine tubes in order to fertilize an egg, provide mechanical protection, nutritional support to the fetus, and remove waste from inside the uterus

PELVIS AND PERINEUM

Key points about the uterine tube	
Definition	10 cm long muscular tubes extending bilaterally from the uterus
Parts	Infundibulum, ampulla, isthmus and intramural part
Ligaments	Broad ligament (specifically the mesosalpinx)
Relations	Ovaries, uterus, appendix (right), sigmoid colon (left), common iliac vessels
Function	Passageway between the ovaries and the uterus

Key points about the ovary	
Definition	Bilateral disc-shaped organs and endocrine glands
Ligaments	Suspensory ligament of ovary, proper ovarian ligament, broad ligament
Relations	Uterine tubes, uterus, appendix (right), sigmoid colon (left)
Function	Production of eggs, secretion of estrogen and progesterone

 Uterus

 The female gonads

 Uterine tubes

PELVIS AND PERINEUM

CERVIX, VAGINA AND VULVA

The **cervix** is a narrow canal about 2.5 cm long that connects the body of the uterus to the vagina. It is divided into a supravaginal part (**endocervix**) found superior to the vagina, and a vaginal part (**ectocervix**) which projects into the vagina. The cervix has many **functions**, such as facilitating passage of sperm, providing a physical barrier from pathogens and foreign objects, and maintaining physical integrity as the uterus enlarges during pregnancy. The cervix directly communicates with the vagina, which is the most distal part of the internal female genitalia.

The **vagina** is a flexible muscular canal that has a variety of functions, including menstruation, childbirth, and sexual intercourse. It is situated in the lesser pelvis, lying between the urinary bladder anteriorly, and the rectum posteriorly. It measures about 8 to 10 cm long, extending from the cervix of the uterus to the external genitalia.

The **vulva** is a collection of structures that represents the external part of the female reproductive system (external genitalia) surrounding the vaginal orifice. It consists of the mons pubis, labia majora, labia minora, clitoris, external orifice of the urethra, vestibule of vagina, vestibular bulb, hymen and vestibular (Bartholin) glands. The vulva plays a role in stimulation and arousal during sexual intercourse, while also protecting the internal organs of the female reproductive system.

PELVIS AND
PERINEUM

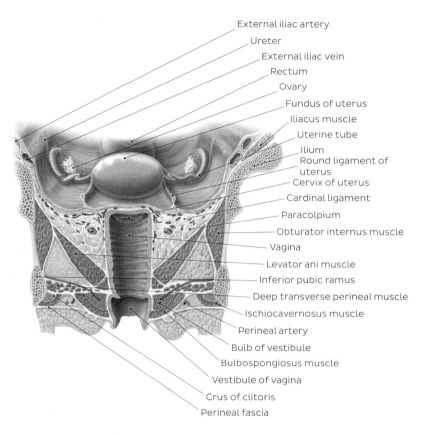

External iliac artery

Ureter

External iliac vein

Rectum

Ovary

Fundus of uterus

Iliacus muscle

Uterine tube

Ilium

Round ligament of uterus

Cervix of uterus

Cardinal ligament

Paracolpium

Obturator internus muscle

Vagina

Levator ani muscle

Inferior pubic ramus

Deep transverse perineal muscle

Ischiocavernosus muscle

Perineal artery

Bulb of vestibule

Bulbospongiosus muscle

Vestibule of vagina

Crus of clitoris

Perineal fascia

FIGURE 7.12. Uterus and vagina. The image above shows a coronal section of the female perineum. The inferior end of the cervix is seen projecting into the vagina, known as the vaginal part of the cervix. This protrusion forms a dome-shaped recess in the vaginal wall around the cervix called the **vaginal fornix**.

The walls of the vagina are covered by many transverse folds called **vaginal rugae**, which contribute to the elasticity and resilience of the vagina during sexual intercourse. The vagina opens into the **vestibule** of vagina, a part of the vulva lying between the labia minora. The vagina is closely related to many organs and structures of the pelvic region. In this coronal section, one can observe its lateral relations with the paracolpium, left and right ureter and levator ani muscle. A part of the levator ani muscle, called the pubovaginalis muscle, provides a U-shaped muscular sling that wraps around the vagina.

PELVIS AND PERINEUM

Key points about the cervix and vagina	
Classification	Internal female genitalia
Definition	**Cervix**: lowermost portion of the uterus approximately 2.5 cm long, connecting the body of uterus to the vagina. **Vagina**: very flexible fibrocartilaginous tube approximately 8–10 cm long, connecting the cervix of the uterus to the external genitalia (vulva)
Parts	**Cervix**: supravaginal and vaginal part
Relations	**Superior**: body of uterus **Anterior**: urinary bladder, urethra **Posterior**: rectum **Lateral**: deep transverse perineal muscle, levator ani muscle, paracolpium, ureter, cardinal ligament.
Functions	**Cervix**: facilitates passage of sperm, maintains sterility of uterus, maintains physical integrity as the uterus enlarges during pregnancy and expands during labor. **Vagina**: menstruation, childbirth, sexual intercourse

Key points about the vulva	
Classification	External female genitalia
Components	Mons pubis, labia majora, labia minora, clitoris Vaginal opening: external orifice of the vagina and urethra
Relations	Bulb of vestibule, artery of bulb of vestibule, bulbospongiosus muscle, perineal fascia
Functions	Sexual function: arousal and stimulation Protection of the internal female genitalia

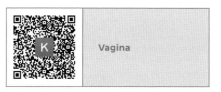

Vagina

Female reproductive organs

PELVIS AND PERINEUM

FETUS IN UTERO

The **fetus** is a term that describes an unborn baby from the **8th week** after fertilization until birth. In the uterus (i.e., *in utero*) the fetus is surrounded by an **amniotic sac**, a membranous sac which provides protection to the fetus.

The **placenta** is a temporary organ for gas, nutrient and substance exchange between mother and fetus. This exchange is mediated by the **umbilical cord**, a structure developed from the fetal tissue. It contains one vein and two arteries, which carry oxygen and nutrients to the fetus and waste products away from it.

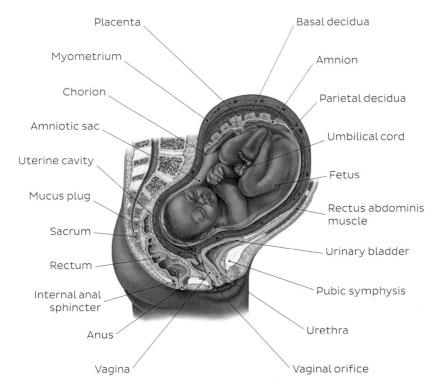

FIGURE 7.13. Fetus in utero. While in the uterus, the fetus is surrounded by a thin double layered membrane called the **amniotic sac**. The inner layer (closer to the fetus) is also known as the **amnion**, while the outer layer (closer to the uterus) is also known as the **chorion**. The amniotic sac is filled with amniotic fluid that surrounds and bathes the fetus during development.

The fetus is connected to the placenta via the **umbilical cord**. The umbilical cord has two **umbilical arteries** that carry the deoxygenated blood from the fetus. In contrast, a single **umbilical vein** carries oxygenated blood, rich in nutrients from the mother to the fetus.

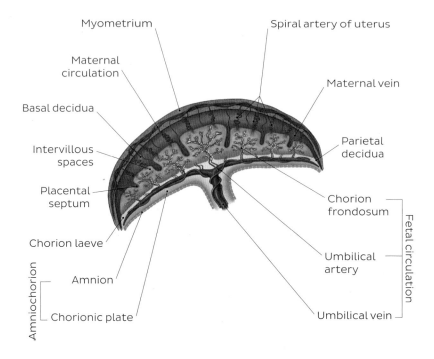

FIGURE 7.14. **Cross-section of the placenta.** At the beginning of the fetal period, the placenta has two components: A **fetal portion**, formed by the chorion frondosum, and a **maternal portion**, formed by the decidua basalis. On the fetal side, the placenta is bordered by the **chorionic plate**. On its maternal side, it is bordered by the **basal decidua**.

The placenta is the meeting point of two circulatory systems: Fetal circulation and maternal circulation. The maternal component of the placenta contains **maternal arteries** and **veins** that feed into the intervillous spaces. On the opposite side, the **umbilical arteries** and **veins** form a tree-like structure within the intervillous space. Here, the fetal and maternal blood comes into close contact separated only by a thin membrane, called the **placental membrane**.

Key points about the placenta	
Definition	The placenta is a highly specialized, temporary organ that develops as a conduit between maternal and fetal tissues.
Portions	**Fetal portion**: chorion frondosum **Maternal portion**: basal decidua
Functions	Exchange of metabolic and gaseous products between maternal and fetal bloodstreams, production of hormones.

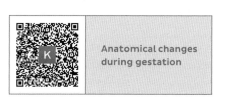

Anatomical changes
during gestation

Embryology 1st week
of development

PELVIS AND
PERINEUM

INTRODUCTION TO THE MALE PELVIC CAVITY

The **male pelvic cavity** is a basin-shaped space formed by bony and musculoligamentous pelvic walls and floor. It contains several organs from the digestive, reproductive and urinary systems, some of which pass into the perineum. These include:

- Terminal part of the sigmoid colon, which continues distally as the rectum
- A pair of seminal vesicles, ductus deferens and the prostate
- Pelvic part of the ureters and urinary bladder

The organs are surrounded by **pelvic visceral fascia** and have the parietal peritoneum of the abdominal cavity reflecting onto their superior surfaces, forming **pouches** in between adjacent organs. The **pelvic floor** is formed by the levator ani and coccygeus muscles (collectively known as the pelvic diaphragm) which separate the pelvic cavity above from the perineum below.

The male pelvic cavity is supplied by various branches of the internal iliac arteries, the superior [ano]rectal artery and the median sacral artery. The organs within the pelvic cavity are innervated by various visceral plexuses that carry both sympathetic and parasympathetic fibers as well as visceral afferent fibers which generally carry pain sensation to the central nervous system.

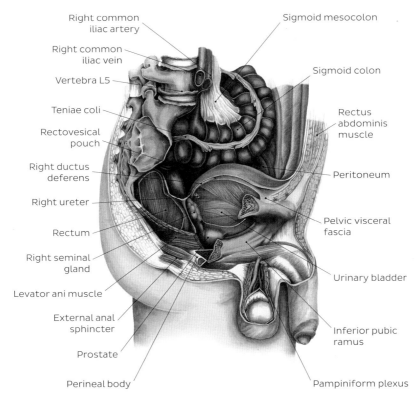

FIGURE 7.15. Male pelvis and perineum (parasagittal section). Parasagittal section of the male pelvis and perineum (right view) with parts of the right pelvic wall and fascia removed to show the relations

of the male pelvic organs. The **urinary bladder** (depicted as full of urine) is located anteriorly within the pelvic cavity, posterior to the pubic bone. The **prostate** sits immediately inferior to the urinary bladder. The terminal part of the **sigmoid colon** continues distally as the rectum, both of which are located in the posterior aspect of the pelvic cavity, anterior to the sacrum and coccyx. The **pelvic part of the ureter**, **ductus deferens** and **seminal vesicle** are centrally located in the image, between the urinary bladder and the rectum.

Key points about the male pelvic cavity	
Walls and floors	**Bones**: hip bone (ilium, ischium, pubis), sacrum, coccyx
	Ligaments: sacroiliac, sacrospinous, and sacrotuberous
	Muscles: levator ani, coccygeus, piriformis, obturator internus
Digestive organs	**Organs**: sigmoid colon, rectum
	Functions: absorption of minerals, vitamins, water and electrolytes, temporary storage of fecal matter and elimination during defecation
Reproductive organs	**Organs**: prostate, seminal vesicles, ductus deferens
	Functions: secretion of protein and nutrient rich fluid that contributes to volume of semen, transport of semen
Urinary organs	**Organs**: pelvic part of ureter, urinary bladder
	Functions: transport and elimination of urine from from the body
Peritoneal pouches	Rectovesical pouch (between the rectum and urinary bladder)
Blood supply	**Internal iliac artery**: superior vesical arteries, inferior vesical artery, internal pudendal artery, middle [ano]rectal artery
	Superior [ano]rectal artery (from inferior mesenteric artery)
	Median sacral artery (from aortic bifurcation)
Innervation	**Sympathetic**: lumbar splanchnic nerves, hypogastric and pelvic plexuses
	Parasympathetic: pelvic splanchnic nerves, left and right inferior hypogastric plexuses, and rectal (pelvic) plexus

 Pelvis and perineum

 Male reproductive organs

TESTIS AND EPIDIDYMIS

The **testes** (sing. testis) are the male gonads which are composed of lobules containing convoluted seminiferous tubules, where sperm production (**spermatogenesis**) occurs. Supporting cells within the testes secrete hormones, primarily androgens such as **testosterone**. The testes reside within connective tissue layers known as the tunica albuginea and tunica vaginalis which are further enveloped by the layers of the spermatic cord.

Efferent ductules from the testis join to form the **epididymis** (pl. epididymides). These ductules unite within the head and body of the epididymis to form a single duct in the tail of the epididymis before becoming the ductus (or vas) deferens. Within the lumens of the ductules in the epididymis, sperm maturation is completed, although they remain immotile.

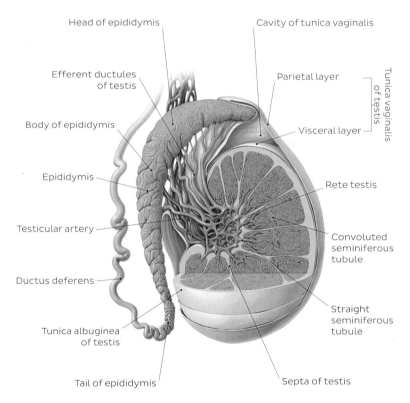

FIGURE 7.16. Lateral view of testis, epididymis and ductus deferens (removed from scrotum). A section of the testis and surrounding connective tissue layers has been removed in order to visualize the internal structure of the testis.

The **convoluted seminiferous tubules** form the bulk of the testis and converge to become the **straight seminiferous tubules** as they approach the hilum, where they form the **rete testis**. The efferent ductules arise from the rete testis and converge to form the **head** and **body of the epididymis**.

The ductules continue to unite within the epididymis, forming a single duct, known as the tail of the epididymis, which continues as the **ductus deferens**. The testis is enveloped by the **tunica vaginalis** and the **tunica albuginea**. The tunica vaginalis has two layers: A visceral layer and parietal layer between which is a potential space known as the **cavity of the tunica vaginalis**. The tunica albuginea envelopes only the testis while the tunica vaginalis envelops the testes and much of the epididymis.

Key points about testis and epididymis	
Testis	**Contents**: lobules, septa, mediastinum of testis, seminiferous tubules (convoluted/straight), rete testis, efferent ductules.
	Coverings: tunica vaginalis (composed of parietal and visceral layers), tunica albuginea, tunica vasculosa.
	Functions: production of sperm, hormone production and secretion.
Epididymis	**Location**: overlies superoposterior aspect of testis.
	Structure: formed by efferent ductules from testis → join together in head and body → become single duct in tail → continues as ductus deferens.
	Function: maturation of sperm.

 Testes

 Epididymis

 Neurovascular supply of the testes

 Ductus defererns

SCROTUM AND SPERMATIC CORD

The **scrotum** is a cutaneous fibromuscular sac composed of thin, pigmented skin and multiple layers of fascia and smooth muscle. The structures contained in the scrotal sac are the testes, epididymis, and lower parts of the spermatic cord. The **function** of the scrotum is to facilitate the positioning of the testes external to the pelvis. This is fundamental for maintaining the **optimal temperature for spermatogenesis**, which is several degrees below normal body temperature.

The testis is suspended in the scrotum by the **spermatic cord**. The spermatic cord is a collection of vessels, nerves, and ducts surrounded by muscle and fascia, that run to and from the testis. Its component layers arise from the deep inguinal ring and inguinal canal, ultimately exiting at the superficial inguinal ring to terminate in the scrotum, at the posterior aspect of the testis. The fascial coverings of the spermatic cord are derived from the anterior abdominal wall, which is explained as the testes 'dragging' the layers of the abdominal wall during their descent into the scrotum during fetal life. Each testis resides in its own compartment, which are separated by a vertical fibrous scrotal septum.

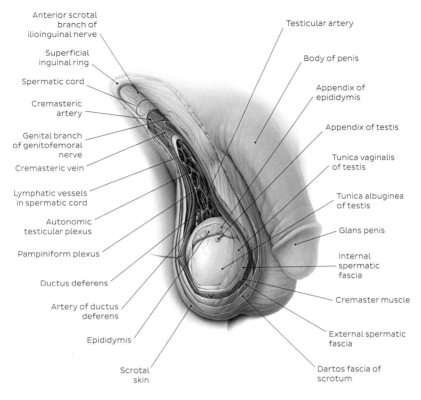

Anterior scrotal branch of ilioinguinal nerve
Superficial inguinal ring
Spermatic cord
Cremasteric artery
Genital branch of genitofemoral nerve
Cremasteric vein
Lymphatic vessels in spermatic cord
Autonomic testicular plexus
Pampiniform plexus
Ductus deferens
Artery of ductus deferens
Epididymis
Scrotal skin

Testicular artery
Body of penis
Appendix of epididymis
Appendix of testis
Tunica vaginalis of testis
Tunica albuginea of testis
Glans penis
Internal spermatic fascia
Cremaster muscle
External spermatic fascia
Dartos fascia of scrotum

FIGURE 7.17. Scrotum and spermatic cord. The **scrotum** consists of several layers: Skin, dartos fascia (with dartos muscle), external spermatic fascia, cremasteric fascia (with cremaster muscle) and internal spermatic fascia. The internal spermatic fascia is loosely attached to the parietal layer of tunica vaginalis of the testis.

Structures in the **spermatic cord** include the ductus deferens, artery to ductus deferens, testicular artery, pampiniform plexus, cremasteric artery and vein, genital branch of the genitofemoral nerve, autonomic testicular plexus and lymphatic vessels. The fascial coverings of the spermatic cord are the internal spermatic fascia, cremasteric fascia (with cremaster muscle), and external spermatic fascia.

Key points about the scrotum	
Contents	Testes, epididymis, lower parts of spermatic cords
Layers	Skin, dartos fascia (dartos muscle), external spermatic fascia, cremasteric fascia (cremaster muscle) and internal spermatic fascia
Function	Maintains optimal temperature for spermatogenesis

Key points about the spermatic cord	
Contents	Ductus deferens, artery to ductus deferens, testicular artery, pampiniform plexus (testicular veins), cremasteric artery and vein, genital branch of the genitofemoral nerve, autonomic testicular plexus, and lymphatic vessels
Coverings	Internal spermatic fascia, cremasteric fascia (cremaster muscle), external spermatic fascia
Function	Contains structures running to and from the testis; suspends the testis in the scrotum

PELVIS AND PERINEUM

Scrotum

 Male reproductive organs

URINARY BLADDER AND URETHRA

The **urinary bladder** is a hollow distensible muscular organ which functions to temporarily store urine. When empty, the urinary bladder is shaped like a pyramid and lies entirely within the lesser pelvis. As the bladder begins to fill, it becomes ovoid and expands in an upward direction to occupy a part of the greater pelvis.

Both male and female urinary bladders consist of **four parts** (apex, body, fundus and neck) and **three surfaces** (superior surface and two inferolateral surfaces). Extending from the neck of the bladder in both sexes is the urethra. The differences between the male and female bladders are within their respective relations with other pelvic organs. The urethrae, however, have major structural differences.

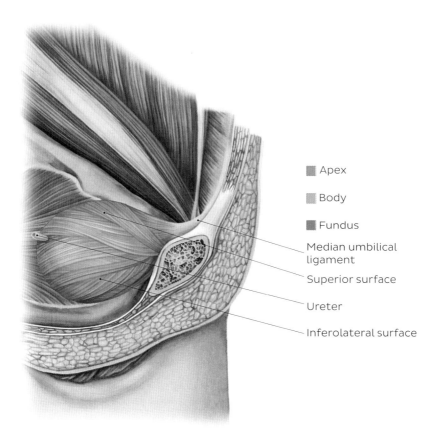

Apex

Body

Fundus

Median umbilical ligament

Superior surface

Ureter

Inferolateral surface

FIGURE 7.18. **Urinary bladder (lateral view).** Urinary bladder shown full of urine, within the female pelvis. Three out of four main parts of the bladder are shown: The apex, body and fundus. The fourth part, the neck of bladder, is not visible on this image as it extends from the undersurface of the bladder. The bladder is held in place by the median umbilical ligament.

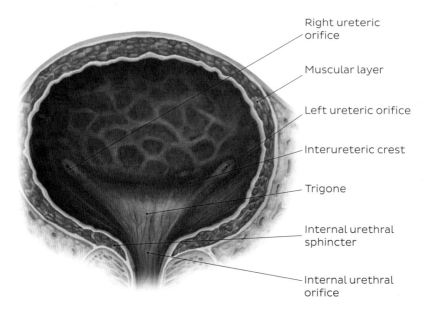

Right ureteric orifice

Muscular layer

Left ureteric orifice

Interureteric crest

Trigone

Internal urethral sphincter

Internal urethral orifice

FIGURE 7.19. Urinary bladder (coronal section). This section displays several main internal features of the urinary bladder, such as the trigone, left and right ureteric orifices and interureteric crest. The **trigone** is a triangular area of the bladder between the left and right ureteric orifices and internal urethral orifice. This region is particularly sensitive to the increase of pressure resulting from the urine accumulation and retention. Urine is delivered to the kidneys via the ureters which empty into the organ via the **ureteric orifices**. A slightly curved ridge called the **interureteric crest** connects the two orifices, at the same time defining the upper margin of the trigone of the bladder.

MALE URINARY BLADDER AND URETHRA

The **male urinary bladder** is located just inferior to the peritoneum and lies anterior to the rectum, anterosuperior to the prostate and posterior to the pubic symphysis.

The **male urethra** is a roughly 20 cm long tube and extends from the internal urethral orifice at the neck of the bladder to the external urethral orifice of the glans penis. From proximal to distal, it is divided into intramural/preprostatic, prostatic, membranous and spongy parts and features openings for prostatic fluid, semen from the testes and excretions of the bulbourethral glands.

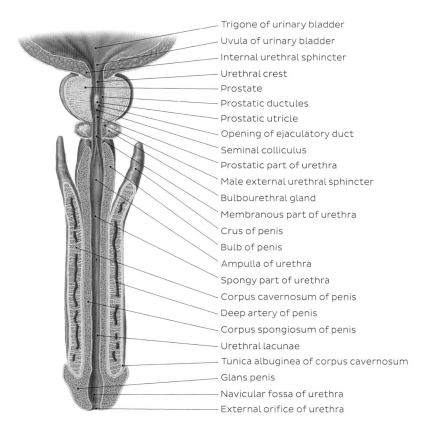

Trigone of urinary bladder
Uvula of urinary bladder
Internal urethral sphincter
Urethral crest
Prostate
Prostatic ductules
Prostatic utricle
Opening of ejaculatory duct
Seminal colliculus
Prostatic part of urethra
Male external urethral sphincter
Bulbourethral gland
Membranous part of urethra
Crus of penis
Bulb of penis
Ampulla of urethra
Spongy part of urethra
Corpus cavernosum of penis
Deep artery of penis
Corpus spongiosum of penis
Urethral lacunae
Tunica albuginea of corpus cavernosum
Glans penis
Navicular fossa of urethra
External orifice of urethra

FIGURE 7.20. **Penis and male urethra.** Longitudinal section through the male urogenital tract showing the structural components of the penis and the male urethra. Urine enters the **intramural/preprostatic part** of the male urethra through the internal urethral sphincter and is transported towards the external urethral orifice at the end of the glans penis. Prostatic fluid enters the prostatic part of the urethra via the **prostatic ductules** and semen from the testes via the opening of the **ejaculatory duct**. Bulbourethral glands secrete lubricating mucus into the spongy part of the urethra just proximal to the ampulla and navicular fossa of the urethra.

Key points about the male urinary bladder	
Surfaces	Superior, left inferolateral and right inferolateral
Parts	Apex, body, fundus and neck
Lining/wall	Peritoneum (superior surface only), pelvic visceral fascia Bladder wall: serosa (reflection of peritoneum), detrusor vesicae muscle, subserosa and mucosa
Internal features	Right ureteral orifice, left ureteral orifice, interureteric crest, trigone, uvula of bladder, internal urethral orifice
Neurovascular supply	**Arterial**: superior vesical artery, inferior vesical artery **Venous**: vesical venous plexus (vesical veins) **Nerve**: vesical plexus, inferior hypogastric plexus
Surrounding structures and spaces	**Superior**: pelvic visceral fascia, peritoneal membrane, sigmoid colon **Anterior**: retropubic space, pubic symphysis **Posterior**: seminal gland, rectoprostatic fascia, rectovesical pouch, rectum **Inferior**: prostate, levator ani muscle

Key points about the male urethra	
Begins	Internal urethral orifice (of urinary bladder)
Ends	External urethral orifice (glans penis)
Parts	Preprostatic/intramural part, prostatic part (crest of urethra, prostatic ducts, seminal colliculus, opening of ejaculatory ducts), membranous part and spongy part (bulbourethral glands, ampulla of urethra, navicular fossa)
Neurovascular supply	**Arterial**: inferior vesical artery, artery of bulb of penis **Venous**: prostatic venous plexus **Nerve**: prostatic plexus, pudendal nerve
Surrounding structures	Prostate, external urethral sphincter, corpus spongiosum, bulbospongiosus muscle, corpus cavernosum

Urinary bladder and urethra

Development of the urinary system

PELVIS AND PERINEUM

FEMALE URINARY BLADDER AND URETHRA

The **female urinary bladder** is located posterior to the pubic symphysis in the retropubic space and lies just anterior to the vagina. Similar to its male counterpart, the female urinary bladder has three **surfaces**: A superior surface and two inferolateral surfaces. It consists of four distinct **parts**: Apex, body, fundus and neck of the urinary bladder.

The **female urethra**, which is much shorter than that found in males, extends from the neck of the urinary bladder at the internal urethral orifice and measures approximately 5 cm in length.

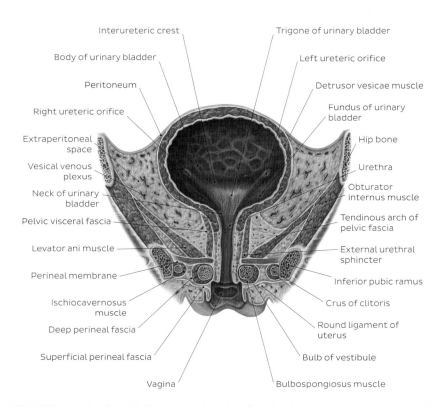

FIGURE 7.21. Female urinary bladder. A coronal section of the female urinary bladder and urethra. This section displays the body, fundus and neck of the bladder as well as the main internal features of the urinary bladder: The trigone, left and right ureteric orifices and interureteric crest of the urinary bladder. The female urethra begins as a continuation of the neck of the bladder at the internal urethral orifice and terminates as the external orifice of the female urethra. The urethra is located just anterior to the vagina and is surrounded by the external urethral sphincter along its proximal two-thirds. Distally, it is encircled by a muscular sling formed by the compressor urethrae muscle as well as the urethrovaginal sphincter (not shown).

Key points about the female urinary bladder	
Surfaces	Superior, left inferolateral and right inferolateral
Parts	Apex, body, fundus and neck
Lining/wall	Peritoneum (superior surface only), pelvic visceral fascia
	Bladder wall: serosa (reflection of peritoneum), detrusor vesicae muscle and mucosa
Internal features	Right ureteric orifice, left ureteric orifice, interureteric crest, trigone and internal urethral orifice
Neurovascular supply	**Arterial**: superior vesical artery, vaginal artery
	Venous: vesical venous plexus (vesical veins)
	Nerve: vesical plexus, inferior hypogastric plexus
Surrounding structures and spaces	**Superior**: pelvic visceral fascia, peritoneal membrane and sigmoid colon
	Anterior: retropubic space and pubic symphysis
	Posterior: vesicouterine pouch and vagina
	Inferior: pelvic diaphragm

Key points about the female urethra	
Begins	Internal urethral orifice of urinary bladder
Ends	External urethral orifice [vestibule of vagina]
Neurovascular supply	**Arterial**: internal pudendal artery, vaginal artery
	Venous: vesical venous plexus (vesical veins)
	Nerve: vesical plexus, pudendal nerve
Surrounding structures	Pelvic diaphragm, external urethral sphincter, compressor urethrae, sphincter urethrovaginalis, perineal membrane, and urethral glands

Development of the urinary system

Urethral sphincters

PENIS

The **penis** is a male external genital organ which functions as part of the reproductive and urinary systems. It becomes erect to facilitate sexual intercourse, acts as a conduit for the passage of semen and facilitates the transport of urine from the urinary bladder to the external environment.

From proximal to distal, the penis consists of a root, body and glans which are composed of 3 erectile bodies: Two bilateral **corpora cavernosa** and one median **corpus spongiosum**.

- The **root** of the penis is made up of the bulb of the penis (proximal expanded part of the corpus spongiosum), the crura (sing.: Crus, proximal tapering parts of the corpora cavernosa which are fixed to the ischiopubic rami) which are surrounded by the bulbospongiosus and ischiocavernosus muscles, respectively.
- The **body** of the penis consists of the free portions of the corpus spongiosum (which contains the urethra), located ventrally, and corpora cavernosa found on the dorsolateral aspect of the penis.
- The **glans penis** is formed by the bulbous extension of the corpus spongiosum distally.

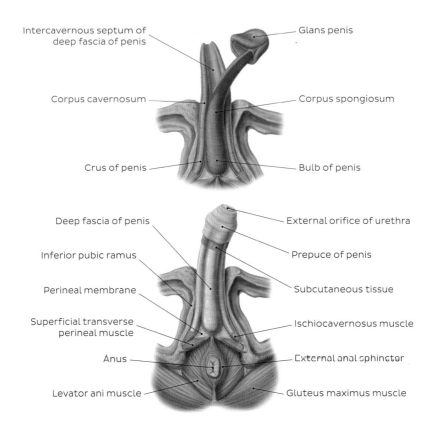

Intercavernous septum of deep fascia of penis

Glans penis

Corpus cavernosum

Corpus spongiosum

Crus of penis

Bulb of penis

Deep fascia of penis

External orifice of urethra

Inferior pubic ramus

Prepuce of penis

Perineal membrane

Subcutaneous tissue

Superficial transverse perineal muscle

Ischiocavernosus muscle

Anus

External anal sphincter

Levator ani muscle

Gluteus maximus muscle

FIGURE 7.22. Penis (inferior view). The **root** forms the fixed or anchored portion of the penis, while the **body** and **glans** forms the free, pendulous part. The **bulb** of the penis, which consists of the proximal portion of the corpus spongiosum, lies firmly anchored to the perineal membrane/body, while the **crura** of the penis are fixed to the ischiopubic rami of the pelvic girdle.

The penis is further stabilized by the **suspensory** and **fundiform ligaments** (not seen in this image). Enveloping the bulb and crura of the penis are the **bulbospongiosus** (removed) and **ischiocavernosus muscles**. These muscles aid in emptying the urethra and stabilizing the erect penis. Surrounding the structure of the penis and erectile tissues is the deep and superficial fascia/subcutaneous tissue of the penis. The **deep fascia** lies just superficial to the tunica albuginea of the penis and surrounds all three erectile tissues. As its name suggests, the **superficial fascia** is located most superficially and is continuous with the superficial fascia/subcutaneous tissue of the perineum (Colles' fascia).

Key points about the penis	
Parts	**Root**: bulb of penis, crura, ischiocavernosus muscles, bulbospongiosus muscle
	Body: distal parts of corpora cavernosa and corpus spongiosum
	Glans: neck and corona of glans
Erectile bodies	Corpora cavernosa (x2), corpus spongiosum (x1)
Fasciae	Tunica albuginea, deep fascia of penis (Buck's fascia) and superficial fascia/subcutaneous tissue of penis (Colles' fascia)
Ligaments	Suspensory and fundiform ligaments
Functions	**Reproductive**: becomes erect to facilitate sexual intercourse
	Urinary: passage of urine from urinary bladder to external environment

PELVIS AND PERINEUM

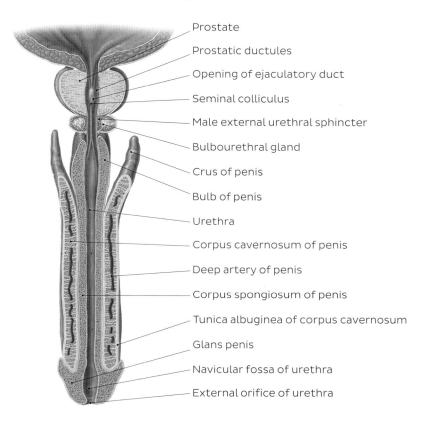

Prostate

Prostatic ductules

Opening of ejaculatory duct

Seminal colliculus

Male external urethral sphincter

Bulbourethral gland

Crus of penis

Bulb of penis

Urethra

Corpus cavernosum of penis

Deep artery of penis

Corpus spongiosum of penis

Tunica albuginea of corpus cavernosum

Glans penis

Navicular fossa of urethra

External orifice of urethra

FIGURE 7.23. Penis. Longitudinal cross-section of the male urogenital tract showing the structural components of the penis and male urethra. The **spongy part** of the male urethra is surrounded in its entirety by corpus spongiosum. The distal portions of the corpus spongiosum and corpora cavernosa form the body of the penis. The head of the penis, known as the **glans** penis is formed by the distal expansion of the corpus spongiosum as it wraps around the ends of the corpora cavernosa.

The base of the glans projects posteriorly, forming a rounded margin known as the **corona** of the glans which overhangs a groove known as the neck of the glans. This forms the boundary between the body and glans penis. Located at the tip of the glans is the opening for the spongy urethra, the **external urethral orifice**.

Male reproductive organs

The male urethra

FEMALE PERINEUM

The **perineum** is a diamond shaped compartment which sits just inferior to the pelvic cavity, forming the lowest portion of the trunk in the human body.

The female perineum is bounded superiorly (internally) by the **pelvic dia-phragm** and inferiorly (externally) by the **perineal skin** and **fascia**. It is occupied by muscles, erectile and cavernous tissues which facilitate excretion, egestion and reproduction. A transverse line, known as the **interischial line**, stretches between the two ischial tuberosities dividing the perineum into two regions:

- The **urogenital triangle**, which is located anteriorly, is further subdivided by the perineal membrane into superficial and deep perineal spaces. The female urogenital triangle contains muscles, fasciae, erectile tissues and spaces associated with the female urogenital system. It also functions as an anchor-ing point for the external female genitalia.
- The **anal triangle**, located posteriorly, houses the anal canal and the internal and external anal sphincters. These are all surrounded by a fat-filled space known as the ischioanal fossa.

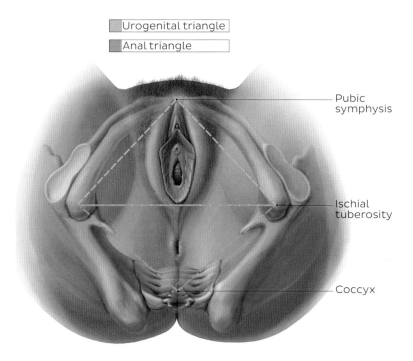

Urogenital triangle
Anal triangle

Pubic symphysis

Ischial tuberosity

Coccyx

FIGURE 7.24. Female perineum (inferior view). The image demonstrates the boundaries of the perineum represented by imaginary lines that connect the pubic symphysis, ischial tuberosities and coccyx. A transverse line that extends between the two ischial tuberosities divides the perineum into the **urogenital** (anterior) and **anal** (posterior) triangles.

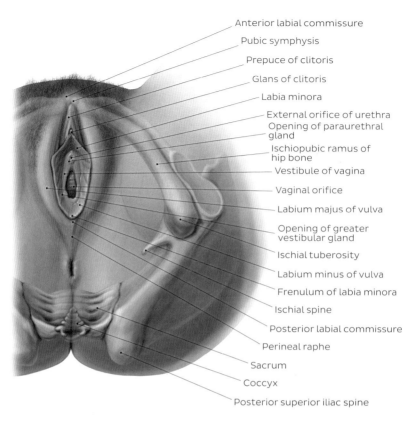

Anterior labial commissure
Pubic symphysis
Prepuce of clitoris
Glans of clitoris
Labia minora
External orifice of urethra
Opening of paraurethral gland
Ischiopubic ramus of hip bone
Vestibule of vagina
Vaginal orifice
Labium majus of vulva
Opening of greater vestibular gland
Ischial tuberosity
Labium minus of vulva
Frenulum of labia minora
Ischial spine
Posterior labial commissure
Perineal raphe
Sacrum
Coccyx
Posterior superior iliac spine

FIGURE 7.25. **Surface anatomy of the female perineum.** An overview of the borders and external features of the female perineum in the lithotomy position. The female perineum is bordered by the **pubic symphysis** anteriorly, the **ischiopubic rami** anterolaterally, the **sacrotuberous ligaments** posterolaterally and the **sacrum** and **coccyx** posteriorly.

Visible in this illustration is the surface anatomy of the female **urogenital triangle** that is defined by the vulva. The **vulva** represents the external female genitalia that include the mons pubis, labia majora, labia minora, clitoris, vestibule of the vagina, vaginal orifice and external orifice of the urethra. Posterior to the urogenital triangle is the **anal triangle**, containing the **anal aperture**. Not visible in this illustration are the internal structures of the female perineum which include the female urethra, vaginal canal, anal canal, perineal muscles and fascia.

Key points about the female perineum	
Borders	**Internal (roof):** pelvic diaphragm (levator ani and coccygeus muscles)
	External (floor): fascia and skin
	Anterior: pubic symphysis
	Posterior: sacrum and coccyx
	Anterolateral: ischiopubic rami
	Posterolateral: sacrotuberous ligaments
Divisions	1. Urogenital triangle (deep perineal space and superficial perineal space)
	2. Anal triangle
	Divided by: interischial line
	Structures between triangles: perineal body and perineal raphe

PELVIS AND PERINEUM

Key points about the urogenital triangle	
Boundaries	**Superiorly**: pelvic diaphragm (levator ani and coccygeus muscles) **Inferiorly**: fascia and skin **Anteriorly**: pubic symphysis **Posteriorly**: interischial line **Laterally**: ischiopubic rami and ischial tuberosities
Divisions	Deep perineal space and superficial perineal space
Layers and contents	From deep to superficial: 1. Inferior fascia of pelvic diaphragm 2. Deep perineal space: deep transverse perineal muscle, compressor urethrae muscle, sphincter urethrovaginalis muscle, external urethral sphincter, parts of urethra and vagina and anterior recess of the ischioanal fossa 3. Perineal membrane 4. Superficial perineal space: crus of clitoris, ischiocavernosus muscle, bulb of vestibule, bulbospongiosus muscle 5. Fascia: perineal fascia and subcutaneous tissue of perineum
Surface anatomy	Mons pubis, labium majus of vulva, anterior labial commissure, posterior labial commissure, cleft of vulva, labium minus of vulva, glans of clitoris, vestibule of vagina (external urethral orifice, opening of paraurethral glands and vaginal orifice)

Key points about the anal triangle	
Boundaries	**Superiorly**: pelvic diaphragm (levator ani and coccygeus muscles) **Inferiorly**: fascia and skin **Anteriorly**: interischial line **Posteriorly**: coccyx and sacrum **Laterally**: sacrotuberous ligament and ischial tuberosities
Contents	External anal sphincter, internal anal sphincter, anal canal, anal aperture, anococcygeal ligament and ischioanal fossa

 External female genitalia

 Female reproductive organs

NEUROVASCULATURE OF THE FEMALE PERINEUM

The main neurovascular structures of the female perineum emerge from the **pudendal canal** and include the internal pudendal artery and vein, and the pudendal nerve.

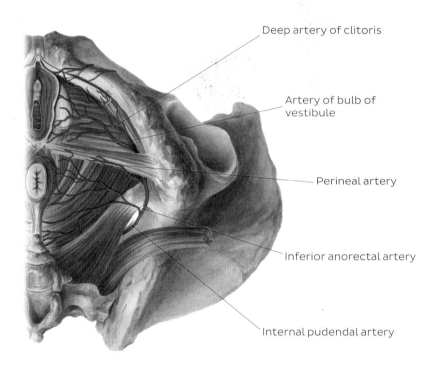

Deep artery of clitoris

Artery of bulb of vestibule

Perineal artery

Inferior anorectal artery

Internal pudendal artery

FIGURE 7.26. Arteries of the female perineum (inferior view). The **internal pudendal artery** is the main artery supplying the structures of the female perineum. It gives off four branches: The inferior [ano]rectal and perineal artery, the artery of vestibular bulb and the deep artery of clitoris.

Key points about the arteries of the female perineum	
Main artery	Internal pudendal artery
Branches	Inferior [ano]rectal artery, perineal artery, artery of vestibular bulb, deep artery of clitoris
Supply area	**Inferior [ano]rectal artery**: anal canal, internal and external anal sphincter, perianal skin
	Perineal artery: transverse perineal muscles, perineal body and posterior part of the labia
	Artery of vestibular bulb: vestibular bulb, erectile tissue of the vagina
	Deep artery of clitoris: corpus cavernosum of the clitoris

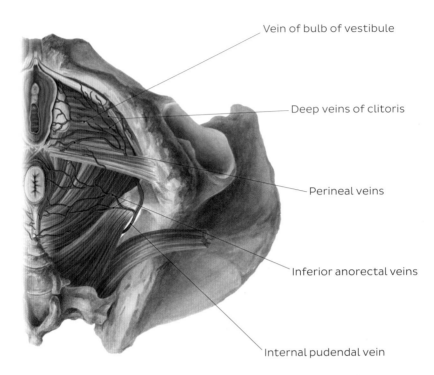

Vein of bulb of vestibule

Deep veins of clitoris

Perineal veins

Inferior anorectal veins

Internal pudendal vein

FIGURE 7.27. **Veins of the female perineum (inferior view).** The **internal pudendal vein** is the main vein draining the venous blood from the female perineum. The venous return is similar to the arterial homolog, as the internal pudendal vein receives the blood of all four sets of veins of the female perineum: The deep veins of clitoris, veins of vestibular bulb, perineal veins and the inferior [ano]rectal veins.

Key points about the veins of the female perineum	
Main vein	Internal pudendal vein
Branches	Deep veins of clitoris, veins of vestibular bulb, perineal veins, inferior [ano]rectal veins
Drainage area	**Deep veins of clitoris**: corpora cavernosa of the clitoris
	Veins of vestibular bulb: vestibular bulb, erectile tissue of vagina
	Perineal veins: transverse perineal muscles, perineal body, posterior part of the labia
	Inferior [ano]rectal veins: inferior part of the rectum

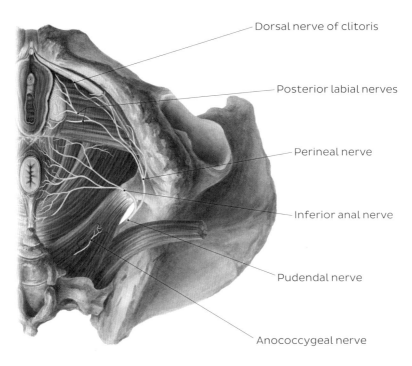

Dorsal nerve of clitoris

Posterior labial nerves

Perineal nerve

Inferior anal nerve

Pudendal nerve

Anococcygeal nerve

FIGURE 7.28. **Nerves of the female perineum (inferior view).** The **pudendal nerve** is the main nerve of the female perineum, providing sensory as well as motor innervation. It gives off the inferior anal nerve, dorsal nerve of clitoris and the perineal nerve.

Key points about the nerves of the female perineum	
Main nerve	Pudendal nerve
Branches	Inferior anal nerve, dorsal nerve of clitoris, perineal nerve (giving off posterior labial nerves)
Supply area	**Inferior anal nerve**: motor innervation to the external anal sphincter, sensory innervation to the skin of the anal canal inferior to the pectinate line
	Dorsal nerve of clitoris: sensory innervation to the corpus cavernosum of clitoris
	Perineal nerve: motor innervation to the superficial and deep perineal muscles (muscular branches), sensory innervation to the skin of the labia majora (posterior labial nerves)

Perineal region

Pelvis and perineum

SACRAL PLEXUS

The **sacral plexus** is a nerve network composed of the anterior rami of the spinal nerves L4-L5 (lumbosacral trunk) and spinal nerves S1-S4 which exit the vertebral column either through the lowest two intervertebral foramina or anterior sacral foramina. The plexus is located posterior to the internal iliac artery and vein and anterior to the piriformis muscle.

The numerous branches of the plexus can be divided into **posterior branches**, arising from the posterior divisions of the anterior rami, **anterior branches**, from the anterior division, and one **terminal branch**. The main function of the plexus is to innervate the majority of muscles of the hip and gluteal region, lower limbs, pelvis and perineum. Additionally, the sacral plexus provides sensory innervation to the lower limb except for the anterior, medial and lateral parts of the thigh. Due to its connection via the lumbosacral trunk, the sacral plexus is often described together with the lumbar plexus under a combined name **lumbosacral plexus**.

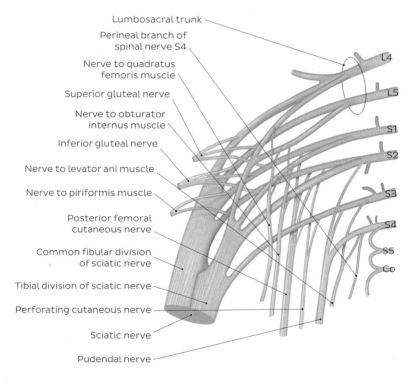

Lumbosacral trunk
Perineal branch of spinal nerve S4
Nerve to quadratus femoris muscle
Superior gluteal nerve
Nerve to obturator internus muscle
Inferior gluteal nerve
Nerve to levator ani muscle
Nerve to piriformis muscle
Posterior femoral cutaneous nerve
Common fibular division of sciatic nerve
Tibial division of sciatic nerve
Perforating cutaneous nerve
Sciatic nerve
Pudendal nerve

L4
L5
S1
S2
S3
S4
S5
Co

FIGURE 7.29. Sacral plexus. The spinal nerves L4—S5 are shown on the right hand side, each giving an anterior and a posterior ramus. The plexus is formed by the **anterior rami of the L4—S4** spinal nerves, while the S5 root joins the coccygeal (Co) root to form the coccygeal plexus.

The anterior rami of spinal nerves further split into **anterior** and **posterior divisions** and numerous branches arise from each division. They then join together to form the nerves of the sacral plexus, which can be divided into **anterior** and **posterior branches**. The anterior branches are the nerve to quadratus femoris, nerve to obturator internus, pudendal nerve, nerves to levator ani and coccygeus. The posterior branches are the nerve to piriformis, superior gluteal nerve, inferior gluteal nerve, posterior femoral cutaneous nerve, perforating cutaneous nerve and pelvic splanchnic nerves. Continuations of spinal nerves L4–S3 converge together to form a single **terminal branch,** known as the sciatic nerve. It splits into the tibial and common fibular nerves to supply structures of the thigh, leg and foot.

Key points about the sacral plexus	
Origin	L4, L5, S1, S2, S3, S4
Branches	**Anterior branches**: nerve to quadratus femoris, nerve to obturator internus, pudendal nerve, nerves to levator ani and coccygeus
	Posterior branches: nerve to piriformis, superior gluteal nerve, inferior gluteal nerve, posterior femoral cutaneous nerve, perforating cutaneous nerve, pelvic splanchnic nerves
	Terminal branch: sciatic nerve (divides into tibial and common fibular nerves)
Function	Motor and sensory innervation to the posterior thigh, leg, foot and part of the pelvis
Mnemonic for main branches	Superior gluteal nerve, inferior gluteal nerve, posterior cutaneous nerve of thigh, pudendal nerve, sciatic nerve (SIPPS)

Sacral plexus

The sciatic nerve

NERVES OF THE MALE PELVIS

The nervous supply to the male pelvis includes both **somatic innervation** (motor and sensory) of the skin and skeletal muscles, and **autonomic (visceral) innervation** of the pelvic organs and glands.

Somatic innervation to the male pelvis stems from the lumbar, sacral and coccygeal plexuses. The nerves that arise from these plexuses, including the pudendal nerve, scrotal nerves, and dorsal penis nerve, provide innervation to the muscles of the pelvis and skin of the penis and scrotum.

Autonomic innervation is provided by both sympathetic and parasympathetic fibers. **Sympathetic** innervation stems from the lumbar and sacral splanchnic nerves, while the **parasympathetic** supply comes from the pelvic splanchnic nerves. These nerves and their branches form the superior and inferior hypogastric plexuses, which then divide into several smaller plexuses. Fibers from these plexuses innervate the blood vessels, glands and organs of the male pelvis including the rectum, urinary bladder, urethra, testis, epididymis, prostate, seminal and bulbourethral glands.

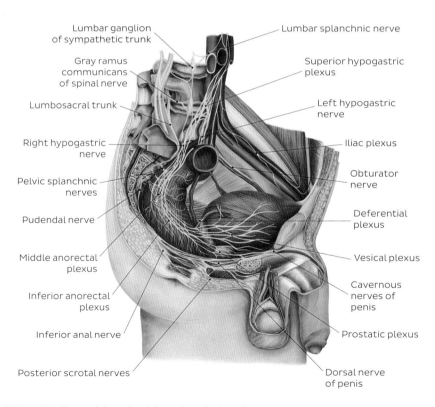

Lumbar ganglion of sympathetic trunk

Gray ramus communicans of spinal nerve

Lumbosacral trunk

Right hypogastric nerve

Pelvic splanchnic nerves

Pudendal nerve

Middle anorectal plexus

Inferior anorectal plexus

Inferior anal nerve

Posterior scrotal nerves

Lumbar splanchnic nerve

Superior hypogastric plexus

Left hypogastric nerve

Iliac plexus

Obturator nerve

Deferential plexus

Vesical plexus

Cavernous nerves of penis

Prostatic plexus

Dorsal nerve of penis

FIGURE 7.30. Nerves of the male pelvis (sagittal view). The **lumbar**, **sacral** and **coccygeal plexuses** give off several pelvic branches such as the obturator nerve, pudendal nerve, rectal nerves, scrotal nerves, and dorsal penis nerve. These nerves provide **motor** and **sensory innervation** to the muscles and skin of the pelvis.

PELVIS AND PERINEUM

Lumbar and sacral splanchnic nerves provide the pelvis with autonomic innervation via the superior hypogastric plexus. This plexus gives off the left and right hypogastric nerves that merge with the pelvic splanchnic nerves to form the inferior hypogastric plexus. The superior and inferior hypogastric plexus further divide into smaller plexuses, forming the[ano]rectal plexuses, vesical plexus, deferential plexus, and prostate plexus. These subplexuses provide autonomic innervation to the male pelvic viscera and glands including the rectum, urinary bladder, testis, epididymis, prostate and seminal glands.

Key points about innervation of the male pelvis	
Somatic innervation	Plexus: lumbar plexus, sacral plexus, coccygeal plexus.
	Nerves: obturator nerve, pudendal nerve, rectal nerves, scrotal nerves, dorsal nerve of penis.
	Function: sensory innervation of penis, scrotum, perineum; motoric innervation of muscles of the pelvis.
Autonomic innervation	Plexus: superior hypogastric plexus, inferior hypogastric plexus, rectal plexus, vesical plexus, deferential plexus, prostate plexus.
	Nerves: lumbar splanchnic nerves, sacral splanchnic nerves, hypogastric nerves, pelvic splanchnic nerves
	Function: sympathetic and parasympathetic innervation of rectum, urinary bladder, urethra, testis, epididymis, deferent duct, prostate, seminal and bulbourethral glands, corpora cavernosa of penis

Neurovascular supply of the pelvis

Male reproductive organs

NERVES OF THE FEMALE PELVIS

The nervous supply to the female pelvis involves both **somatic innervation** (motor and sensory) of the skin and skeletal muscle, and **autonomic (visceral) innervation** of the pelvic organs and glands.

Somatic innervation to the female pelvis stems from the lumbar, sacral and coccygeal plexus. The nerves arising from them provide sensory as well as motor innervation to the skin and muscles of the pelvis.

Autonomic innervation is provided by both sympathetic and parasympathetic nervous systems. **Sympathetic** innervation is carried by the lumbar and sacral splanchnic nerves, which go on to form the superior hypogastric plexus. **Parasympathetic** innervation is carried by the pelvic splanchnic nerves, which merge with a branch of the superior hypogastric plexus to form the inferior hypogastric plexus. These in turn divide into several smaller plexuses that are close to the target organs, collectively known as pelvic plexuses. Fibers from these plexuses innervate the blood vessels, glands and organs of the female pelvis.

PELVIS AND PERINEUM

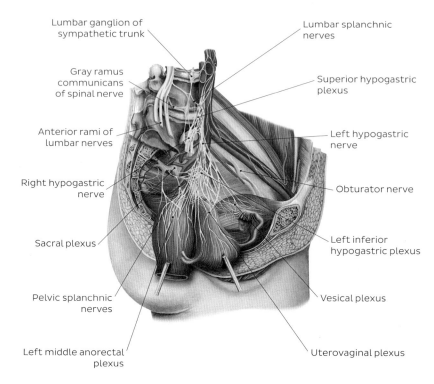

Lumbar ganglion of sympathetic trunk

Gray ramus communicans of spinal nerve

Anterior rami of lumbar nerves

Right hypogastric nerve

Sacral plexus

Pelvic splanchnic nerves

Left middle anorectal plexus

Lumbar splanchnic nerves

Superior hypogastric plexus

Left hypogastric nerve

Obturator nerve

Left inferior hypogastric plexus

Vesical plexus

Uterovaginal plexus

FIGURE 7.31. Nerves of the female pelvis (sagittal view). The **lumbar**, **sacral** and **coccygeal plexus** give off several pelvic branches such as the obturator nerve, pudendal nerve and anococcygeal nerves. These nerves provide **motor** and **sensory innervation** to the muscles of the pelvic floor and perineum.

Lumbar and **sacral splanchnic nerves** provide the pelvis with **autonomic innervation** via the **superior hypogastric plexus**. This plexus gives off the left and right hypogastric nerves that merge with the pelvic splanchnic nerves to form the **inferior hypogastric plexus**. The superior and inferior hypogastric plexus further divide into smaller plexuses, forming the vesical plexus, uterovaginal plexus and [ano]rectal plexuses.These subplexuses provide autonomic innervation to the female pelvic viscera, glands and blood vessels, including the rectum, urinary bladder, urethra, uterus, ovaries and vagina.

Key points about innervation of the female pelvis		
Somatic innervation	**Plexus**: lumbar plexus, sacral plexus, coccygeal plexus.
	Nerves: obturator nerve, pudendal nerve, anococcygeal nerves.
	Function: sensory innervation of vulva and perineum, motoric innervation of muscles of the pelvic floor.
Autonomic innervation	**Plexus**: superior hypogastric plexus, inferior hypogastric plexus, vesical plexus, uterovaginal plexus, rectal plexus.
	Nerves: lumbar splanchnic nerves, sacral splanchnic nerves, hypogastric nerves, pelvic splanchnic nerves.
	Function: sympathetic and parasympathetic innervation of rectum, vesica urinaria, urethra, uterus, ovaries, vagina.

Neurovascular supply of the pelvis

Female reproductive organs

BLOOD SUPPLY OF THE MALE PELVIS

The arterial blood supply of the male pelvis stems mainly from the **internal** and **external iliac arteries** which originate from the abdominal aorta via the common iliac artery.

The **external iliac artery** travels anteriorly, inferiorly and laterally in the pelvis giving off two branches before continuing its course to the thigh as the femoral artery: The inferior epigastric and deep circumflex iliac arteries. The **internal iliac artery** is the main artery of the pelvis and with its branches supplies the walls and viscera of the pelvis, reproductive organs, buttocks and the thigh. A notable *exception* are the testes (which are supplied by the testicular artery that arises directly from the abdominal aorta), and the rectum which is largely supplied by the superior [ano]rectal branch of the inferior mesenteric artery.

Venous drainage of the male pelvis generally follows a course similar to its arterial counterparts.

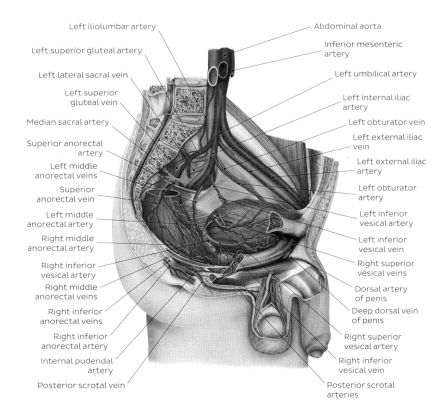

Left iliolumbar artery	Abdominal aorta
Left superior gluteal artery	Inferior mesenteric artery
Left lateral sacral vein	Left umbilical artery
Left superior gluteal vein	Left internal iliac artery
Median sacral artery	Left obturator vein
Superior anorectal artery	Left external iliac vein
Left middle anorectal veins	Left external iliac artery
Superior anorectal vein	Left obturator artery
Left middle anorectal artery	Left inferior vesical artery
Right middle anorectal artery	Left inferior vesical vein
Right inferior vesical artery	Right superior vesical veins
Right middle anorectal veins	Dorsal artery of penis
Right inferior anorectal veins	Deep dorsal vein of penis
Right inferior anorectal artery	Right superior vesical artery
Internal pudendal artery	Right inferior vesical vein
Posterior scrotal vein	Posterior scrotal arteries

FIGURE 7.32. Blood supply of the male pelvis (sagittal view). At the level of the sacroiliac joint, the bilateral common iliac artery bifurcates into the external and internal iliac arteries. The **external iliac artery** courses towards the thigh to continue as the femoral artery, whereas the **internal iliac artery** courses towards the greater sciatic foramen and gives off multiple branches to supply the pelvic wall and organs. These can be divided into an anterior and a posterior division.

PELVIS AND PERINEUM

Branches of the **posterior division** are the iliolumbar, superior gluteal and lateral sacral arteries. The **anterior division** gives off the obturator, umbilical, superior and inferior vesical, internal pudendal, middle [ano]rectal and inferior gluteal arteries.

The veins of the male pelvis collect blood from the urogenital organs and the rectum and drain into the **internal iliac vein** (or inferior mesenteric vein in the case of the superior [ano]rectal vein). From the internal iliac vein, the blood is transported to the common iliac vein and from there into the inferior vena cava. The right and left testicular veins drain directly to the **inferior vena cava** and **left renal vein**, respectively.

Key points about the arteries and veins of the male pelvis	
Internal iliac artery	**Supply area**: pelvic wall and organs, gluteal region and medial compartment of thigh (except for superior part of rectum – supplied via superior [ano]rectal branch of inferior mesenteric artery) **Branches**: · **Posterior division**: iliolumbar, superior gluteal, lateral sacral arteries · **Anterior division**: obturator, umbilical, superior and inferior vesical, internal pudendal, middle [ano]rectal and inferior gluteal arteries
External iliac artery	**Supply area**: lower limb, muscles and skin of the lower abdominal wall **Branches**: inferior epigastric, deep circumflex iliac arteries
Other arteries	Superior [ano]rectal artery (from inferior mesenteric artery); Testicular artery (from abdominal aorta)
Veins	Most veins drain to internal iliac vein → inferior vena cava **Exceptions**: · Superior [ano]rectal vein → inferior mesenteric vein · Right/left testicular veins → inferior vena cava/left renal vein

Male reproductive organs

Pelvis and perineum

PELVIS AND PERINEUM

BLOOD SUPPLY OF THE FEMALE PELVIS

The female pelvis receives the majority of its arterial supply from the **external** and **internal iliac arteries**, both of which originate from the common iliac artery.

A notable *exception* are the ovaries (as well as parts of the uterine tube/uterus) which are supplied by the **ovarian artery** that arises directly from the abdominal aorta and the rectum which is largely supplied by the superior [ano]rectal branch of the inferior mesenteric artery.

For the most part, **venous drainage** of the female pelvis follows a course similar to that of its arterial counterparts.

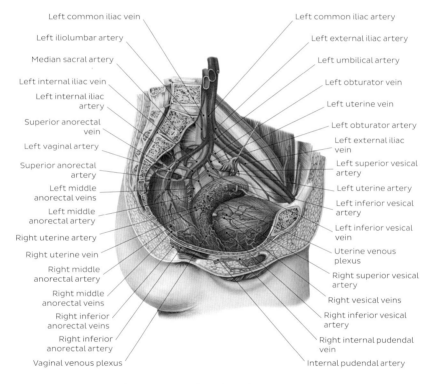

FIGURE 7.33. Blood supply of the female pelvis (sagittal view). At the level of the sacroiliac joint, the bilateral common iliac artery bifurcates into the external and internal iliac arteries. The **external iliac artery** courses towards the thigh to continue as the femoral artery, whereas the **internal iliac artery** gives off multiple branches to supply the pelvic wall and viscera. It can be divided into anterior and posterior divisions.

The branches of the **posterior division** are the iliolumbar, superior gluteal and lateral sacral arteries. The **anterior division** gives off the uterine, obturator, umbilical, vaginal, superior vesical, internal pudendal, middle [ano]rectal and inferior gluteal arteries.

The **veins** of the female pelvis collect blood from the urogenital organs and the rectum and drain into the **internal iliac vein** (or inferior mesenteric vein in the case of the superior [ano]rectal vein. From the internal iliac vein, the blood is transported to the common iliac vein and from there to the inferior vena cava. The **right** and **left ovarian veins** directly drain directly to the **inferior vena cava** and **left renal vein**, respectively.

Key points about the arteries and veins of the male pelvis	
Internal iliac artery	**Supply area**: pelvic wall and organs, gluteal region and medial compartment of thigh (except for superior part of rectum – supplied via superior [ano]rectal branch of inferior mesenteric artery) **Branches**: • **Posterior division**: iliolumbar, superior gluteal, lateral sacral arteries • **Anterior division**: uterine, obturator, umbilical, vaginal, superior vesical, internal pudendal, middle [ano]rectal and inferior gluteal arteries
External iliac artery	**Supply area**: lower limb, muscles and skin of the lower abdominal wall **Branches**: inferior epigastric, deep circumflex iliac arteries
Other arteries	Superior [ano]rectal artery (from inferior mesenteric artery); Ovarian artery (from abdominal aorta)
Veins	Most veins drain to internal iliac vein → inferior vena cava **Exceptions**: • Superior [ano]rectal vein → inferior mesenteric vein • Right/left ovarian veins → inferior vena cava/left renal vein

Arterial supply of the pelvis

Iliac artery

LYMPHATICS OF THE URINARY ORGANS

Lymphatic drainage of the urinary system, as occurs with many other systems, is carried out to **regional lymph nodes** found around its organs, which then drain into larger lymphatic vessels and more **central lymph node groups**.

The main lymphatic drainage routes of the urinary system are centered around the common, internal and external iliac lymph nodes, as well as the lumbar (aortic and caval) lymph nodes. These in turn drain into the left and right lumbar lymph trunks, which join together to form the cisterna chyli, which continues as the thoracic duct. In the case of the urinary bladder, lymph collected from this organ is drained to **paravesical** lymph nodes which feed into the larger groups mentioned above.

PELVIS AND
PERINEUM

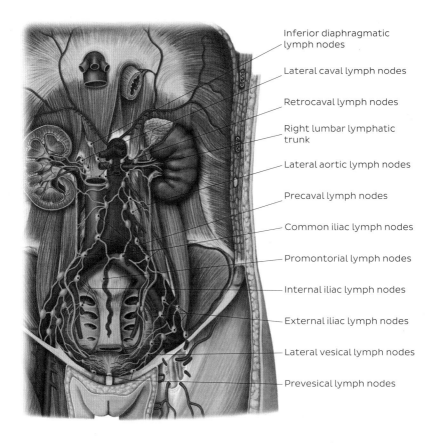

Inferior diaphragmatic lymph nodes

Lateral caval lymph nodes

Retrocaval lymph nodes

Right lumbar lymphatic trunk

Lateral aortic lymph nodes

Precaval lymph nodes

Common iliac lymph nodes

Promontorial lymph nodes

Internal iliac lymph nodes

External iliac lymph nodes

Lateral vesical lymph nodes

Prevesical lymph nodes

FIGURE 7.34. Lymph nodes of the urinary organs. Retroperitoneal compartment exposed, showing the urinary system (kidneys, ureters and urinary bladder), and the major abdominal and pelvic vessels. The main groups of pelvic lymph nodes of the pelvis and posterior abdominal wall can be seen. Lymph from the paravesical, common, internal and external lymph nodes ultimately converge to the **lumbar lymph nodes**. Those in turn drain to the left and right **lumbar lymph trunks**, which along with the intestinal lymph trunk converge to form the **cisterna chyli**.

Key points about the lymphatics of the urinary organs	
Kidney	Three plexuses of lymphatic vessels: parenchymal, subcapsular, perirenal fat; All three drain to lumbar (caval and aortic) lymph nodes.
Ureters	**Superior abdominal part**: lumbar lymph nodes **Inferior abdominal part**: common iliac lymph nodes **Pelvic part**: external iliac lymph nodes
Bladder	Lymph drains into paravesical (prevesical, lateral vesical and retrovesical) lymph nodes **Superolateral part**: common iliac lymph nodes **Fundus**: external and internal iliac lymph nodes
Urethra	Lymph drains to common, internal and external lymph nodes **Males**: the spongy part of urethra drains to prepubic lymph node and superomedial superficial inguinal lymph nodes before draining to external iliac lymph nodes

Lymphatics of abdomen and pelvis

Lymphatic vessels and nodes of the pelvis

LYMPHATICS OF THE MALE GENITALIA

There are five main groups of lymph nodes that lymph from the external and internal male genitalia drain to:

- The skin of the scrotal sac, perineum, skin of the penis, cavernous bodies of the penis, glans penis, and distal spongy urethra drain into the **superficial and deep inguinal lymph nodes**.
- The ductus deferens, ejaculatory ducts, bulbourethral glands, seminal glands, membranous and proximal spongy urethra, as well as the prostate drain into the **external iliac and internal iliac lymph nodes**. The external iliac lymph nodes also receive lymph drained via the inguinal nodes. Lymph then travels to the common iliac lymph nodes.
- Finally, the last major group draining the male genitalia of lymph are the **lumbar lymph nodes** (a.k.a. aorticocaval nodes). They drain lymph directly from the testes, epididymis, and proximal portion of the ductus deferentes while also receiving afferent vessels from the common iliac lymph nodes. Lymph then travels to the cisterna chyli.

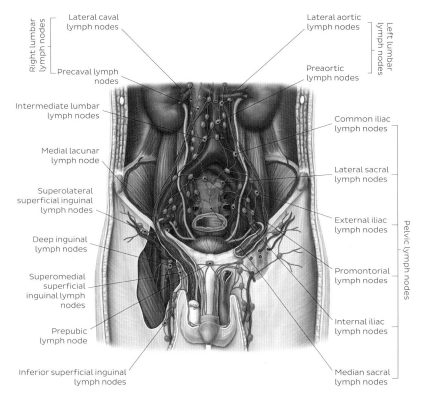

FIGURE 7.35. **Lymph nodes of the male genitalia.** The external male genitalia (skin of scrotum, penis) are primarily drained by the **superficial** and **deep inguinal lymph nodes.** Lymph from the inguinal nodes is then drained to the external iliac nodes, which in addition to the internal iliac nodes, also drain the internal male genitalia (prostate, seminal glands etc...)

The *exceptions* of this are the testes, epididymides and proximal ductus deferens which drain directly to the lumbar lymph nodes, via vessels along the testicular arteries.

Key points about the lymphatics of the male genitalia	
Superficial and deep inguinal lymph nodes	**Receive from**: skin of scrotal sac, perineum, skin of penis, cavernous bodies of penis, glans penis, distal spongy urethra. **Drain to**: external iliac lymph nodes
External and internal iliac lymph nodes	**Receive from**: ductus deferens, ejaculatory ducts, bulbourethral glands, seminal glands, membranous urethra, proximal spongy urethra, prostate. **Drain to**: common iliac lymph nodes
Lumbar lymph nodes	**Receive from**: testes, epididymis, ductus deferens, common iliac lymph nodes. **Drain to**: cisterna chyli

Lymphatic system

Lymphatics of abdomen and pelvis

LYMPHATICS OF THE FEMALE GENITALIA

The lymphatic drainage of the female reproductive organs is carried by the three major groups of lymph nodes:

- **Superficial** and **deep inguinal lymph** nodes drain the clitoris, skin of the vulva and vestibule of the vagina.
- **Internal** and **external iliac nodes** drain the remainder of vagina and part of the uterus. The external iliac nodes also receive lymph from the inguinal nodes. The **common iliac lymph nodes**, in turn, receive lymph from the internal and external iliac nodes.
- **Lumbar (aorticocaval) lymph nodes** directly receive lymph drained from much of the uterus and uterine tubes as well as the ovaries. They also drain lymph from the common iliac lymph nodes. Finally, lymph drained by the lumbar nodes is then carried to the cisterna chyli via the left and right lumbar lymphatic trunks.

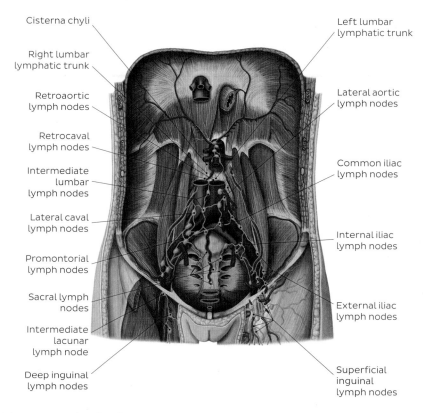

FIGURE 7.36. Lymph nodes of the female genitalia. Lymph drained from the ovaries, as well as much of the uterine tube and body of the uterus is drained by a number of collecting vessels which bypass the pelvic lymph nodes to empty directly into the ipsilateral **lumbar lymph nodes** (via a collateral pathway of the ovarian arteries).

Lymph from the cervix is largely drained to the **external iliac lymph nodes**, however collecting vessels from the lateral and posterior aspects of the cervix may drain to the **internal iliac** and/or **sacral lymph nodes**.

The upper half of the vagina is largely drained by the external iliac lymph nodes, while lymph drained from the lower half of the vagina (except the vestibule) is received by the internal iliac nodes. The vestibule of the vagina, as well as skin of the vulva is drained by collecting vessels which terminate in the **superficial inguinal lymph nodes**, while those of the clitoris are largely received by the **deep inguinal lymph nodes**.

From here the general pathway is as follows: Inguinal lymph nodes → iliac lymph nodes → lumbar lymph nodes → cisterna chyli.

Key points about the lymphatics of the female genitalia	
Superficial and deep inguinal lymph nodes	**Receive from**: clitoris, skin of the vulva and vestibule of vagina **Drain to**: external iliac lymph nodes
External and internal iliac lymph nodes	**Receive from**: vagina, uterus (partly), external iliac lymph nodes **Drain to**: common iliac lymph nodes
Lumbar lymph nodes	**Receive from**: ovaries, uterine tubes, uterus common iliac lymph nodes **Drain to**: cisterna chyli

Lymphatics of abdomen and pelvis

PELVIS AND PERINEUM

HEAD AND NECK

REGIONS OF THE HEAD AND FACE

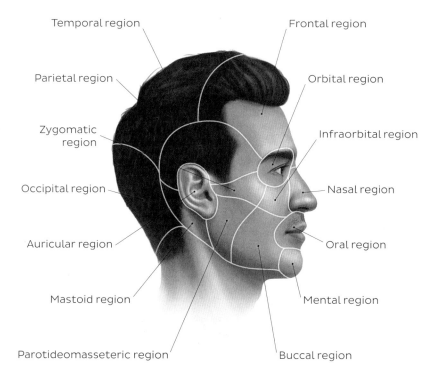

Temporal region

Frontal region

Parietal region

Orbital region

Zygomatic region

Infraorbital region

Occipital region

Nasal region

Auricular region

Oral region

Mastoid region

Mental region

Parotideomasseteric region

Buccal region

FIGURE 8.1. **Regions of the head and face.** Most of the regions in the neurocranial portion correspond to underlying bones/landmarks of the same name. The exception to this is the **auricular region**, that contains the external ear/auricle. The regions of the viscerocranium are named according to bony or soft tissue structures of the face. The **orbital region** contains the organs, bones and soft tissue of the orbit. Inferior to this is the infraorbital region, overlying the maxilla, and the **zygomatic region**, named after the zygomatic bone (commonly referred to as the cheek bone). The **nasal region** contains the bone, cartilage and other tissues of the nose, while the **oral region** below contains the structures of the oral cavity. The **buccal region** is named after the latin term 'bucca', which refers to the cheek (largely comprised by the buccinator muscle), while **parotidomasseteric region** is named after the underlying parotid gland and masseter muscle. The inferior-most region of the face is the **mental region**, demarcating the chin (Latin = mentus).

Human anatomy terminology

Regions of the head and neck

The human skull consists of **22 bones** which are mostly connected together by ossified joints, called sutures. The skull is divided into the braincase (**neuro-cranium**) and the facial skeleton (**viscerocranium**). Neurocranium provides the protection of the most important organ in the human body: The brain, while viscerocranium supports all of the facial structures.

ANTERIOR VIEW OF THE SKULL

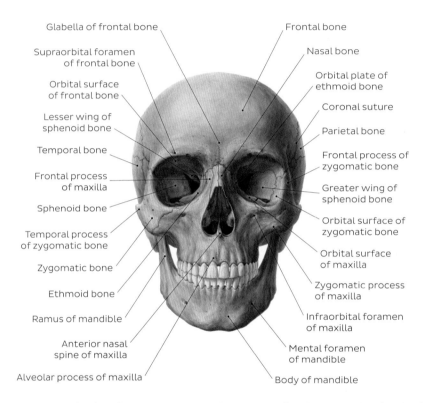

Glabella of frontal bone
Supraorbital foramen of frontal bone
Orbital surface of frontal bone
Lesser wing of sphenoid bone
Temporal bone
Frontal process of maxilla
Sphenoid bone
Temporal process of zygomatic bone
Zygomatic bone
Ethmoid bone
Ramus of mandible
Anterior nasal spine of maxilla
Alveolar process of maxilla

Frontal bone
Nasal bone
Orbital plate of ethmoid bone
Coronal suture
Parietal bone
Frontal process of zygomatic bone
Greater wing of sphenoid bone
Orbital surface of zygomatic bone
Orbital surface of maxilla
Zygomatic process of maxilla
Infraorbital foramen of maxilla
Mental foramen of mandible
Body of mandible

FIGURE 8.2. Anterior view of the skull. Two **temporal** bones, two **parietal** bones, the **sphenoid**, **ethmoid** and the **frontal** bone can be observed from this perspective. These are all **bones of the neurocranium**. Most bones of the viscerocranium are visible: The vomer, two inferior nasal conchae, two nasal bones, two maxillae, mandible, two zygomatic bones, and two lacrimal bones. The skull bones form two anatomical spaces, the bony orbit which houses the eyeballs and the nasal cavity.

Key points about the anterior view of the skull	
Bones	Frontal bone, nasal bones (2), maxillae (2), lacrimal bones (2), ethmoid bone, zygomatic bones (2), sphenoid bone, parietal bones (2), temporal bones (2), mandible
Sutures	**Frontonasal suture**: joins frontal and nasal bones
	Frontozygomatic suture: joins frontal and zygomatic bone
	Zygomaticomaxillary suture: joins zygoma and maxilla
	Intermaxillary suture: joins the two maxillae

Anterior and lateral
views of the skull

 Viscerocranium

LATERAL AND POSTERIOR VIEWS OF THE SKULL

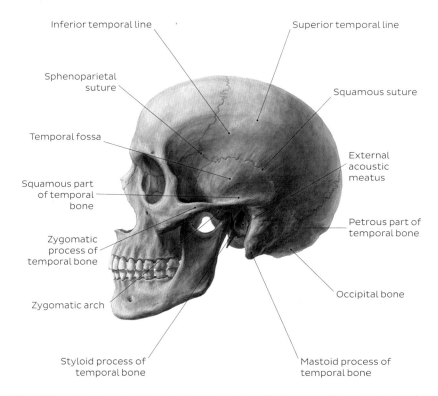

Inferior temporal line

Superior temporal line

Sphenoparietal suture

Squamous suture

Temporal fossa

External acoustic meatus

Squamous part of temporal bone

Zygomatic process of temporal bone

Petrous part of temporal bone

Zygomatic arch

Occipital bone

Styloid process of temporal bone

Mastoid process of temporal bone

FIGURE 8.3. **Skull (lateral view).** The **frontal bone** articulates with the zygomatic bone (frontozygomatic suture), the greater wing of the sphenoid bone (sphenofrontal suture) and the parietal bones (coronal suture).

From this lateral perspective, the squamous and petrous part of the **temporal bone** are visible and are separated from each other by the zygomatic process. This zygomatic process unites with the temporal process of the zygomatic bone to form the zygomatic arch. The squamous part of the temporal bone articulates with the **parietal bone** superiorly (squamous suture) and with the greater wing of the **sphenoid bone** anteriorly (sphenosquamosal suture). The squamous part of the temporal bone and the greater wing of the sphenoid bone together form the majority of the temporal fossa. The external acoustic meatus is part of the tympanic portion of the temporal bone with the styloid process situated inferior, and the mastoid process posterior to it. The pterion is a point of intersection of frontal, sphenoid, parietal, and temporal bones.

On this view, the **occipital bone** is seen articulating with the parietal bone superiorly and the petrous part of the temporal bone inferiorly.

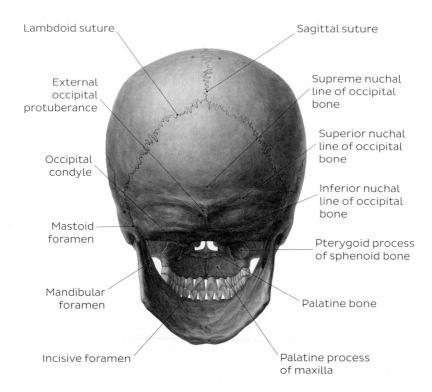

Lambdoid suture

Sagittal suture

External occipital protuberance

Supreme nuchal line of occipital bone

Superior nuchal line of occipital bone

Occipital condyle

Inferior nuchal line of occipital bone

Mastoid foramen

Pterygoid process of sphenoid bone

Mandibular foramen

Palatine bone

Incisive foramen

Palatine process of maxilla

FIGURE 8.4. Skull (posterior view). The posterior view is mostly occupied by the squamous part of the **occipital bone** and the posterior aspect of the **parietal bones**. The two parietal bones meet in the midline and form the sagittal suture. Each parietal bone also articulates with the occipital bone to form the lambdoid suture. The main features of the occipital bone are visible on this view, primarily the supreme, superior and inferior nuchal lines, the external occipital protuberance and the occipital condyles. The rest of the posterior skull is occupied by the posterior aspects of the **maxillae** and **mandible**, and parts of the **palatine** and **sphenoid bones**.

Key points	Lateral view	Posterior view
Bones	Nasal bone, lacrimal bone, frontal bone, maxilla, mandible, zygomatic, sphenoid, temporal, parietal and occipital bone	Occipital bone, parietal bones, palatine bone, sphenoid bone, temporal bone, maxilla, mandible
Sutures	**Squamous suture**: joins the parietal and the temporal bones **Sphenofrontal suture**: joints frontal and the sphenoid bones **Sphenoparietal suture**: joins sphenoid and the parietal bones **Occipitomastoid suture**: joins occipital bone and the mastoid process of the temporal bone **Temporozygomatic suture**: joins temporal and the zygomatic bones	**Sagittal suture**: joins the two parietal bones **Lambdoid suture**: joins parietal and occipital bones The sagittal and lambdoid sutures converge into a **lambda**

CALVARIA

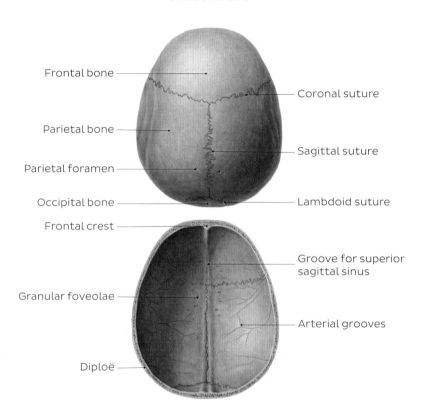

Frontal bone

Coronal suture

Parietal bone

Sagittal suture

Parietal foramen

Occipital bone

Lambdoid suture

Frontal crest

Groove for superior sagittal sinus

Granular foveolae

Arterial grooves

Diploë

FIGURE 8.5. **Superior and inferior views of the calvaria.** The superior surface features the sutures that connect the bones of the calvaria: The sagittal, coronal and lambdoid **sutures**. Each parietal bone contains a **parietal foramen** that forms a channel for the emissary vein. The most prominent feature on the inferior view of the calvaria called the **groove for superior sagittal sinus** can be seen right in the middle. Anteriorly, the edges of this groove unite to form a bony ridge called the **frontal crest**. On either side of the groove for superior sagittal sinus there are several round pits called the **granular foveolae**, which house the arachnoid granulations. Moving further laterally, there are many branching grooves, called **arterial grooves**, in which the meningeal arteries course.

Key points about the calvaria	
Bones	Frontal bone, parietal bone (2), occipital bone
Sutures	**Sagittal suture**: parietal bones Coronal suture: frontal bone and parietal bones Lambdoid suture: parietal bones and occipital bone
Bony features	**Superior view**: cranial sutures, parietal foramina **Inferior view**: frontal crest, groove for superior sagittal sinus, granular foveolae, arterial grooves, diploë

HEAD AND NECK

Calvaria

Cranial sutures

INFERIOR VIEW OF THE CRANIUM

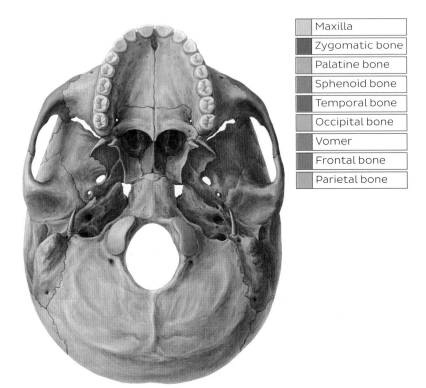

	Maxilla
	Zygomatic bone
	Palatine bone
	Sphenoid bone
	Temporal bone
	Occipital bone
	Vomer
	Frontal bone
	Parietal bone

FIGURE 8.6. **Base of the cranium (inferior view).** The temporal bones articulate with the zygomatic bones anteriorly, forming the zygomatic arches. Posterior to them is the occipital bone which occupies most of the posterior aspect on the inferior side of the cranium. The sphenoid bone can be identified centrally articulating with the maxillae and palatine bones anterior to it; these form the hard palate while the former also houses the maxillary/upper dentition.

HEAD AND NECK

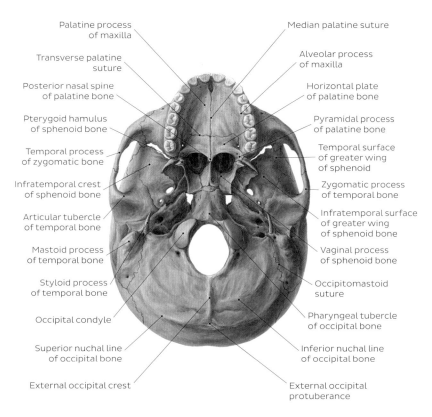

Palatine process of maxilla

Transverse palatine suture

Posterior nasal spine of palatine bone

Pterygoid hamulus of sphenoid bone

Temporal process of zygomatic bone

Infratemporal crest of sphenoid bone

Articular tubercle of temporal bone

Mastoid process of temporal bone

Styloid process of temporal bone

Occipital condyle

Superior nuchal line of occipital bone

External occipital crest

Median palatine suture

Alveolar process of maxilla

Horizontal plate of palatine bone

Pyramidal process of palatine bone

Temporal surface of greater wing of sphenoid

Zygomatic process of temporal bone

Infratemporal surface of greater wing of sphenoid bone

Vaginal process of sphenoid bone

Occipitomastoid suture

Pharyngeal tubercle of occipital bone

Inferior nuchal line of occipital bone

External occipital protuberance

FIGURE 8.7. **Prominent landmarks.** The external surface of the occipital bone is defined by several well defined ridges and crests, namely the external occipital crest as well as the superior and inferior occipital lines. Also visible are the occipital condyles, which articulate with the atlas (vertebra C1). The temporal bone presents more prominent landmarks compared to its posterior neighbor, the largest of which being the mastoid, styloid and zygomatic processes. Important landmarks of the sphenoid bone from this perspective include pterygoid process (located centrally); this is formed of medial and lateral plates, the former of which bears a hooked shaped extremity known as the pterygoid hamulus. The horizontal plates of the palatine bones along with the palatine processes of the maxillae form the hard palate.

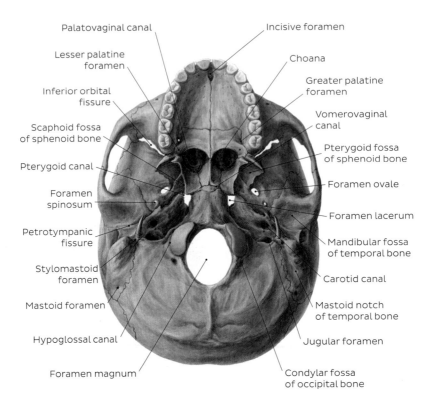

Palatovaginal canal
Lesser palatine foramen
Inferior orbital fissure
Scaphoid fossa of sphenoid bone
Pterygoid canal
Foramen spinosum
Petrotympanic fissure
Stylomastoid foramen
Mastoid foramen
Hypoglossal canal
Foramen magnum

Incisive foramen
Choana
Greater palatine foramen
Vomerovaginal canal
Pterygoid fossa of sphenoid bone
Foramen ovale
Foramen lacerum
Mandibular fossa of temporal bone
Carotid canal
Mastoid notch of temporal bone
Jugular foramen
Condylar fossa of occipital bone

FIGURE 8.8. **Foramina and fissures.** The most prominent feature from this perspective is foramen magnum of the occipital bone, which gives passage to the spinal cord from the brainstem. Notable foramina which give passage to cranial nerves include the foramen rotundum (maxillary nerve (CN V_2)), foramen ovale (mandibular nerve (CN V_3), jugular foramen (glossopharyngeal, vagus and accessory nerves (CN IX–XI), internal jugular vein) and the hypoglossal canal (hypoglossal nerve (CN XII).

Anterior to the jugular foramen, the carotid canal which gives passage to the internal carotid artery can be seen. The foramen spinosum transmits the middle meningeal artery and vein, while the inferior orbital fissure gives passage to several structures including the infraorbital nerve and artery, zygomatic nerve and a branch of the inferior ophthalmic vein.

Foramina, fissures, canals and contents	
Incisive foramen	Nasopalatine nerve, sphenopalatine artery
Greater palatine foramen	Greater palatine nerves, arteries and veins
Lesser palatine foramen	Lesser palatine nerves, arteries and veins
Foramen ovale	Mandibular nerve (CN V_3), accessory meningeal artery, lesser petrosal nerve, emissary veins
Foramen spinosum	Middle meningeal artery and vein, meningeal branch of mandibular nerve (CN V_3)
Jugular foramen	Internal jugular vein, inferior petrosal sinus, posterior meningeal artery, glossopharyngeal nerve, vagus nerve, accessory nerve (CN IX, X, XI)
Stylomastoid foramen	Stylomastoid artery, facial nerve (CN VII)
Foramen magnum	Medulla oblongata, vertebral arteries
Inferior orbital fissure	Infraorbital nerve, zygomatic nerve, artery and vein, inferior branch of inferior ophthalmic vein
Petrotympanic fissure	Chorda tympani, anterior tympanic artery
Carotid canal	Internal carotid artery, internal carotid nerve plexus
Condylar canal	Emissary veins, meningeal branch of occipital artery

Inferior view of the base of the skull

Skull

CRANIAL FOSSAE

The base of the skull, or the cranial floor, is the inferior wall of the cranial cavity. It comprises parts of the frontal, sphenoid, temporal, and occipital bones. These bones form the three **cranial fossae**: Anterior, middle and posterior.

The base of the skull features many openings that are traversed by nerves, arteries and veins traveling between the brain and the neck.

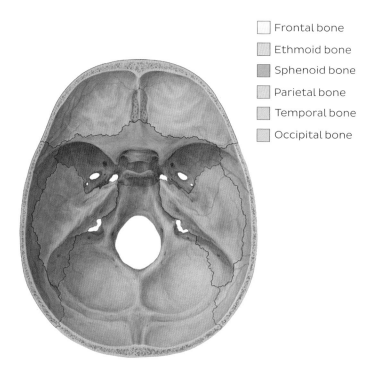

☐ Frontal bone

☐ Ethmoid bone

☐ Sphenoid bone

☐ Parietal bone

☐ Temporal bone

☐ Occipital bone

FIGURE 8.9. **Superior view of the base of the skull.** The bones that comprise the base of the skull are the frontal, ethmoid, sphenoid, temporal and occipital bones. The frontal and sphenoid bone, as well as a small part of ethmoid bone, join to form the anterior cranial fossa; the sphenoid and temporal bones together form the middle cranial fossa, while the temporal and occipital bones form the posterior cranial fossa.

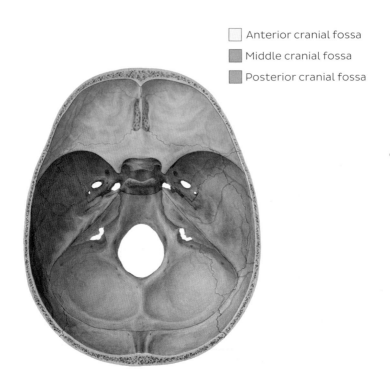

☐ Anterior cranial fossa
▨ Middle cranial fossa
▨ Posterior cranial fossa

FIGURE 8.10. **Cranial fossae.** The **anterior cranial fossa** is the anteriormost area of the cranial floor, formed by the orbital surface of the frontal bone, cribriform plate of the ethmoid bone, and part of the lesser wing of the sphenoid bone. The **middle cranial fossa** is composed of the body and greater wings of sphenoid bone, as well as the squama and anterior surface of the petrous part of temporal bone. The **posterior cranial fossa** is formed by the posterior surface of the petrous part of temporal bone and the occipital bone.

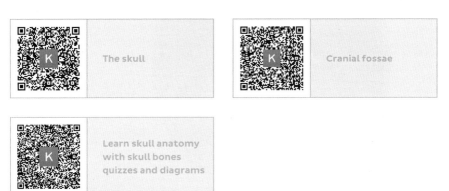

The skull

Cranial fossae

Learn skull anatomy
with skull bones
quizzes and diagrams

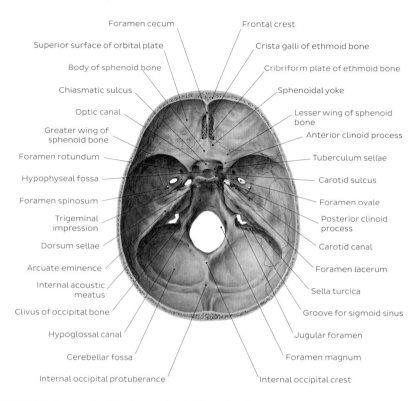

Foramen cecum
Superior surface of orbital plate
Body of sphenoid bone
Chiasmatic sulcus
Optic canal
Greater wing of sphenoid bone
Foramen rotundum
Hypophyseal fossa
Foramen spinosum
Trigeminal impression
Dorsum sellae
Arcuate eminence
Internal acoustic meatus
Clivus of occipital bone
Hypoglossal canal
Cerebellar fossa
Internal occipital protuberance

Frontal crest
Crista galli of ethmoid bone
Cribriform plate of ethmoid bone
Sphenoidal yoke
Lesser wing of sphenoid bone
Anterior clinoid process
Tuberculum sellae
Carotid sulcus
Foramen ovale
Posterior clinoid process
Carotid canal
Foramen lacerum
Sella turcica
Groove for sigmoid sinus
Jugular foramen
Foramen magnum
Internal occipital crest

FIGURE 8.11. Landmarks of the base of the skull (superior view). There are many foramina, canals, sulci and other structures seen on the superior view of the base of the skull. The **anterior cranial fossa** features several landmarks, such as the cribriform foramina, foramen cecum, sphenoidal yoke and frontal crest. The **middle cranial fossa** contains a higher number of landmarks compared to the anterior cranial fossa e.g. clinoid processes, sella turcica, carotid sulcus, foramen ovale and trigeminal impression. The **posterior cranial fossa** features structures such as the clivus, foramen magnum, internal acoustic meatus, jugular foramen and hypoglossal canal.

Key points	Anterior cranial fossa	Middle cranial fossa	Posterior cranial fossa
Bones	Orbital surface of frontal bone, lesser wing of sphenoid bone	Body and greater wings of sphenoid bone, squama and anterior surface of petrous part of temporal bone	Posterior surface of petrous part of temporal bone, occipital bone
Landmarks	Anterior ethmoidal foramen, cribriform foramina, sphenoidal yoke, foramen caecum, frontal crest	Chiasmatic sulcus, tuberculum sellae, anterior clinoid process, sella turcica, middle clinoid process, carotid sulcus, foramen lacerum, foramen spinosum, superior orbital fissure, foramen rotundum, foramen ovale, trigeminal impression, internal opening of carotid canal	Clivus, foramen magnum, internal acoustic meatus, jugular foramen, hypoglossal canal
Contents	Frontal lobe of cerebrum, olfactory bulb, olfactory tract	Temporal lobe of cerebrum, pituitary gland	Brainstem, cerebellum

MIDSAGITTAL SKULL

The midsagittal section of the skull enables us to understand the structure of the two main parts of the skull:

- **Neurocranium**, or the brain case, which houses the brain
- **Viscerocranium**, which houses the structures of the face, oral, nasal and orbital cavities

The bones of the skull not only form and enclose these spaces, but they also feature numerous passageways for neurovascular structures to pass in and out of the cranial cavity.

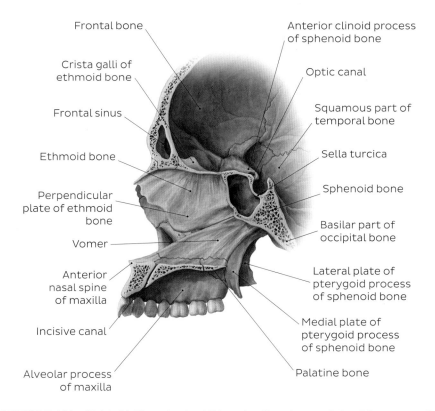

Frontal bone

Anterior clinoid process of sphenoid bone

Crista galli of ethmoid bone

Optic canal

Frontal sinus

Squamous part of temporal bone

Ethmoid bone

Sella turcica

Perpendicular plate of ethmoid bone

Sphenoid bone

Vomer

Basilar part of occipital bone

Anterior nasal spine of maxilla

Lateral plate of pterygoid process of sphenoid bone

Incisive canal

Medial plate of pterygoid process of sphenoid bone

Alveolar process of maxilla

Palatine bone

FIGURE 8.12. **Midsagittal skull (with nasal septum).** This section allows the appreciation of the structure of the bony nasal septum, which is composed of the perpendicular plate of ethmoid bone and vomer joining the maxilla and palatine bones. The latter two bones are seen comprising the floor of the nasal cavity, separating it from the oral cavity. At the roof of the nasal cavity there is the ethmoid bone which encloses it towards the anterior cranial fossa. Below, there is a hollow cavity which represents the sphenoidal sinus.

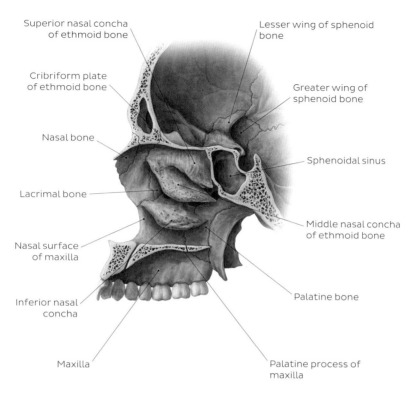

Superior nasal concha
of ethmoid bone

Cribriform plate
of ethmoid bone

Nasal bone

Lacrimal bone

Nasal surface
of maxilla

Inferior nasal
concha

Maxilla

Lesser wing of sphenoid
bone

Greater wing of
sphenoid bone

Sphenoidal sinus

Middle nasal concha
of ethmoid bone

Palatine bone

Palatine process of
maxilla

FIGURE 8.13. **Midsagittal skull (septum removed).** With nasal septum removed, a better view on the lateral wall of the nasal cavity is possible. The wall shows three bony projections called the superior, middle and inferior nasal conchae (turbinates). The superior and middle conchae are parts of the ethmoid bone, while the inferior nasal concha is an individual bone that attaches to the ethmoid, maxilla, lacrimal and palatine bones.

Key points about the midsagittal skull	
Bones	**Neurocranium**: frontal bone, ethmoid bone, sphenoid bone, parietal bone, temporal bone, occipital bone
	Viscerocranium: nasal bone, inferior nasal concha, lacrimal bone, maxilla, palatine bone, vomer
	Sutures: coronal suture, lambdoid suture, squamous suture, occipitomastoid suture, sphenofrontal suture
Frontal bone	Frontal sinus
Ethmoid bone	Crista galli, cribriform plate, perpendicular plate, superior nasal concha, middle nasal concha
Sphenoid bone	Greater wing, lesser wing, anterior clinoid process, optic canal, sella turcica, sphenoidal sinus, medial pterygoid plate, lateral pterygoid plate, pterygoid hamulus
Maxilla	Anterior nasal spine, incisive canal, palatine process, alveolar process
Palatine bone	Perpendicular plate, horizontal plate
Parietal bone	Groove for middle meningeal artery
Temporal bone	Squamous part, petrous part, internal acoustic meatus, groove for superior petrosal sinus, external opening of vestibular aqueduct, groove for sigmoid sinus
Occipital bone	Basilar part, groove for transverse sinus, external occipital protuberance (inion), jugular foramen, groove for inferior petrosal sinus, hypoglossal canal, foramen magnum, occipital condyle

HEAD AND NECK

ETHMOID BONE

The **ethmoid** is a small fragile bone located in the midline of the anterior skull. It sits in the anterior cranial fossa, medial to the orbits and slightly superoposterior to the nasal cavity. Due to its position, it contributes to forming the medial orbital walls, the nasal septum, as well as the roof and lateral walls of the nasal cavity.

The ethmoid bone is a **pneumatized bone**, meaning that it is full of air cells (spaces), and has been compared to an ice cube, in size, shape and weight. It is a complex shaped bone with a number of named parts.

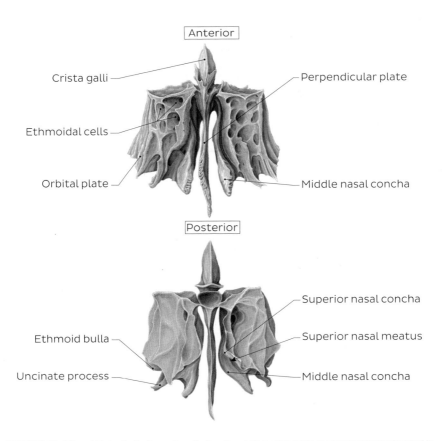

FIGURE 8.14. Ethmoid bone (anterior and posterior views). The ethmoid is an unpaired bone situated in the midline of the skull. It consists of a centrally positioned **crista galli**, which is continued inferiorly by the **perpendicular plate**.

On each side of the midline there is a spongy lateral mass, often referred to as the ethmoidal labyrinth. Each mass consists of numerous air-filled **ethmoidal cells**. Thus, each mass is known as the **ethmoidal paranasal sinus**. The lateral wall of the sinus presents a saccular extension called the **ethmoid bulla**, one of the largest of ethmoidal cells. Ethmoidal masses feature a hook-like projection pointing inferiorly called the **uncinate process**. This process forms a part of the wall of the maxillary sinus and is often confused as a part of the maxilla rather than of ethmoid.

The lateral surface of ethmoidal masses faces the orbit, forming a part of its medial wall. The medial surface of each mass faces the perpendicular plate. From an anterior view, it is visible how a separate bony lamina called the **middle nasal concha** extends inferiorly from the root of each mass. The posterior view allows the appreciation of the **superior nasal concha** as well. The conchae project into the nasal cavity increasing its surface. Between the conchae is the **middle nasal meatus**, which drains the ethmoidal sinuses into the nasal cavity.

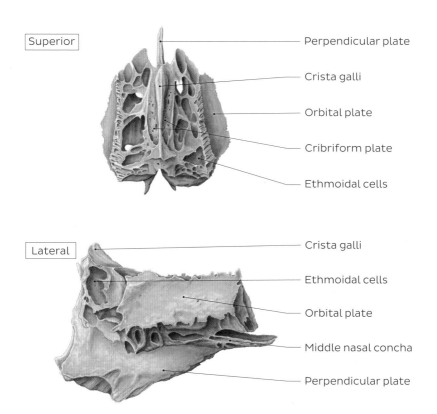

Superior

Perpendicular plate

Crista galli

Orbital plate

Cribriform plate

Ethmoidal cells

Lateral

Crista galli

Ethmoidal cells

Orbital plate

Middle nasal concha

Perpendicular plate

FIGURE 8.15. **Ethmoid bone (superior and lateral views).** The superior view allows the appreciation of one of the most unique landmarks of the ethmoid bone: The **cribriform plate**. The cribriform plate is split into left and right halves by the crista galli. The plate shows multiple openings through which the fibers of the olfactory nerve (CN I) pass. The fibers converge into the olfactory bulbs, each resting on the respective surfaces of the cribriform plate.

The lateral view provides a better visualization of the **perpendicular plate**. It forms a part of the nasal septum and articulates with the vomer.

Key points about the ethmoid bone	
Location	Anterior cranial fossa, medial to the orbits and slightly superoposterior to the nasal cavity.
Landmarks	Crista galli, ala of crista galli, cribriform plate of ethmoid bone, perpendicular plate of ethmoid bone, ethmoidal labyrinth, cells of ethmoid bone, orbital plate of ethmoid bone, ethmoid bulla, uncinate process of ethmoid bone, supreme nasal concha, superior nasal concha, middle nasal concha, ethmoidal infundibulum
Articulating bones	Frontal, sphenoid, nasals (2), maxillae (2), lacrimals (2), palatines (2), inferior nasal conchae (2) and the vomer.

Ethmoid bone

SPHENOID BONE

The **sphenoid bone** is one of the most complex bones of the skull. It comprises most of the middle part of the base of the skull, contributes to the floor of the middle cranial fossa of the skull, and forms a small portion of the bony orbit.

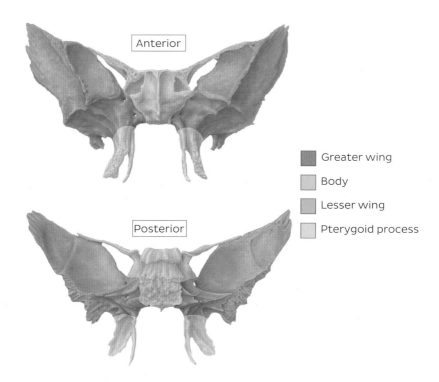

FIGURE 8.16. Parts of the sphenoid bone. The sphenoid bone consists of a centrally positioned **body** from which the two pairs of wings arise: **Greater wings** and **lesser wings**. The bifid **pterygoid process** arises from each greater wing and points inferiorly.

HEAD AND NECK

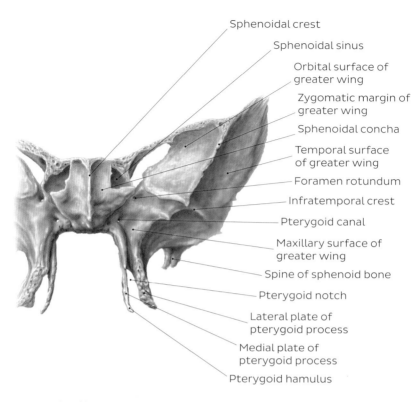

Sphenoidal crest

Sphenoidal sinus

Orbital surface of
greater wing

Zygomatic margin of
greater wing

Sphenoidal concha

Temporal surface
of greater wing

Foramen rotundum

Infratemporal crest

Pterygoid canal

Maxillary surface of
greater wing

Spine of sphenoid bone

Pterygoid notch

Lateral plate of
pterygoid process

Medial plate of
pterygoid process

Pterygoid hamulus

FIGURE 8.17. **Sphenoid bone (anterior view).** The anterior surface of the sphenoid body features the **sphenoidal crest** in the midline via which it articulates with the perpendicular plate of the ethmoid bone, contributing to the formation of the nasal septum. On each side of the crest is the **sphenoidal concha** which partially encloses the **sphenoidal sinus**. The superolateral part of the sinus remains open and communicates with the nasal cavity.

The root of the greater wing features two openings: The foramen rotundum and pterygoid canal. The **foramen rotundum** is traversed by the maxillary branch of trigeminal nerve (CN V_2), while the **pterygoid (Vidian) canal** transmits the artery and nerve of pterygoid canal. From an anterior perspective the orbital, temporal and maxillary surfaces of the greater wing are visible. The **orbital surface** contributes to the lateral part of the orbit. The **temporal surface** faces laterally and is divided by the **infratemporal crest** into superior and inferior portions. The superior portion contributes to the wall of the temporal fossa, while the inferior portion forms a part of the infratemporal fossa. The **maxillary surface** faces the maxilla.

The **spine of sphenoid bone** points inferiorly from the lower margin of the temporal surface, providing the attachment site for the sphenomandibular ligament.

The pterygoid process extends inferiorly from the root of the greater wing. It bifurcates into the **lateral** and **medial plates**, between which is a space called the **pterygoid notch**. The very tip of the medial plate is called the **pterygoid hamulus**.

Sphenoid bone

HEAD AND NECK

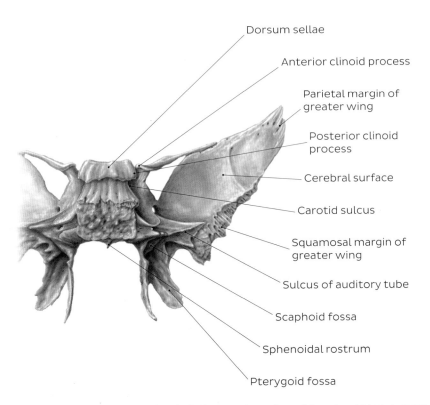

Dorsum sellae

Anterior clinoid process

Parietal margin of greater wing

Posterior clinoid process

Cerebral surface

Carotid sulcus

Squamosal margin of greater wing

Sulcus of auditory tube

Scaphoid fossa

Sphenoidal rostrum

Pterygoid fossa

FIGURE 8.18. **Sphenoid bone (posterior view).** The posterior surface of the sphenoid body is rough, featuring a prominent landmark: Dorsum sellae. The **dorsum sellae** articulates with the occipital bone and forms the clivus. The inferolateral angles of the dorsum present small posterior clinoid processes, which forms one of the attachment points for the tentorium cerebelli. In the midline, the body presents a triangular process called the **sphenoidal rostrum** which points towards the ala of vomer.

The posterior view allows a better appreciation of the root of the **lesser wing**. This bony process spirals from the sphenoid body, forming the **anterior clinoid process**, after which it continues laterally and fuses with the greater wing.

The irregular appearance of the root of the greater wing is also noticeable from this perspective. This area features the **sulcus of auditory tube** which houses the cartilaginous auditory tube. The **cerebral surface** of greater wing contributes to the middle cranial fossa, lodging a part of the temporal lobe of the brain. The ridged **parietal** and **squamosal margins** of the greater wings are visible, which serve for the articulations with the parietal and temporal bones respectively.

From this aspect, the plates of the pterygoid process present as concave. At their origin there is a shallow **scaphoid fossa** which serves as the attachment site for the tensor veli palatini muscle. The very concavity of the lateral plate comprises an obtuse-angled **pterygoid fossa** which provides the attachment site for the medial pterygoid muscle.

Key points about the sphenoid bone	
Parts	Body (median portion)
	Greater wing (lateral portion)
	Lesser wings (anterior portion)
	Pterygoid processes (directed inferiorly)
Sutures	Sphenofrontal suture with frontal bone
	Sphenoparietal suture with parietal bone
	Sphenosquamosal suture with temporal bone
	Spheno-occipital suture with occipital bone (disappears by age 25 as bones fuse together)

TEMPORAL BONE

The **temporal bone** is a complex cranial bone that constitutes a large portion of the lateral wall and base of the skull. There are a number of openings and canals in the temporal bone through which structures enter and exit the cranial cavity. The temporal bone also houses the structures forming the middle and inner ear.

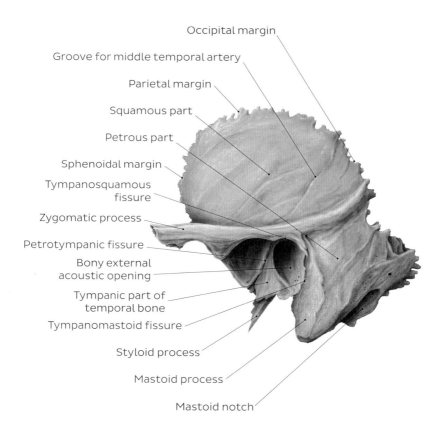

Occipital margin

Groove for middle temporal artery

Parietal margin

Squamous part

Petrous part

Sphenoidal margin

Tympanosquamous fissure

Zygomatic process

Petrotympanic fissure

Bony external acoustic opening

Tympanic part of temporal bone

Tympanomastoid fissure

Styloid process

Mastoid process

Mastoid notch

FIGURE 8.19. Temporal bone (lateral view). The temporal bone is a bone located bilaterally on either side of the skull. The image above shows the temporal bone from a lateral perspective, which allows the appreciation of the main parts of the temporal bone: The **petrous** part, **squamous** part and **tympanic** part. These are demarcated by several **fissures**, such as the petrosquamous fissure, which separates the squamous and petrous part; the tympanosquamous fissure, separating the tympanic and squamous parts, and others. Some notable features of the temporal bone are seen from this perspective, such as the mastoid process, zygomatic process and groove for the middle temporal artery.

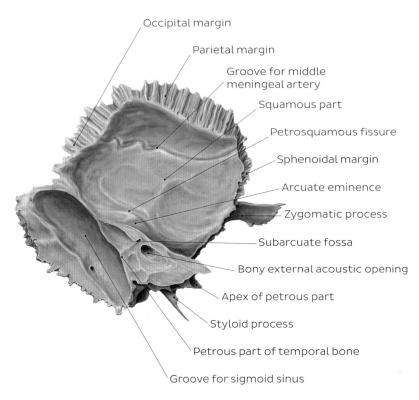

Occipital margin

Parietal margin

Groove for middle
meningeal artery

Squamous part

Petrosquamous fissure

Sphenoidal margin

Arcuate eminence

Zygomatic process

Subarcuate fossa

Bony external acoustic opening

Apex of petrous part

Styloid process

Petrous part of temporal bone

Groove for sigmoid sinus

FIGURE 8.20. **Temporal bone (medial view).** The medial view of the temporal bone provides a visual of its internal features. Some of these are formed by the imprinting of the passing intracranial structures, such as the groove for middle meningeal artery and groove for sigmoid sinus. The tympanic part houses the structures of the middle and inner ear. The temporal bone has three margins, which denote the bones it articulates with: **Sphenoidal**, **parietal** and **occipital margins**.

Temporal bone

Mastoid process

HEAD AND NECK

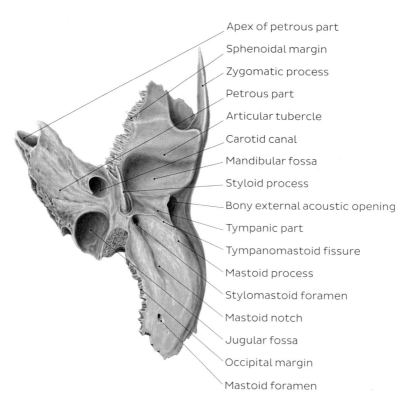

Apex of petrous part

Sphenoidal margin

Zygomatic process

Petrous part

Articular tubercle

Carotid canal

Mandibular fossa

Styloid process

Bony external acoustic opening

Tympanic part

Tympanomastoid fissure

Mastoid process

Stylomastoid foramen

Mastoid notch

Jugular fossa

Occipital margin

Mastoid foramen

FIGURE 8.21. **Temporal bone (inferior view).** On the inferior side, the temporal bone provides a clear visual of the several landmarks not seen on other views. These are the **styloid process, mandibular fossa** and **articular tubercle** of the temporal bone. This view also gives the best visual of several openings (foramina) in the temporal bone through which structures enter and exit the cranial cavity. These include the carotid canal, for the passage of the internal carotid artery, the stylomastoid foramen transmitting the facial nerve (CN VII) and stylomastoid artery, and the mastoid foramen for the passage of the emissary veins.

Key points about the temporal bone	
Main parts	Petrous part
	Tympanic part
	Squamous part
Articulations	Occipital bone, parietal bone, sphenoid bone, zygomatic bone and mandible
Fissures	Petrotympanic fissure
	Petrosquamous fissure
	Tympanosquamous fissure
	Tympanomastoid fissure
Bony features	**Petrous part**: occipital margin, mastoid process, mastoid notch, mastoid foramen, apex of petrous part, carotid canal, tegmen tympani, arcuate eminence, bony labyrinth, internal acoustic meatus, subarcuate fossa, jugular fossa, styloid process, stylomastoid foramen, groove for sigmoid sinus, tympanic cavity
	Tympanic part: bony external acoustic opening, bony external acoustic meatus
	Squamous part: sphenoidal margin, parietal margin, parietal notch, groove for middle temporal artery, zygomatic process, mandibular fossa, articular tubercle, groove for middle meningeal artery

MANDIBLE

The **mandible** is the largest bone of the human head. It is the only mobile bone of the skull (not including the auditory ossicles). The mandible is technically not part of the viscerocranium, however is sometimes still considered as such by some texts. It connects to the maxilla (part of the viscerocranium) via the teeth when the jaw is closed, and with the temporal bone (part of the neurocranium) via the temporomandibular joint. Due to its mobility, the prime function of the mandible is to assist in mastication.

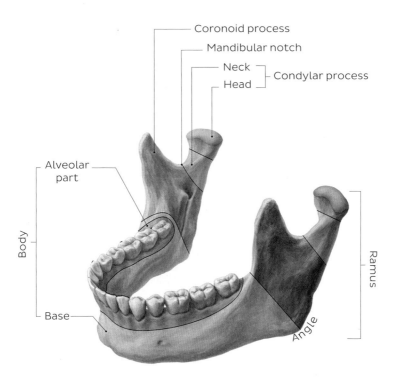

FIGURE 8.22. Parts of the mandible. The mandible is composed of two main parts: The body and ramus. The point at which the ramus and body of the mandible unite is known as the angle of mandible.

The **body** is the horizontal portion of the mandible that creates the jawline. It is subdivided into the base and alveolar part. The **base** forms the lower portion of the mandible and provides the structural integrity of the jaw, while the **alveolar part** holds the mandibular teeth.

The **rami** are the two vertical processes that are connected to the body at the **mandibular angle**. The superior portion of each is composed of two bony processes (**coronoid** and **condylar processes**) separated by the **mandibular notch**. The condylar process consists of the head (also known as the mandibular condyle) and neck of the mandible. The rounded head of the mandible articulates with the temporal bone on each side to create the temporomandibular joint which provides mobility to the mandible and allows mastication.

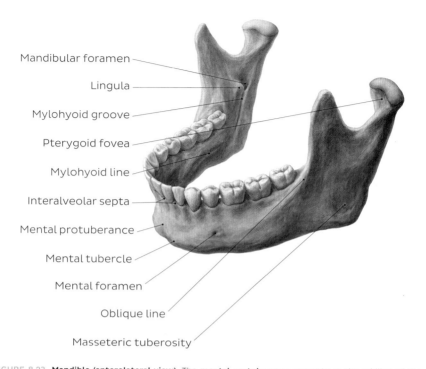

Mandibular foramen

Lingula

Mylohyoid groove

Pterygoid fovea

Mylohyoid line

Interalveolar septa

Mental protuberance

Mental tubercle

Mental foramen

Oblique line

Masseteric tuberosity

FIGURE 8.23. **Mandible (anterolateral view).** The **mental protuberance** presents at the midline of the base of the external surface of the mandible and is continuous laterally on either side with the **mental tubercles**. Collectively these structures form the prominence of the chin.

Inferior to the mandibular premolar teeth, along the external surface of the base of the mandible is a small, round opening known as the **mental foramen**, which allows for the passage of the mental branch of inferior alveolar artery, mental vein and mental nerve. The **oblique lines** of the body of the mandible are continuous superiorly with the anterior border of the ramus of the mandible and extend anteroinferiorly towards the mental tubercles. They form the lateral boundary of the retromolar fossa and provide an origin site for the depressor anguli oris muscle.

The external surface of the angle of mandible presents with a roughening for the attachment of the masseter muscle known as the **masseteric tuberosity**.

Along the anterior aspect of each neck of mandible are two small, shallow depressions known as the **pterygoid foveae**, which provide an insertion site for the lateral pterygoid muscle on each side. The internal surface of the ramus of the mandible presents with the **mandibular foramen** (also known as the inferior alveolar foramen) which houses the inferior alveolar artery, vein and nerve. The opening has a prominent ridge in its front known as the **lingula** of mandible for the attachment of the sphenomandibular ligament. The **mylohyoid groove** runs in an anteroinferior direction from this point and contains the mylohyoid nerve.

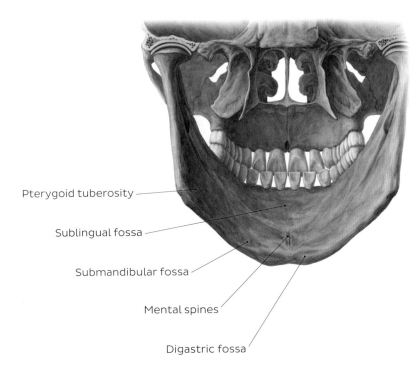

Pterygoid tuberosity ———

Sublingual fossa ———

Submandibular fossa ———

Mental spines ———

Digastric fossa ———

FIGURE 8.24. **Mandible (posterior view).** The internal surface of the body, angle and ramus of the mandible can be seen from this posterior view. The midline of the internal surface of the body of the mandible presents with two bony indentenations known as the **sublingual** and **submandibular fossae**. These structures house the sublingual and submandibular salivary glands, respectively. The **mental spines** (superior and inferior) are small midline processes on the body of the mandible which act as an attachment site for the genioglossus muscle.

Along the base of the mandible are two rough, shallow depressions known as the **digastric fossae** which serve as an origin site for the anterior belly of the digastric muscle.

The internal surface of the angle of the mandible presents with a roughening for the attachment of the medial pterygoid muscle, known as the **pterygoid tuberosity**.

Key points about the mandible	
Main parts	Body, ramus
Articulations	Maxilla (via teeth), temporal bone (via temporomandibular joint)
Bony features	**Body**: mental protuberance, mental tubercle, mental foramen, oblique line of mandible, sublingual fossa, mylohyoid line, submandibular fossa, mental spines, digastric fossa, alveolar part, interalveolar septa **Ramus**: coronoid process, mandibular notch, condylar process, head of mandible, neck of mandible, pterygoid fovea, pterygoid tuberosity, masseteric tuberosity, angle of mandible, mandibular foramen, lingula, mylohyoid groove

Mandible

Temporomandibular joint

HEAD AND NECK

MUSCLES OF FACIAL EXPRESSION

The muscles of the facial expression are a group of approximately 20 superficial skeletal muscles of the face and scalp which originate from the bony and fibrous structures of the skull and insert into the skin. These attachments give them an important role in showing emotions through facial expressions.

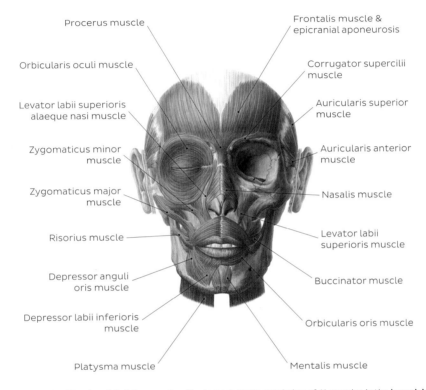

Procerus muscle

Orbicularis oculi muscle

Levator labii superioris alaeque nasi muscle

Zygomaticus minor muscle

Zygomaticus major muscle

Risorius muscle

Depressor anguli oris muscle

Depressor labii inferioris muscle

Platysma muscle

Frontalis muscle & epicranial aponeurosis

Corrugator supercilii muscle

Auricularis superior muscle

Auricularis anterior muscle

Nasalis muscle

Levator labii superioris muscle

Buccinator muscle

Orbicularis oris muscle

Mentalis muscle

FIGURE 8.25. **Muscles of facial expression.** The largest group consisting of 11 muscles is the **buccolabial group**. The majority of the mouth muscles are connected by a fibromuscular hub (**modiolus**) at each angle of the mouth into which these muscles insert. This group is in charge of the shape and movements of the mouth and lips. The next group is the nasal group that consists of two muscles (nasalis and procerus muscles). Next, the **orbital group** consists of three muscles (orbicularis oculi, corrugator supercilii, depressor supercilii muscles) that are responsible for opening and closing the eyes and moving the eyebrows. The **auricular group** is a group of three fan-shaped muscles (auricularis anterior, auricularis posterior and auricularis superior muscles) that move the ear lobe/auricle to a small extent. The last group is the **epicranial group** (scalp and neck group) which includes two wide and flat muscles (occipitofrontalis and platysma muscles). The occipitofrontalis muscle consists of two bellies (occipital and frontal) and acts mainly on the forehead, while the platysma mainly acts on the neck and lower lip.

Buccolabial group	Origin	Insertion	Innervation	Function
Orbicularis oris	Medial aspects of maxilla and mandible, Perioral skin and muscles, Modiolus	Skin and mucous membrane of lips	Buccal branch of facial nerve (CN VII)	Closes mouth, Compresses and protrudes lips
Buccinator	(External lateral surface of) Alveolar process of maxilla, Buccinator ridge of mandible, Pterygomandibular raphe	Modiolus, Blends with muscles of upper lip		Compresses cheek against molar teeth
Zygomaticus major	(Posterior part of) Lateral aspect of zygomatic bone			Elevates and everts angle of mouth
Zygomaticus minor	(Anterior part of) Lateral aspect of zygomatic bone	Blends with muscles of upper lip (medial to zygomaticus major muscle)	Zygomatic and buccal branches of facial nerve (CN VII)	Elevates upper lip, Exposes maxillary teeth
Levator labii superioris	Zygomatic process of maxilla, Maxillary process of zygomatic bone	Blends with muscles of upper lip		Elevates and everts upper lip, Exposes maxillary teeth
Levator anguli oris	Canine fossa of maxilla			Elevates angle of mouth
Risorius	Parotid fascia, Buccal skin, Zygomatic bone (variable)	Modiolus	Buccal branch of facial nerve (CN VII)	Extends angle of mouth laterally
Depressor anguli oris	Mental tubercle and oblique line of mandible (continuous with platysma muscle)		Buccal and mandibular branches of facial nerve (CN VII)	Depresses angle of mouth
Depressor labii inferioris	Oblique line of mandible (continuous with platysma muscle)	Skin and submucosa of lower lip	Mandibular branch of facial nerve (CN VII)	Depresses lower lip inferolaterally
Mentalis	Incisive fossa of mandible	Skin of chin (Mentolabial sulcus)		Elevates, everts and protudes lower lip, Wrinkles skin of chin
Levator labii superioris alaeque nasi	Frontal process of maxilla	Lateral crus of major alar cartilage, Blends with fibres of levator labii superioris and orbicularis oris muscles	Zygomatic and buccal branches of facial nerve (CN VII)	Elevates and everts upper lip and nasal ala

HEAD AND NECK

Nasal group	Origin	Insertion	Innervation	Function
Procerus	Nasal bone, (Superior part of) Lateral nasal cartilage	Skin of glabella, Fibres of frontal belly of occipitofrontalis muscle	Temporal, lower zygomatic or buccal branches of facial nerve (CN VII)	Depresses medial end of eyebrow, Wrinkles skin of glabella
Nasalis	**Alar part**: frontal process of maxilla (superior to lateral incisor) **Transverse part**: maxilla (superolateral to incisive fossa)	**Alar part**: skin of ala; **Transverse part**: merges with counterpart at dorsum of nose	Buccal branch of facial nerve (CN VII)	**Alar part**: depresses ala laterally, dilates nostrils **Transverse part**: wrinkles skin of dorsum of nose

Orbital group	Origin	Insertion	Innervation	Function
Orbicularis oculi	Nasal part of frontal bone, Frontal process of maxilla, Medial palpebral ligament, Lacrimal bone	Skin of orbital region, Lateral palpebral ligament, Superior and inferior tarsi	Temporal and zygomatic branches of facial nerve (CN VII)	**Orbital part**: closes eyelids tightly **Palpebral part**: closes eyelids gently **Lacrimal part**: compresses lacrimal sac
Corrugator supercilii	Medial end of superciliary arches, Fibers of orbicularis oculi muscle	Skin above middle of supraorbital margin	Temporal branches of facial nerve (CN VII)	Creates vertical wrinkles over glabella
Depressor supercilii	Medial angle of orbit	Skin of medial end of eyebrow and glabella		Depresses medial portion of eyebrow, Moves skin of glabella

Epicranial group	Origin	Insertion	Innervation	Function
Occipitofrontalis	**Frontal belly (frontalis)**: skin of eyebrow, Muscles of forehead **Occipital belly (occipitalis)**: (Lateral 2/3 of) Superior nuchal line	Epicranial aponeurosis	**Frontal belly**: temporal branches of facial nerve (CN VII) **Occipital belly**: posterior auricular nerve (branch of facial nerve (CN VII))	**Frontal belly**: elevates eyebrows, wrinkles skin of forehead **Occipital belly**: retracts scalp
Temporoparietalis	Auricular muscles		Temporal branches of facial nerve (CN VII)	Tenses fascia of temporal region, assists with movement of auricle

Auricular group	Origin	Insertion	Innervation	Function
Auricularis anterior	Temporal fascia/ Epicranial aponeurosis	Spine of helix	Temporal branches of facial nerve (CN VII)	Draws auricle anteriorly
Auricularis superior	Epicranial aponeurosis	Superior surface of auricle		Draws auricle superiorly
Auricularis posterior	Mastoid process of temporal bone	Ponticulus of conchal eminence	Posterior auricular nerve (branch of facial nerve (CN VII))	Draws auricle posteriorly

Facial muscles

The human face

BLOOD VESSELS OF THE FACE AND SCALP

The arterial supply of the face and scalp originates almost exclusively from the **external carotid artery**. The vast majority of the supply to the skin and muscles of the face originates from the **facial artery**. Additional supply to the face stems from the **maxillary artery**, which is a branch of the external carotid artery. Other branches of the external carotid artery mostly supply the scalp, and include the posterior auricular, occipital and superficial temporal arteries. While most of the face is supplied by the branches of the external carotid, a major contributor to the arterial supply is the **ophthalmic artery**, a branch of the internal carotid artery.

The venous drainage of the face and the scalp is mostly analogue to the arterial supply. The most notable vein is the **facial vein**, that runs a similar course to its arterial counterpart, receives many tributaries along its course, and ultimately drains into the **internal jugular vein**.

HEAD AND NECK

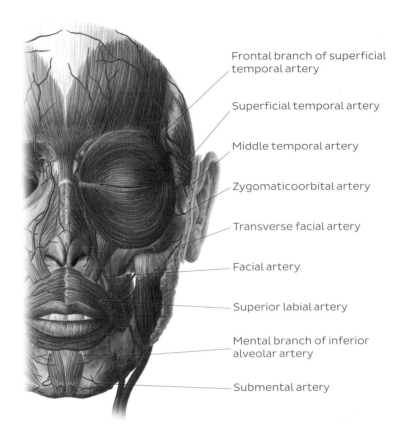

Frontal branch of superficial temporal artery

Superficial temporal artery

Middle temporal artery

Zygomaticoorbital artery

Transverse facial artery

Facial artery

Superior labial artery

Mental branch of inferior alveolar artery

Submental artery

FIGURE 8.26. **Arteries of face and scalp (anterior view: Superficial).** The facial artery arises from the external carotid artery within the neck and continues along the inner surface of the mandible. It then crosses over the inferior aspect of the mandible and continues its course superiorly across the face. The branches of the facial artery which supply the superficial face and scalp are the **submental artery**, supplying the submental area (alongside the mental branch of the inferior alveolar artery), the **superior and inferior labial arteries** (see next image), which supply the upper and lower lip, the **lateral nasal artery**, which supplies the skin of the nose and its terminal branch, the **angular artery** (see next image).

Supplying the superficial aspect of the face and scalp is one of the terminal branches of the external carotid artery, the **superficial temporal artery**. The superficial temporal artery extends through the temporal region and gives rise to its two main branches: The transverse facial and middle temporal arteries. The **zygomaticoorbital artery** is an occasional branch of the middle temporal artery that runs along the upper border of the zygomatic arch. It may also arise from the superficial temporal artery.

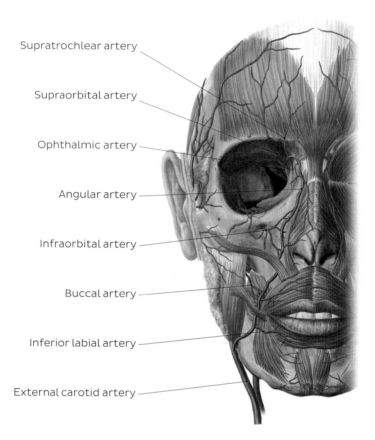

Supratrochlear artery

Supraorbital artery

Ophthalmic artery

Angular artery

Infraorbital artery

Buccal artery

Inferior labial artery

External carotid artery

FIGURE 8.27. Arteries of face and scalp (anterior view: Deep). The **ophthalmic artery** arises within the skull and extends anteriorly to enter the orbit with the optic nerve via the optic foramen. It continues along the medial wall of the orbit where it gives off several branches. Branches of the ophthalmic artery which supply deep structures of the face include the supraorbital, supratrochlear and dorsal nasal arteries. The **supraorbital** and **supratrochlear arteries** extend superiorly to supply the forehead and scalp while the **dorsal nasal artery** extends inferomedially to anastomose with the **angular artery** (terminal branch of facial artery).

The **buccal artery** arises from the 2nd part of the maxillary artery, while the infraorbital artery originates from the 3rd part of the maxillary artery within the pterygopalatine fossa. The buccal artery passes forwards to reach and supply the buccinator muscle and overlying skin. The **infraorbital artery** ascends to the orbit of the eye via the inferior orbital fissure and emerges onto the face through the infraorbital foramen. It supplies the skin of the inferior eyelid, cheek and nose as well as the maxillary teeth via its terminal branches.

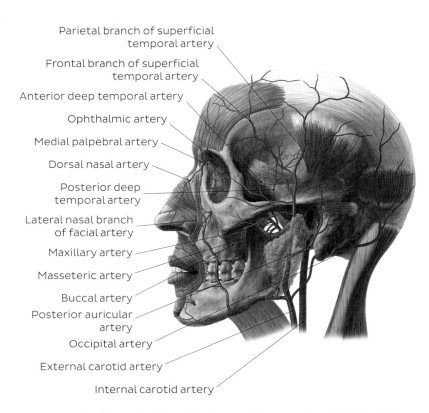

Parietal branch of superficial temporal artery

Frontal branch of superficial temporal artery

Anterior deep temporal artery

Ophthalmic artery

Medial palpebral artery

Dorsal nasal artery

Posterior deep temporal artery

Lateral nasal branch of facial artery

Maxillary artery

Masseteric artery

Buccal artery

Posterior auricular artery

Occipital artery

External carotid artery

Internal carotid artery

FIGURE 8.28. **Arteries of face and scalp (lateral view).** The **maxillary artery** gives off the infraorbital artery, that supplies the area between the eye and upper lip, the buccal artery, supplying the buccinator muscle and skin of the cheek, as well as the inferior alveolar artery, which gives off the mental artery to supply the chin. The scalp receives its vascular supply through branches of the **external carotid artery**: The posterior auricular, superficial temporal and occipital arteries.

Artery	Branches	Supply
Facial artery	Submental artery	Muscles and skin of the submental area
	Inferior labial artery	Lower lip
	Superior labial artery	Upper lip, nasal septum, and ala of the nose
	Angular artery	Orbicularis oris muscle and the lacrimal sac
Maxillary artery	Infraorbital artery	Area between the lower eyelid and upper lip
	Buccal artery	Buccinator muscle and surrounding structures
	Mental branch of the inferior alveolar artery	Chin
Other branches of external carotid artery	Posterior auricular artery	Auricle of the ear and scalp posterior and superior to the auricle
	Occipital artery	Posterior scalp
	Superficial temporal artery	Temporal region of the face and scalp
	Transverse facial artery	Parotid gland and surrounding structures
	Middle temporal artery	Temporal region of the face and scalp
Ophthalmic artery	Supratrochlear artery	Forehead, scalp and superior conjunctiva
	Supraorbital artery	Forehead, scalp and superior conjunctiva

HEAD AND NECK

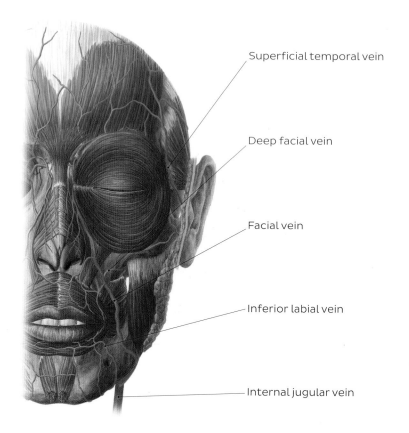

Superficial temporal vein

Deep facial vein

Facial vein

Inferior labial vein

Internal jugular vein

FIGURE 8.29. Veins of face and scalp (anterior view: Superficial). Superficial venous drainage of the face is mainly achieved through tributaries from the retromandibular and facial veins. The **superficial temporal veins** pass laterally from the temporal region over the zygomatic arch and enter the parotid gland. Within the parotid gland, the superficial temporal veins join with the maxillary veins to form the **retromandibular vein**. The superficial temporal veins drain the muscles and skin of the temporal region.

The **deep facial vein** drains the rostral aspect of the pterygoid plexus to the facial vein, while the **inferior labial veins** courses laterally along the lower lip, draining structures of this region into the facial vein. The **retromandibular** and **facial veins** extend inferiorly and drain to the **internal jugular vein**.

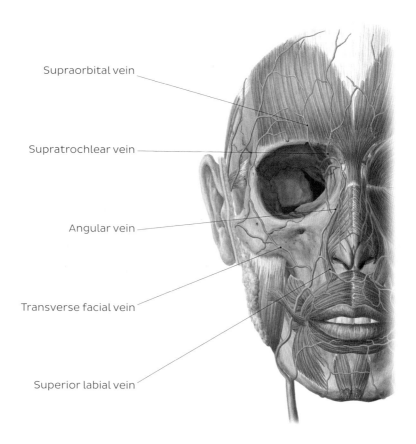

Supraorbital vein

Supratrochlear vein

Angular vein

Transverse facial vein

Superior labial vein

FIGURE 8.30. **Veins of face and scalp (anterior view: Deep).** The main vein draining the deep structures of the face is the **facial vein**, which receives various tributaries that run a similar course to their arterial counterparts and are therefore identically named. The facial vein originates at the lower margin of the orbit as a continuation of the **angular vein**, which is formed by the junction of the supratrochlear and supraorbital veins. The facial vein courses inferolaterally, directly posterior to the facial artery. It receives the superior labial, inferior labial and deep facial vein (previous image) as tributaries, and terminates by draining into the **internal jugular vein**.

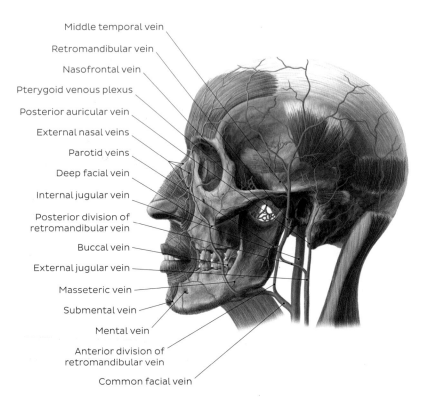

Middle temporal vein

Retromandibular vein

Nasofrontal vein

Pterygoid venous plexus

Posterior auricular vein

External nasal veins

Parotid veins

Deep facial vein

Internal jugular vein

Posterior division of retromandibular vein

Buccal vein

External jugular vein

Masseteric vein

Submental vein

Mental vein

Anterior division of retromandibular vein

Common facial vein

FIGURE 8.31. Veins of face and scalp (lateral view). The veins of the scalp are named by their arterial counterparts; the posterior auricular, superficial temporal and middle temporal veins. These drain into the **retromandibular vein**, which courses just posterior to the mandible and anastomoses with the facial vein prior to draining into the **internal jugular vein**.

Region	Veins	Drainage area
Face	Supratrochlear and supraorbital veins	Forehead and anterior scalp
	Angular vein	Anterior scalp, forehead, eyelids and conjunctiva
	Inferior labial, superior labial and facial veins	Anterior scalp, forehead, eyelids, external nose, anterior cheek, lips, chin and submandibular gland
	Deep facial vein	Structures of the infratemporal fossa
Scalp	Superficial temporal vein	Temporal scalp, temporal muscle and ear
	Middle temporal vein	Temporal scalp
	Posterior auricular vein	Scalp posterior to the ear

Superficial arteries and veins of the face and scalp

Facial artery

NERVES OF THE FACE AND SCALP

The nerves responsible for the motor innervation of the face and scalp originate mainly from the **facial nerve (CN VII)**. The sensory innervation occurs mainly through branches of the **trigeminal nerve (CN V)**. This large cranial nerve divides into three branches, the ophthalmic (CN V₁), maxillary (CN V₂) and mandibular (CN V₃) nerves. These are responsible for the sensory innervation of three distinct dermatomes on the face, with the mandibular nerve (CN V₃) also carrying additional motor fibers to the muscles of mastication. The skin of the scalp anterior to the ears is innervated by branches of the trigeminal nerve, while the posterior scalp is supplied by branches arising from the upper cervical spinal nerves.

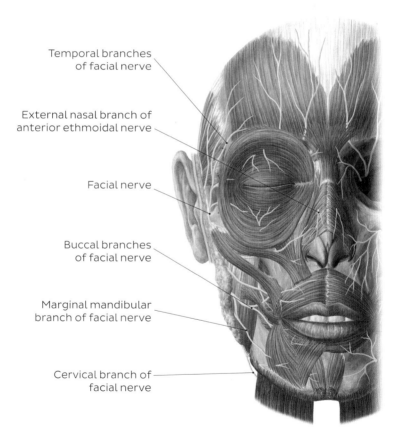

Temporal branches
of facial nerve

External nasal branch of
anterior ethmoidal nerve

Facial nerve

Buccal branches
of facial nerve

Marginal mandibular
branch of facial nerve

Cervical branch of
facial nerve

FIGURE 8.32. **Nerves of face and scalp (anterior view: Superficial).** The **facial nerve (CN VII)** provides motor innervation to the muscles of the face via the temporal, zygomatic, buccal, mandibular and cervical branches. More specifically, these branches supply the stapedius, posterior belly of digastric, the stylohyoid muscle and all the muscles of facial expression. The facial nerve also conveys preganglionic parasympathetic fibers to the geniculate ganglion to innervate all the major glands of the face, except the parotid gland.

HEAD AND NECK

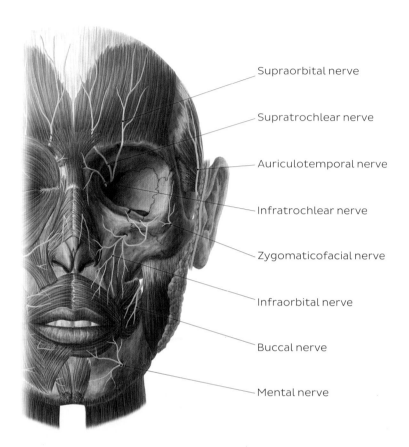

Supraorbital nerve

Supratrochlear nerve

Auriculotemporal nerve

Infratrochlear nerve

Zygomaticofacial nerve

Infraorbital nerve

Buccal nerve

Mental nerve

FIGURE 8.33. **Nerves of face and scalp (anterior view: Deep).** The sensory innervation to the face and scalp arises from the **trigeminal nerve (CN V)** (not visible). The trigeminal nerve divides to give off three branches (ophthalmic (V_1), maxillary (VII) and mandibular (VIII)) which supply sensory innervation to corresponding regions of the face and scalp. The **ophthalmic nerve (CN V.)** gives off the supraorbital, supratrochlear, external nasal branch of anterior ethmoidal nerve (see previous image) and infratrochlear nerve to innervate the area from the anterior scalp down to the upper eyelid. The **maxillary nerve (CN V_2)** gives off the infraorbital, zygomaticofacial and zygomaticotemporal nerve to supply the area from the lower eyelid to the upper lip. The **mandibular nerve (CN V_3)** gives off the auriculotemporal nerve, buccal nerve and mental nerve to innervate the lower lip, chin and jaw.

Nerve	Branches	Supply
Facial nerve (CN VII)	Posterior auricular nerve, temporal branches, zygomatic branches, buccal branches, marginal mandibular branch, cervical branch	Muscles of facial expression
Mandibular nerve (V_3)	Motor branches	Muscles of mastication, mylohyoid muscle, anterior belly of digastric muscle
Ophthalmic nerve (V_1)	Supraorbital nerve, supratrochlear nerve, external nasal branch of anterior ethmoidal nerve, infratrochlear nerve, lacrimal nerve	Anterior scalp, forehead, upper eyelid, conjunctiva and nose
Maxillary nerve (V_2)	Infraorbital nerve, zygomaticofacial nerve, zygomaticotemporal nerve	Area over the zygomatic bone, anterior temple, lower eyelid, side of the nose and upper lip

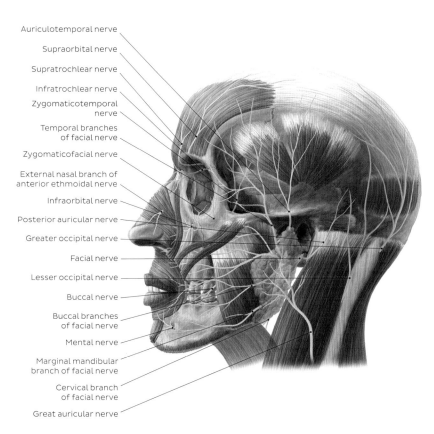

Auriculotemporal nerve

Supraorbital nerve

Supratrochlear nerve

Infratrochlear nerve

Zygomaticotemporal nerve

Temporal branches of facial nerve

Zygomaticofacial nerve

External nasal branch of anterior ethmoidal nerve

Infraorbital nerve

Posterior auricular nerve

Greater occipital nerve

Facial nerve

Lesser occipital nerve

Buccal nerve

Buccal branches of facial nerve

Mental nerve

Marginal mandibular branch of facial nerve

Cervical branch of facial nerve

Great auricular nerve

FIGURE 8.34. **Nerves of face and scalp (lateral view).** The nerves providing sensory innervation to the area of the scalp posterior to the ear are the **great auricular** and **lesser occipital nerves** (via the cervical plexus/anterior rami of spinal nerves C2/C3), as well as the **greater** and **third occipital nerves** (which arise from posterior ramus of spinal nerve C2). The area of the scalp anterior to the ears is innervated by the **zygomaticotemporal nerve**, a branch of the maxillary nerve (CN V$_2$) and the **auriculotemporal nerve**, which is a branch of the mandibular nerve (CN V$_3$). As discussed in the last image, the anterior scalp is innervated by the supratrochlear and supraorbital nerves, which are branches of the ophthalmic nerve (CN V$_1$).

Nerve	Branches	Supply
Mandibular nerve (V$_3$)	Auriculotemporal nerve, buccal nerve, mental nerve	Temple, external acoustic meatus, tympanic membrane, buccinator muscle, lower lip and chin
Spinal nerves C2/C3	Great auricular nerve (C2–C3), lesser occipital nerve (C2) (via cervical plexus); greater occipital nerve, third occipital nerve (posterior ramus spinal nerve C3)	Skin of the posterior scalp

Superficial nerves of the face and scalp

Facial nerve

ARTERIES OF THE HEAD: LATERAL VIEW

The arteries of the head can be divided didactically according to the branches of three main arteries:

- External carotid artery
- Internal carotid artery
- Vertebral artery

The **external carotid artery** supplies most of the structures located outside the cranial vault, i.e. muscles, viscera and skin of the scalp, face and neck. The **internal carotid artery** is the most important artery for the anterolateral aspects of the brain, while the **vertebral artery** supplies most of the posterior structures of the brain, as well as some muscles and skin of the posterior neck.

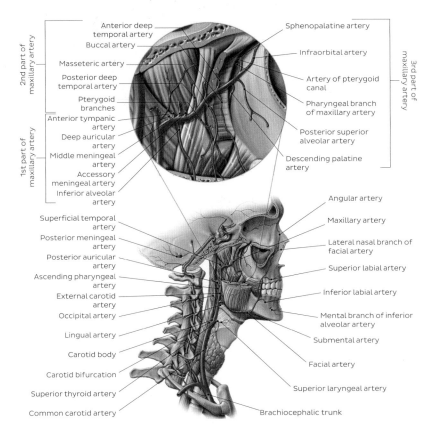

2nd part of maxillary artery
- Anterior deep temporal artery
- Buccal artery
- Masseteric artery
- Posterior deep temporal artery
- Pterygoid branches

1st part of maxillary artery
- Anterior tympanic artery
- Deep auricular artery
- Middle meningeal artery
- Accessory meningeal artery
- Inferior alveolar artery

3rd part of maxillary artery
- Sphenopalatine artery
- Infraorbital artery
- Artery of pterygoid canal
- Pharyngeal branch of maxillary artery
- Posterior superior alveolar artery
- Descending palatine artery

- Superficial temporal artery
- Posterior meningeal artery
- Posterior auricular artery
- Ascending pharyngeal artery
- External carotid artery
- Occipital artery
- Lingual artery
- Carotid body
- Carotid bifurcation
- Superior thyroid artery
- Common carotid artery

- Angular artery
- Maxillary artery
- Lateral nasal branch of facial artery
- Superior labial artery
- Inferior labial artery
- Mental branch of inferior alveolar artery
- Submental artery
- Facial artery
- Superior laryngeal artery
- Brachiocephalic trunk

FIGURE 8.35. **External carotid artery and its branches.** After bifurcating from the common carotid artery, the external carotid artery courses superiorly along the neck, giving branches to supply the muscles, viscera and skin of the head, neck and face. There are **eight major branches** emerging directly from the external carotid artery: The superior thyroid, ascending pharyngeal, lingual, facial, occipital and posterior auricular arteries, as well as two terminal branches, the maxillary and superficial temporal arteries. The image shows the three parts of the maxillary artery and its branches, which supply many structures of the face, ear, skull, meninges, oral cavity and oropharynx.

HEAD AND NECK

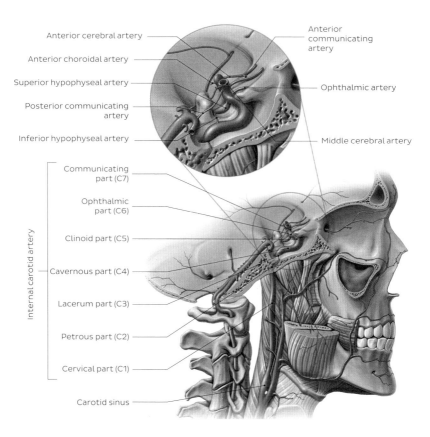

Anterior cerebral artery

Anterior choroidal artery

Superior hypophyseal artery

Posterior communicating artery

Inferior hypophyseal artery

Anterior communicating artery

Ophthalmic artery

Middle cerebral artery

Internal carotid artery

Communicating part (C7)

Ophthalmic part (C6)

Clinoid part (C5)

Cavernous part (C4)

Lacerum part (C3)

Petrous part (C2)

Cervical part (C1)

Carotid sinus

FIGURE 8.36. **Internal carotid artery and its branches.** All **seven segments** of the internal carotid artery can be seen in this image. From proximal to distal these are the cervical (C1), petrous (C2), lacerum (C3), cavernous (C4), clinoid (C5), ophthalmic (C6) and communicating (C7) parts. Except for C7, the odd numbered parts usually do not give off any branches. The most important branches can be seen originating from the **cavernous segment** (meningohypophyseal and inferolateral trunks), ophthalmic segment (ophthalmic and superior hypophyseal arteries) and communicating segment (posterior communicating and anterior choroidal arteries). The termination of the internal carotid artery can also be observed where it bifurcates into the **anterior** and **middle cerebral arteries**.

External carotid artery and its branches

Internal carotid artery

HEAD AND NECK

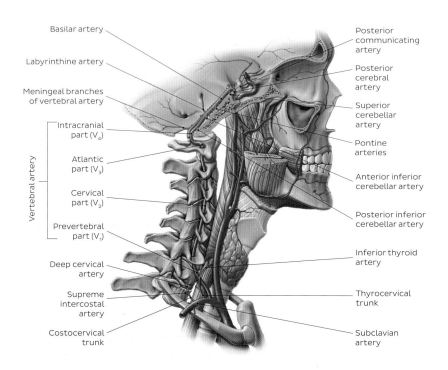

FIGURE 8.37. Vertebral artery and its branches. The vertebral artery can be seen in its totality with **four parts**: Prevertebral (V$_1$), cervical (V$_2$), atlantic (V$_3$) and intracranial (V$_4$). The most important branches originate in the **intracranial segment**: Meningeal branches (that supply the meninges of the posterior fossa), posterior inferior cerebellar artery (a.k.a. PICA). The vertebral artery terminates by merging with the contralateral vertebral artery to form the **basilar artery**. Some branches of the basilar artery should also be recognized: The labyrinthine and pontine arteries can be noted, as well as the anterior inferior cerebellar arteries (a.k.a. AICA), the superior cerebellar arteries and the posterior cerebral arteries, which are its terminal branches.

Artery	Branches	Supply
External carotid artery	Superior thyroid, ascending pharyngeal, lingual, facial, occipital, posterior auricular, maxillary and superficial temporal arteries	Muscles, viscera and skin of the scalp, face and neck
Internal carotid artery	Meningohypophyseal trunk, ophthalmic, superior hypophyseal, posterior communicating, anterior choroidal, anterior cerebral, anterior communicating and middle cerebral arteries	Anterolateral aspect of the brain
Vertebral artery	Muscular, spinal, meningeal branches; Posterior inferior cerebellar, basilar, anterior inferior cerebellar, superior cerebellar, pontine, posterior cerebral arteries	Posterior parts of the brain, muscles and skin of the posterior neck

Vertebral artery

MUSCLES OF MASTICATION

The muscles of mastication are the temporalis, masseter, medial pterygoid and lateral pterygoid. These muscles produce movements of the mandible, or lower jaw, at the temporomandibular joints, thus enabling functions such as chewing and grinding.

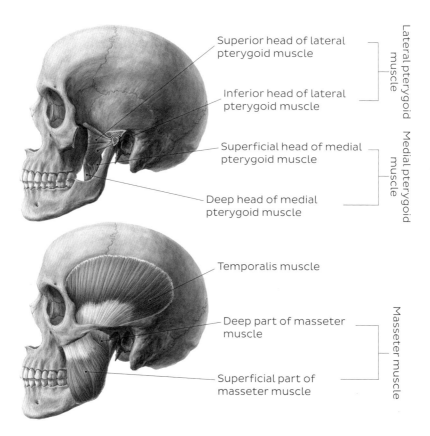

FIGURE 8.38. **Overview of the muscles of mastication.** The muscles of mastication originate from different bones of the skull and insert into the mandible. **Temporalis muscle** is located in the temporal fossa. **Masseter muscle** can be found on the face, superficial to the lateral surface of the ramus of the mandible. This muscle has a superficial and a deep layer. The **medial** and **lateral pterygoids** are found in the infratemporal fossa. Each muscle consists of two heads. The medial pterygoid has a deep and a superficial head, while the lateral pterygoid has a superior and an inferior head.

Muscles of mastication	Origin	Insertion	Innervation	Function
Temporalis muscle	Temporal fossa (up to inferior temporal line), Temporal fascia	Apex and medial surface of coronoid process of mandible	Deep temporal branches (of mandibular nerve [CN V$_3$])	**Anterior part:** elevates mandible **Posterior part:** retracts mandible
Masseter muscle	**Superficial part:** maxillary process of zygomatic bone, Inferior border of zygomatic arch (anterior 2/3's) **Deep part:** deep/inferior surface of zygomatic arch (posterior 1/3)	Lateral surface of ramus and angle of mandible	Masseteric nerve (of mandibular nerve [CN V$_3$])	Elevates and protrudes mandible
Lateral pterygoid muscle	**Superior head:** infratemporal crest of greater wing of sphenoid bone **Inferior head:** lateral surface of lateral pterygoid plate of sphenoid bone	**Superior head:** joint capsule of temporomandibular joint **Inferior head:** pterygoid fovea on neck of condyloid process of mandible	Lateral pterygoid nerve (of mandibular nerve [CN V$_3$])	**Bilateral contraction –** Protrudes and depresses mandible, Stabilizes condylar head during closure; **Unilateral contraction –** Medial movement (rotation) of mandible
Medial pterygoid muscle	**Superficial part:** tuberosity of maxilla, Pyramidal process of palatine bone; **Deep part:** medial surface of lateral pterygoid plate of sphenoid bone	Medial surface of ramus and angle of mandible	Medial pterygoid nerve (of mandibular nerve [CN V$_3$])	**Bilateral contraction –** Elevates and protrudes mandible **Unilateral contraction –** Medial movement (rotation) of mandible

Muscles of mastication

Temporomandibular joint

TEMPOROMANDIBULAR JOINT

The temporomandibular joint (TMJ) connects the skull to the mandible. It is located between the mandibular fossa and articular tubercle of the temporal bone and the condylar process of the mandible. It is classified as a synovial-type joint, however, is atypical in that its articular surfaces are lined by fibrocartilage rather than hyaline cartilage and that it contains a fibrocartilaginous disc. The TMJs facilitate a range of movements of the lower jaw namely depression/elevation, lateral deviation (left or right), and protraction/retraction.

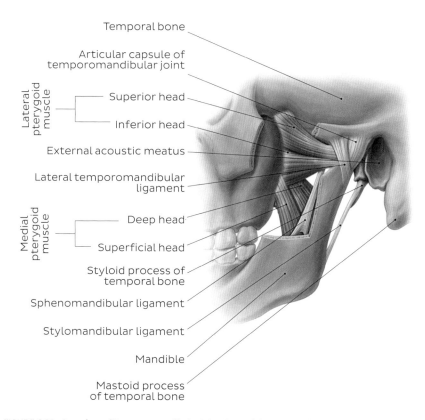

Temporal bone

Articular capsule of temporomandibular joint

Lateral pterygoid muscle
— Superior head
— Inferior head

External acoustic meatus

Lateral temporomandibular ligament

Medial pterygoid muscle
— Deep head
— Superficial head

Styloid process of temporal bone

Sphenomandibular ligament

Stylomandibular ligament

Mandible

Mastoid process of temporal bone

FIGURE 8.39. **Overview of temporomandibular joint.** Part of the ramus of the mandible and zygomatic arch have been removed to expose the infratemporal fossa, where two muscles of mastication are located: The medial and lateral pterygoid muscles. Three major ligaments are associated with this joint. The **lateral temporomandibular ligament** is a thickening of the joint capsule and strengthens it laterally. The **sphenomandibular ligament** is located medial to the joint, running from the spine of the sphenoid bone to the lingula on the medial side of the ramus of the mandible. The **stylomandibular ligament** passes from the styloid process of the temporal bone to the posterior margin and angle of the mandible.

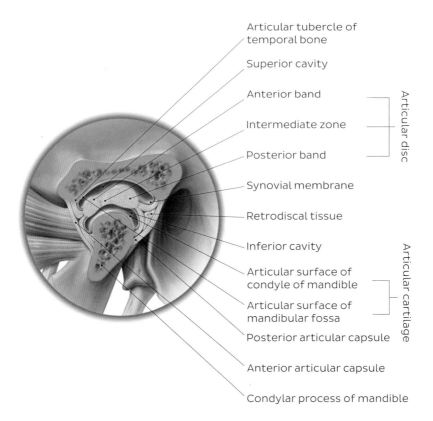

Articular tubercle of temporal bone

Superior cavity

Anterior band

Intermediate zone — Articular disc

Posterior band

Synovial membrane

Retrodiscal tissue

Inferior cavity

Articular surface of condyle of mandible

Articular surface of mandibular fossa — Articular cartilage

Posterior articular capsule

Anterior articular capsule

Condylar process of mandible

FIGURE 8.40. Capsule of temporomandibular joint. Magnification of the TMJ with the capsule opened. In this sagittal view, details of the anatomy of the joint are illustrated. The joint cavity is divided into **two cavities** (superior and inferior) by an articular disc. In the sagittal section, the disc has a thin **intermediate zone** which is bounded by thickened anterior and posterior bands. The disc stabilizes the condyle of the mandible within the joint, reduces frictional forces between the articular surfaces and may aid lubrication of the joint.

Key points about the temporomandibular joint	
Articular surfaces	**Temporal bone**: mandibular fossa and articular tubercle
	Mandible: condylar process
Components	Joint capsule
	Synovial membrane
	Articular disc (anterior/posterior bands, intermediate zone)
Cavities	Superior (discotemporal) cavity (translational movement)
	Inferior (discomandibular) cavity (rotational movement)
Ligaments	**Major**: lateral temporomandibular ligament (thickened lateral portion of capsule, strengthens TMJ laterally)
	Minor: stylomandibular ligament, sphenomandibular ligament

HEAD AND NECK

Key points about the movements of mandible at the TMJ	
Rotational movements	**Elevation**: temporalis, masseter and medial pterygoid muscles
	Depression: lateral pterygoid, digastric, geniohyoid and mylohyoid muscles
Translational movements	**Protrusion**: lateral pterygoid and medial pterygoid muscles
	Retraction: posterior fibers of temporalis, deep part of masseter, geniohyoid and digastric muscles
	Lateral deviation (left or right): posterior fibers of temporalis, digastric, mylohyoid and geniohyoid muscles (ipsilateral movement); lateral and medial pterygoid muscles (contralateral movement)

Temporomandibular joint

Mandible

PTERYGOPALATINE FOSSA

The **pterygopalatine fossa** is a small cone-shaped space located between the pterygoid process of the sphenoid posteriorly, the posterior aspect of the maxilla anteriorly and the lateral surface of the palatine bone medially. Despite its small size, this region is **anatomically strategic** because of its communications with different intra and extracranial spaces: The middle cranial fossa, pharyngeal vault, infratemporal fossa, lateral nasal cavity, floor of the orbit and tissues of soft and hard palates.

The **main contents** of the pterygopalatine fossa are the maxillary nerve (CN V_2) and its branches as well as the pterygopalatine ganglion, formed by preganglionic fibers of the nerve of the pterygoid canal. Additionally, it contains the pterygopalatine part of the maxillary artery, its branches and accompanying veins.

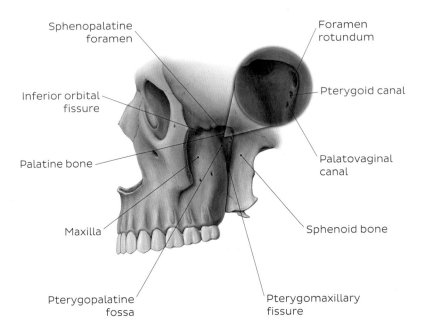

Sphenopalatine foramen

Foramen rotundum

Inferior orbital fissure

Pterygoid canal

Palatine bone

Palatovaginal canal

Maxilla

Sphenoid bone

Pterygopalatine fossa

Pterygomaxillary fissure

FIGURE 8.41. **Structure of pterygopalatine fossa.** Left lateral view of the cranium with the zygomatic arch removed to expose the pterygopalatine fossa located between the maxilla, sphenoid and palatine bones. Posteriorly the pterygopalatine fossa communicates with the middle cranial fossa via the **foramen rotundum** and **pterygoid canal** as well as with the nasopharynx, via the **palatovaginal canal** (pharyngeal canal). Medially the **inferior orbital fissure** can be seen, communicating with the floor of the orbit, while laterally the **pterygomaxillary fissure** connects the pterygopalatine fossa with the infratemporal fossa. The **sphenopalatine foramen** found on the medial wall of the pterygopalatine fossa opens into the lateral mucosa of the nasal cavity.

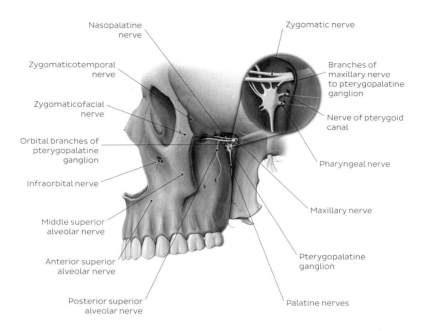

Nasopalatine nerve

Zygomatic nerve

Zygomaticotemporal nerve

Branches of maxillary nerve to pterygopalatine ganglion

Zygomaticofacial nerve

Nerve of pterygoid canal

Orbital branches of pterygopalatine ganglion

Pharyngeal nerve

Infraorbital nerve

Middle superior alveolar nerve

Maxillary nerve

Anterior superior alveolar nerve

Pterygopalatine ganglion

Posterior superior alveolar nerve

Palatine nerves

FIGURE 8.42. **Nerves of pterygopalatine fossa.** The **maxillary nerve (CN V$_2$)** is seen entering the pterygopalatine fossa posteriorly through the foramen rotundum, before it gives off the zygomatic and the posterior superior alveolar nerves. Both the maxillary and zygomatic nerves continue anteriorly to enter the inferior orbital fissure.

Some ganglionic branches also emerge from the maxillary nerve in the pterygopalatine fossa, where they join the **pterygopalatine ganglion**, a parasympathetic ganglion which also receives preganglionic fibers via the **nerve of pterygoid canal** (from facial nerve [CN VII]). Apart from the pharyngeal nerve that exits the fossa via the palatovaginal canal, the main nerves branching from the pterygopalatine ganglion are the **nasopalatine nerve** (courses medially through the sphenopalatine foramen), **orbital branches of maxillary nerve**, **posterior superior lateral nasal branches** (not shown) and **greater** and **lesser palatine nerves** (which course inferiorly to the greater and lesser palatine foramina, respectively).

Key points about pterygopalatine fossa		
Borders	Anterior	Posterior surface of maxilla
	Posterior	Pterygoid process of sphenoid bone
	Superior	Greater wing of sphenoid bone
	Inferomedial	Palatine bone
	Lateral	Opening into infratemporal fossa via pterygomaxillary fissure
Gateways	Foramen rotundum and pterygoid canal	→ middle cranial fossa
	Palatovaginal canal	→ mucosa of pharyngeal vault
	Pterygomaxillary fissure	→ infratemporal fossa
	Sphenopalatine foramen	→ mucosa of lateral nasal cavity
	Inferior orbital fissure	→ floor of the orbit
	Lesser palatine canal	→ mucosa of the soft palate
	Greater palatine canal	→ mucosa of the hard palate

HEAD AND NECK

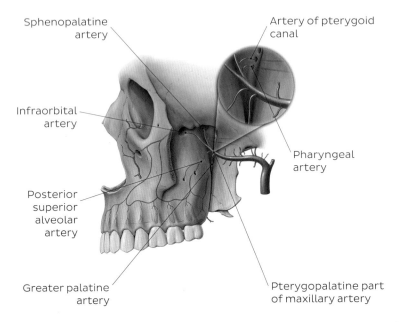

Sphenopalatine artery

Artery of pterygoid canal

Infraorbital artery

Pharyngeal artery

Posterior superior alveolar artery

Greater palatine artery

Pterygopalatine part of maxillary artery

FIGURE 8.43. **Arteries of pterygopalatine fossa.** The main artery to be found in the pterygopalatine fossa is the third (pterygopalatine) part of the **maxillary artery**. There is a lot of anatomical variation concerning the branches of this part of the maxillary artery. Usually it gives off the greater palatine and posterior superior alveolar arteries inside the pterygopalatine fossa, before it bifurcates in the infraorbital and sphenopalatine arteries.

The **infraorbital artery** enters the inferior orbital fissure anteriorly, while the **sphenopalatine artery** courses medially to enter the sphenopalatine foramen. Two other arteries are worth mentioning here: The pharyngeal artery and the artery of pterygoid canal, both of which course posteriorly to enter respectively the palatovaginal canal and the pterygoid canal.

Key points about pterygopalatine fossa		
Contents	Nerves	Maxillary nerve (CN V$_2$) and its branches: zygomatic nerve and branches to the pterygopalatine ganglion
		Pterygopalatine ganglion afferent nerves: branches from maxillary nerve, nerve of pterygoid canal
		Pterygopalatine ganglion efferent nerves: pharyngeal nerve, greater and lesser palatine nerves, orbital branches, posterior superior lateral nasal branches, nasopalatine nerve
	Arteries	Pterygopalatine part (3rd part) of maxillary artery and its branches: greater palatine, posterior superior alveolar, infraorbital, sphenopalatine and pharyngeal arteries and artery of pterygoid canal
	Veins	Pterygoid venous plexus, greater palatine vein, infraorbital vein, deep facial vein → all draining to cavernous sinus, maxillary, or facial veins

HEAD AND NECK

Infraorbital vein

Cavernous sinus

Greater palatine vein

Maxillary vein

Facial vein

Retromandibular vein

Deep facial vein

Pterygoid venous plexus

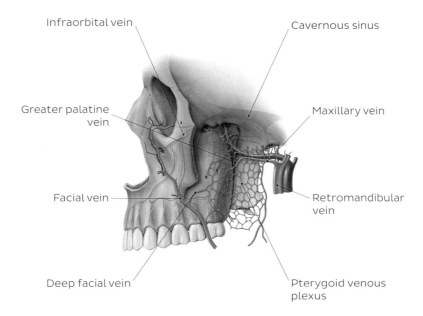

FIGURE 8.44. Veins of pterygopalatine fossa. The main venous structure seen in the pterygopalatine fossa is the **pterygoid venous plexus**. This plexus drains to multiple different venous structures: Posteriorly to the greater palatine vein, that accompanies the course of the maxillary artery; anteroinferiorly to the facial and deep facial veins; and medially to the cavernous sinus, which is an intracranial venous structure located adjacent to the sella turcica.

Anatomy of the pterygopalatine fossa

Pterygopalatine ganglion

HEAD AND NECK

BONES OF THE ORBIT

The orbits are two bony sockets that hold and protect the eyeballs and their associated structures. These structures include the optic nerve, extraocular muscles, the lacrimal apparatus, fascia and neurovasculature that supply them, as well as orbital fat within which these structures are embedded.

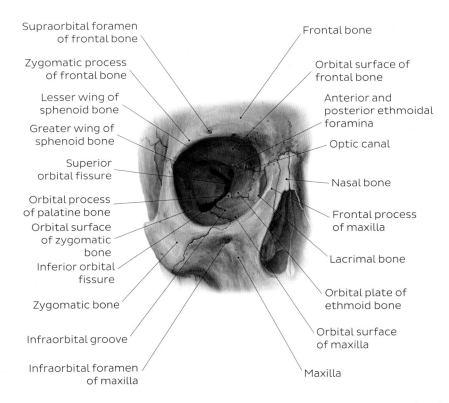

Supraorbital foramen of frontal bone

Zygomatic process of frontal bone

Lesser wing of sphenoid bone

Greater wing of sphenoid bone

Superior orbital fissure

Orbital process of palatine bone

Orbital surface of zygomatic bone

Inferior orbital fissure

Zygomatic bone

Infraorbital groove

Infraorbital foramen of maxilla

Frontal bone

Orbital surface of frontal bone

Anterior and posterior ethmoidal foramina

Optic canal

Nasal bone

Frontal process of maxilla

Lacrimal bone

Orbital plate of ethmoid bone

Orbital surface of maxilla

Maxilla

FIGURE 8.45. Bones of the orbit: Overview. Anterior view of the right orbit showing its bony walls and associated fissures and foramina. The **superior wall** of the orbital cavity is formed mainly by the orbital surface of the frontal bone. The **medial wall** consists of the orbital plate of ethmoid bone, the frontal process of maxilla, the lacrimal and the sphenoid bones. The **inferior wall** of the orbit is formed by the orbital surface of maxilla, orbital process of palatine bone and zygomatic bone, while the lateral wall consists of the frontal process of zygomatic bone and the greater wing of sphenoid bone.

Key points about the bony orbit	
Bones	Maxilla, frontal, zygomatic, ethmoid, lacrimal, sphenoid and palatine bones
Walls	**Roof (superior)**: orbital surface of frontal bone, lesser wing of sphenoid bone
	Medial: orbital plate of ethmoid bone, frontal process of maxilla, lacrimal bone, lesser wing of sphenoid bone
	Floor (inferior): orbital surface of maxilla, orbital process of palatine bone, zygomatic bone
	Lateral: frontal process of zygomatic bone, greater wing of sphenoid bone
Fissures and foramina	Supraorbital foramen, infraorbital groove, infraorbital foramen, anterior and posterior ethmoidal foramina, optic canal, superior orbital fissure, inferior orbital fissure

Bones of the orbit

 Viscerocranium

 Foramina and fissures of the skull

MUSCLES OF THE ORBIT

The muscles of the orbit, also referred to as **extraocular muscles**, or extrinsic muscles of the eyeball, consist of seven skeletal muscles that are located within the orbital cavity, external to the eyeball. Of the seven muscles, the levator palpebrae superioris muscle elevates the upper eyelid. The remaining six are responsible for moving the eyeball in various directions and consist of four recti muscles (superior, inferior, medial and lateral rectus muscles) and two oblique muscles (superior and inferior oblique muscles).

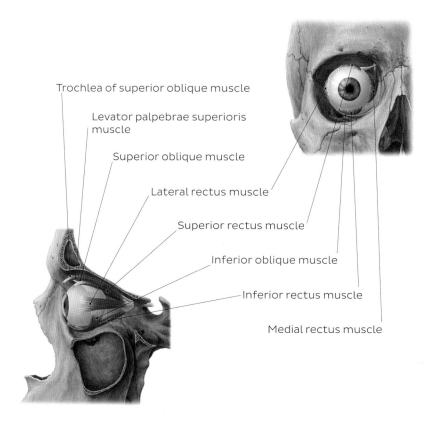

Trochlea of superior oblique muscle

Levator palpebrae superioris muscle

Superior oblique muscle

Lateral rectus muscle

Superior rectus muscle

Inferior oblique muscle

Inferior rectus muscle

Medial rectus muscle

FIGURE 8.46. **Muscles of the orbit.** Lateral view of the left orbit (left image) and anterior view of the right orbit (right image) showing the positions of muscles of the orbit. The most superior muscle is the **levator palpebrae superioris**, originating from the lesser wing of the sphenoid bone and inserting on the superior tarsus and skin of the superior eyelid. Four straplike **recti muscles** (superior, inferior, medial and lateral rectus muscles) all originate from the common tendinous ring and run straight within the orbit to insert on the anterior half of the eyeball. The **superior oblique muscle** arises from the body of sphenoid bone and passes superomedially within the orbit, with its tendon running through the trochlea of the superior oblique, prior to inserting on the superior surface of the eyeball. The **inferior oblique muscle** is seen crossing the floor of the orbit below the inferior rectus muscle after arising from the maxillary bone, to insert on the inferior surface of the eyeball below the lateral rectus muscle.

Extraocular muscles	Origin	Insertion	Innervation	Function
Levator palpebrae superioris	Lesser wing of sphenoid bone	Superior tarsal plate	Oculomotor nerve (CN III)	Elevates superior eyelid
Lateral rectus			Abducens nerve (CN VI)	Abducts eyeball
Medial rectus				Adducts eyeball
Superior rectus	Common tendinous ring (Anulus of Zinn)	Anterior half of eyeball (posterior to corneoscleral junction)		Elevates, adducts, internally rotates eyeball
Inferior rectus			Oculomotor nerve (CN III)	Depresses, adducts, externally rotates eyeball
Inferior oblique	Orbital surface of maxilla	Inferolateral aspect of eyeball (deep to lateral rectus muscle)		Abducts, elevates, externally rotates eyeball
Superior oblique	Body of sphenoid bone	Superolateral aspect of eyeball (deep to rectus superior, via trochlea orbitae)	Trochlear nerve (CN IV)	Abducts, depresses, internally rotates eyeball

 Muscles of the orbit

 Nerves of the orbit

NEUROVASCULATURE OF THE ORBIT

The **ophthalmic artery** provides the main arterial supply to the orbit with minor contributions from the external carotid artery. The principal drainage system of the orbit is by the **ophthalmic veins**.

Facilitating vision, movements of the eye, tear production and general sensation are the nerves of the orbit which include the optic nerve (CN II), oculomotor nerve (CN III), trochlear nerve (CN IV), abducens nerve (CN VI) and autonomic nerves. The ophthalmic (V_1) and maxillary branches (V_2) of the trigeminal nerve (CN V) also supply branches which innervate structures of the orbit.

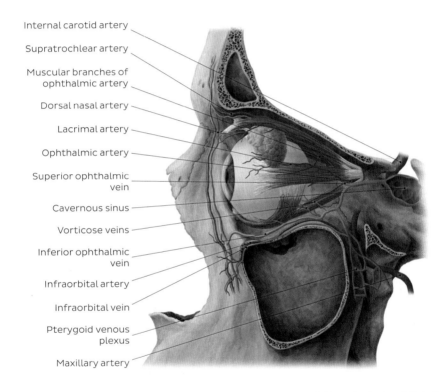

Internal carotid artery
Supratrochlear artery
Muscular branches of ophthalmic artery
Dorsal nasal artery
Lacrimal artery
Ophthalmic artery
Superior ophthalmic vein
Cavernous sinus
Vorticose veins
Inferior ophthalmic vein
Infraorbital artery
Infraorbital vein
Pterygoid venous plexus
Maxillary artery

FIGURE 8.47. Arteries and veins of orbit (lateral view). The main artery of this region is the **ophthalmic artery** (arising from the internal carotid artery), which gives off 10 branches to supply all of the structures of the orbit, in addition to some surrounding structures. The **lacrimal artery** arises from the ophthalmic artery just lateral to the optic nerve and courses anteriorly to supply the lacrimal gland. The muscular branches of the ophthalmic artery supply the intrinsic muscles of the eyeball and give off a small branch, the anterior ciliary artery which supplies the anterior eye.

The **supratrochlear** and **dorsal nasal arteries** travel through and exit the orbit to supply regions of the nose, eyelids, forehead and scalp. Other branches of the ophthalmic artery (central retinal, posterior ciliary, medial palpebral, supraorbital and the anterior and posterior ethmoidal arteries) can be observed from a superior view of the orbit (see next image). Aside from the ophthalmic artery, this region is also supplied by the **maxillary artery** (arising from the external carotid artery), which gives off an infraorbital branch to supply the floor of the orbit.

Venous drainage of the orbit is mainly facilitated by the superior and inferior ophthalmic veins, central retinal vein, vorticose veins and infraorbital vein which drain into the cavernous sinus of the cranial cavity and pterygoid plexus of veins within the infratemporal fossa.

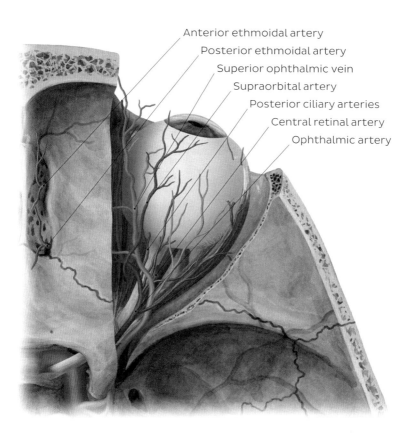

Anterior ethmoidal artery
Posterior ethmoidal artery
Superior ophthalmic vein
Supraorbital artery
Posterior ciliary arteries
Central retinal artery
Ophthalmic artery

FIGURE 8.48. **Arteries and veins of orbit (superior view).** The **central retinal artery** arises from the ophthalmic artery and courses alongside the optic nerve within the dural sheath, to supply the inner layers of the retina of the eyeball. The **long** and **short posterior ciliary arteries** extend anteriorly and supply the choroid, ciliary body and iris of the eyeball. The **supraorbital artery** arises from the ophthalmic artery as it passes medially and crosses the optic nerve in the orbital cavity. It supplies some of the muscles of the eye as well as the skin and muscles of the forehead via superficial and deep branches. The **anterior** and **posterior ethmoidal arteries** arise from the ophthalmic artery within the orbital cavity and pass medially to enter the ethmoidal canal. They supply the nasal cavity and septum.

Venous drainage of the superior orbital region is mainly carried out by the **superior ophthalmic vein** and its associated tributaries. It accompanies the ophthalmic artery along its course, passing through the superior orbital fissure to reach the cavernous sinus.

Key points about the blood vessels of the orbit	
Arteries	**Ophthalmic artery**: lacrimal artery, long and short posterior ciliary arteries, muscular branches of ophthalmic artery (anterior ciliary arteries), central retinal artery, supraorbital artery, anterior and posterior ethmoidal arteries, medial palpebral arteries, supratrochlear artery, dorsal nasal artery
	Maxillary artery: infraorbital artery
Veins	**Superior ophthalmic vein**: tributaries → nasofrontal vein, anterior and posterior ethmoidal veins, lacrimal vein, vorticose veins, ciliary veins, central retinal vein, episcleral veins; drains into cavernous sinus
	Inferior ophthalmic vein: drains into superior ophthalmic vein/cavernous sinus/pterygoid plexus of veins
	Central retinal vein: drains into cavernous sinus but may join superior ophthalmic vein
	Vorticose veins: drain into ophthalmic veins
	Infraorbital vein: drains into pterygoid venous plexus

HEAD AND NECK

Frontal nerve

Oculomotor nerve

Supraorbital nerve

Supratrochlear nerve

Superior branch of oculomotor nerve

Lacrimal nerve

Infratrochlear nerve

Short ciliary nerves

Ciliary ganglion

Branch of nasociliary nerve to ciliary ganglion

Inferior branch of oculomotor nerve

Communicating branch of zygomatic nerve to lacrimal nerve

Infraorbital nerve

Ophthalmic nerve

Zygomatic nerve

Maxillary nerve

Trigeminal nerve

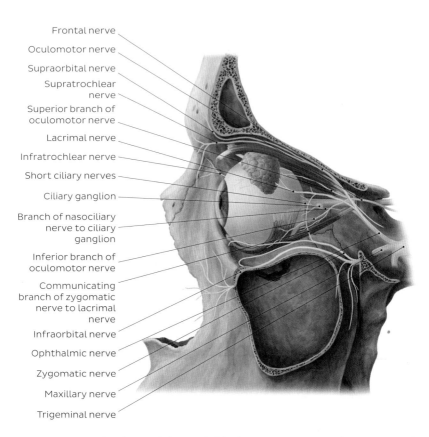

FIGURE 8.49. **Nerves of orbit (lateral view: Eyeball in situ).** The superior and inferior branches of the **oculomotor nerve (CN III)** enter the orbit through the superior orbital fissure to supply the extraocular muscles of the eye. The **ophthalmic nerve** (CN V_1) passes through the cavernous sinus and divides into three branches: The lacrimal, frontal and nasociliary nerves (not visible) before passing through the superior orbital fissure to enter the orbit. The **lacrimal nerve** carries sensory and autonomic nerve fibers to supply the lacrimal gland, eyelids and conjunctiva. The **frontal nerve** divides into supratrochlear and supraorbital branches and conveys general sensation from the forehead, glabella, frontal sinus, skin of the upper eyelid and conjunctiva.

The orbit also receives partial innervation from the **zygomatic** and **infraorbital branches of the maxillary nerve** (CN V_2). Located towards the posterior region of the orbit is the parasympathetic **ciliary ganglion**. The ciliary ganglion relays parasympathetic impulses and transports sympathetic and sensory impulses to structures of the orbit.

HEAD AND NECK

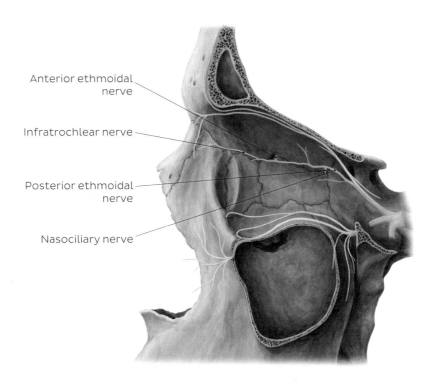

FIGURE 8.50. **Nerves of orbit (lateral view: Eyeball removed).** The **nasociliary nerve** arises from the ophthalmic branch (CN V₁) of the trigeminal nerve and runs obliquely forward through the orbit. Along the way it gives off the long ciliary (not shown), posterior and anterior ethmoidal and infratrochlear nerves, which supply regions of the orbit. The nasociliary nerve conveys sensation from the skin of the dorsum of the nose, eyelids, medial conjunctiva, membranes of the ethmoidal air cell, sphenoid sinus and portions of the nasal cavity. It also transmits sympathetic fibers which supply sensory fibers to the sclera, cornea, iris and ciliary body through the ciliary ganglion.

Key points about the nerves of the orbit	
Oculomotor nerve (CN III)	**Superior branch of oculomotor nerve**
	Inferior branch of oculomotor nerve
	(Branch of oculomotor nerve to ciliary ganglion)
Ophthalmic nerve (V₁)	**Frontal nerve** Supraorbital nerve Supratrochlear nerve
	Nasociliary nerve Posterior ethmoidal nerve Anterior ethmoidal nerve Infratrochlear nerve Long ciliary nerves Branch of nasociliary nerve to ciliary ganglion
	Lacrimal nerve
Maxillary nerve (V₂)	**Zygomatic nerve** Zygomaticotemporal nerve (Communicating branch of zygomaticotemporal nerve to lacrimal nerve)
	Infraorbital nerve

Key points about the nerves of the orbit	
Ciliary ganglion	Parasympathetic ganglion in the orbit; receives preganglionic fibers from the oculomotor nerve, gives off postganglionic branches (short ciliary nerves) to ciliary muscle and sphincter pupillae.
	(Postganglionic sympathetic fibers from internal carotid plexus as well as sensory/afferent fibers also pass through this ganglion)

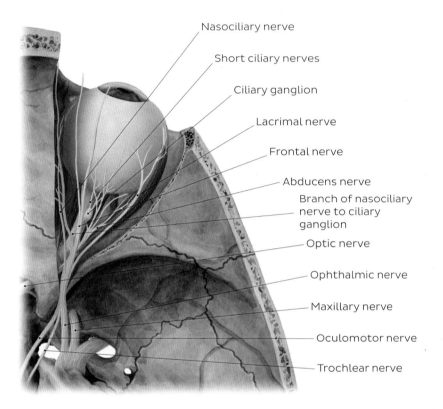

Nasociliary nerve

Short ciliary nerves

Ciliary ganglion

Lacrimal nerve

Frontal nerve

Abducens nerve

Branch of nasociliary nerve to ciliary ganglion

Optic nerve

Ophthalmic nerve

Maxillary nerve

Oculomotor nerve

Trochlear nerve

FIGURE 8.51. **Nerves of orbit (superior view).** The **optic nerve (CN II)** is purely sensory and transmits visual impulses from the eyeball to the brain. The **trochlear nerve (CN IV)** and **abducens nerve (CN VI)** enter the orbit through the superior orbital fissure to supply the extraocular muscles of the eye.

The **ciliary ganglion** is one of the four parasympathetic ganglia of the head and receives preganglionic parasympathetic fibers from the Edinger-Westphal nucleus via the oculomotor nerve (CN III). It supplies structures of the eye (ciliary and sphincter pupillae muscles) via the short ciliary nerves with parasympathetic, sensory and sympathetic fibers, which also pass through the ganglion.

Blood vessels and nerves of the eye

HEAD AND NECK

SUPERIOR AND INFERIOR ORBITAL FISSURES

The superior and inferior orbital fissures are clefts inside the bony orbit. They are located between the lesser and greater wings of the sphenoid bone, and the sphenoid bone and the maxilla, respectively.

The orbit and the middle cranial fossa communicate via the superior orbital fissure, while the inferior orbital fissure connects the pterygopalatine fossa to the bony orbit. Several important neurovascular structures pass through the superior and inferior orbital fissures.

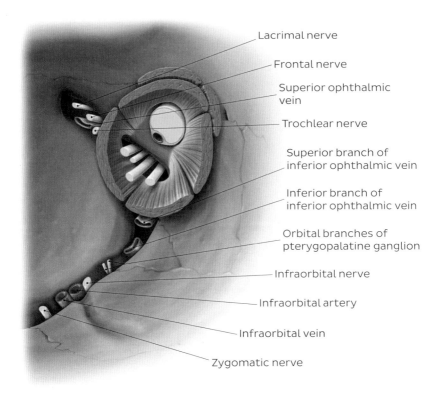

Lacrimal nerve

Frontal nerve

Superior ophthalmic vein

Trochlear nerve

Superior branch of inferior ophthalmic vein

Inferior branch of inferior ophthalmic vein

Orbital branches of pterygopalatine ganglion

Infraorbital nerve

Infraorbital artery

Infraorbital vein

Zygomatic nerve

FIGURE 8.52. **Superior and inferior orbital fissures: Neurovasculature.** The **superior orbital fissure** is located superolateral to the optic canal and positioned between the lesser and greater wings of the sphenoid bone. The **common tendinous ring** is situated along the anteroinferior aspect of the superior orbital fissure. Several nerves and veins pass through the superior orbital fissure with some also extending within the common tendinous ring. From superior to inferior, the **contents** of the superior orbital fissure include the lacrimal nerve, frontal nerve, superior ophthalmic vein, trochlear nerve (CN IV), the superior branch of the oculomotor nerve (CN III), nasociliary nerve, abducens nerve (CN VI), the inferior branch of the oculomotor nerve (CN III) and the superior branch of the inferior ophthalmic vein.

The **inferior orbital fissure** is located between the sphenoid bone and maxilla and lies inferolateral to the optic canal and inferior to the superior orbital fissure. It opens into the posterolateral aspect of the orbital floor and allows the passage of several neurovascular structures. **Contents** of the inferior orbital fissure include the infraorbital nerve, zygomatic nerve, inferior branch of the inferior ophthalmic vein, infraorbital artery and the orbital branches of the pterygopalatine ganglion.

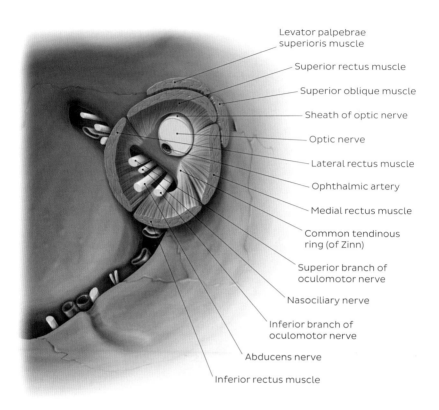

Levator palpebrae superioris muscle

Superior rectus muscle

Superior oblique muscle

Sheath of optic nerve

Optic nerve

Lateral rectus muscle

Ophthalmic artery

Medial rectus muscle

Common tendinous ring (of Zinn)

Superior branch of oculomotor nerve

Nasociliary nerve

Inferior branch of oculomotor nerve

Abducens nerve

Inferior rectus muscle

FIGURE 8.53. **Common tendinous ring: Structure and neurovasculature.** The common tendinous ring of Zinn is a fibrous tissue that serves as a common origin for the four rectus muscles. It encircles the inferolateral part of the superior orbital fissure and surrounds the superior branch of the oculomotor nerve (CN III), nasociliary nerve, abducens nerve (VI) and the inferior branch of the oculomotor nerve (CN III) as they pass through the superior orbital fissure.

Contents of the superior and inferior orbital fissures	
Superior orbital fissure	Lacrimal and frontal nerve (branches of CN V_1), trochlear nerve, superior ophthalmic vein, inferior and superior branches of oculomotor nerve, nasociliary nerve (branch of CN V_1), abducens nerve, and superior branch of inferior ophthalmic vein
Inferior orbital fissure	Inferior branch of inferior ophthalmic vein, orbital branches of pterygopalatine ganglion, infraorbital nerve (branch of CN V_2), infraorbital artery and vein, and zygomatic nerve (branch of CN V_2)

Nerves of the orbit

Arteries and veins of the orbit

HEAD AND NECK

ANATOMY OF THE EYEBALL

The globe shaped eyeball sits within the anterior aspect of the orbit of the skull and contains the optical structures responsible for vision.

The **outer fibrous layer** (external tunic) is formed by the sclera and the protruding translucent cornea. The **middle vascular layer** (middle tunic), also known as the uvea, consists of three connecting layers: The choroid, ciliary body and iris. The **inner layer** (internal tunic) is formed solely by the retina.

Between the cornea and lens are two **chambers** (anterior and posterior) which are separated by the iris. The anterior and posterior chambers communicate with each other via the pupil and are filled with a nutrient rich fluid known as **aqueous humor**. A third, postremal chamber is located posterior to the lens which houses the **vitreous body** of the eye.

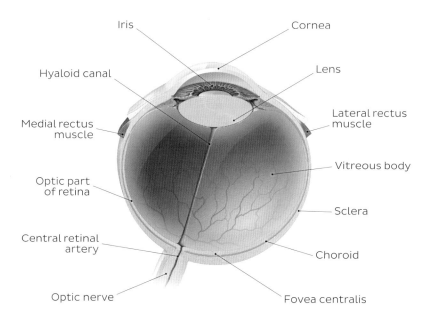

Iris

Cornea

Hyaloid canal

Lens

Medial rectus muscle

Lateral rectus muscle

Optic part of retina

Vitreous body

Central retinal artery

Sclera

Choroid

Optic nerve

Fovea centralis

FIGURE 8.54. **Eyeball (transverse section).** The **choroid** of the eye is located between the sclera and retina and is filled with numerous vascular bundles which supply the outer portion of the retina. Posterior to the iris and anterior portion of the sclera is a thickening of muscular and connective tissue known as the **ciliary body**. The final component of the vascular layer is the pigmented **iris** which contains a central aperture known as the pupil.

The **retina** forms the inner layer of the eye and is composed of non-visual and optic parts. Located posterior to the lens and enveloped by the retina is a compartment known as the **postremal/vitreous chamber** which is occupied by a semi-solid/jelly-like structure known as the vitreous body. Embedded within the meshes of the vitreous body is a fluid-like substance known as vitreous humor. Together these structures allow for the passage of light to the retina and provide structural support to the lens anteriorly.

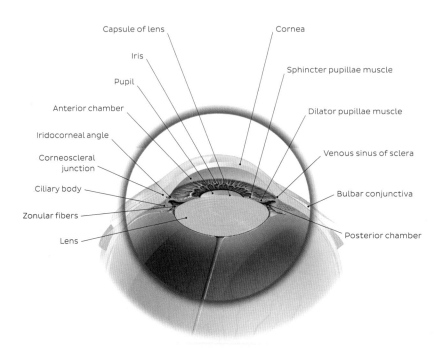

Capsule of lens

Cornea

Iris

Sphincter pupillae muscle

Pupil

Anterior chamber

Dilator pupillae muscle

Iridocorneal angle

Venous sinus of sclera

Corneoscleral junction

Ciliary body

Bulbar conjunctiva

Zonular fibers

Posterior chamber

Lens

FIGURE 8.55. **Anterior part of eyeball (transverse section).** The opaque **sclera** lies just behind the translucent **bulbar conjunctiva** and provides an attachment site for the extrinsic and intrinsic muscles of the eye. Located on the inner portion of the anterior sclera at the **iridocorneal angle** is the **venous sinus of sclera** (canal of Schlemm), which collects aqueous humor from the anterior chamber of the eye, delivering it through a trabecular meshwork into the bloodstream. Forming the transparent part of the fibrous layer is the convex **cornea**. The junction at which the cornea and sclera meet is known as the **corneoscleral junction**.

Key points about the anatomy of the eyeball	
Connective tissue layer	**Anterior**: bulbar conjunctiva **Posterior**: fascial sheath of eyeball
Fibrous layer (External tunic)	**Cornea**: bordered by corneoscleral junction **Sclera**: features venous sinus of sclera, sulcus sclerae, scleral spur
Vascular layer (Middle tunic)	**Iris**: surrounds pupil, contains sphincter pupillae/dilator pupillae muscles **Ciliary body**: corona ciliaris/pars plicata (with ciliary processes and folds), orbiculus ciliaris/pars plana, ciliary muscle, zonular fibres **Choroid**
Inner layer (Internal tunic)	**Retina**: nonvisual retina (iridal and ciliary parts), ora serrata, optic part of retina **Intraocular part of optic nerve**: optic disc
Chambers	Anterior chamber Posterior chamber Postremal chamber: vitreous body (with vitreous humor/membrane, hyaloid canal)
Refractive media	Cornea Aqueous humor Lens Vitreous body (and vitreous humor)

HEAD AND NECK

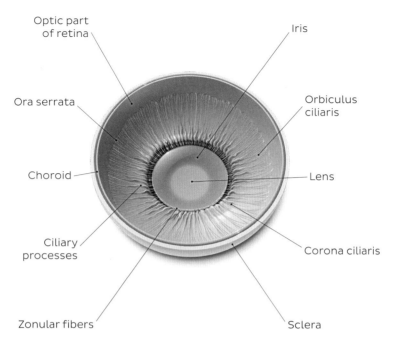

Optic part
of retina

Iris

Ora serrata

Orbiculus
ciliaris

Choroid

Lens

Ciliary
processes

Corona ciliaris

Zonular fibers

Sclera

FIGURE 8.56. **Lens and ciliary body (posterior view).** At the center of this image is the **lens**, located posterior to the iris and anterior to the postremal/vitreous chamber of the eye. The capsule of the lens is anchored to adjacent ciliary processes of the ciliary body by **zonular fibers** which collectively form the suspensory ligament of the lens/ciliary zonule.

The anterior portion of the ciliary body is known as the **corona ciliaris/pars plicata** and is marked by **ciliary processes** (separated by ciliary folds) which function to produce aqueous humor within the posterior chamber providing nutrients for the cornea and lens. The **orbiculus ciliaris/pars plana** forms the posterior portion of the ciliary body and terminates along the **ora serrata**. The optic part of the retina is continuous with the choroid and sclera before terminating anteriorly at the ora serrata while the non-visual part of the retina extends over the ciliary body and iris.

Structure of the
eyeball

Visual pathway

Blood vessels and
nerves of the eye

Arteries and veins of
the orbit

BLOOD VESSELS OF THE EYEBALL

The eyeball receives its main arterial supply via the **ophthalmic artery** that gives off several branches. The **venous drainage** occurs via the central retinal, superior ophthalmic, inferior ophthalmic, and middle ophthalmic veins. The veins drain an intricate venous network located between the different layers of the eyeball.

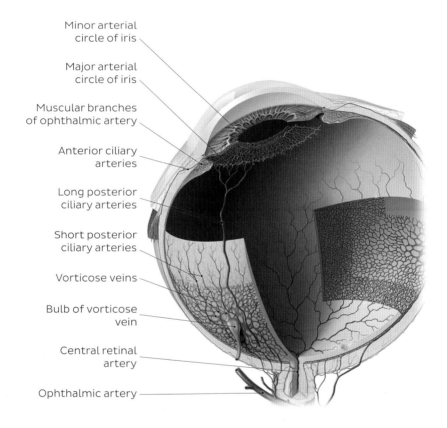

Minor arterial circle of iris

Major arterial circle of iris

Muscular branches of ophthalmic artery

Anterior ciliary arteries

Long posterior ciliary arteries

Short posterior ciliary arteries

Vorticose veins

Bulb of vorticose vein

Central retinal artery

Ophthalmic artery

FIGURE 8.57. **Blood vessels of the eyeball: Overview.** The main arterial supply arises from the **ophthalmic artery**, a branch of the internal carotid artery. It gives rise to several ocular branches, such as the central retinal artery, muscular branches (which give rise to the anterior ciliary arteries), as well as the long and short posterior ciliary arteries. The **central retinal artery** supplies the optic nerve and the innermost layers of the retina. The **ciliary arteries** supply the choroid and the outermost layers of the retina. The anterior ciliary arteries and the posterior ciliary arteries anastomose to form the minor and major arterial circle of the iris. Venous drainage occurs via the **vorticose veins** and the **central retinal vein** into the superior and inferior ophthalmic veins.

Key points about the blood vessels of the eyeball	
Arterial supply	Branches of ophthalmic artery: central retinal, anterior ciliary, short and long posterior ciliary, episcleral artery, muscular branches
Venous drainage	Central retinal vein, vorticose veins, anterior ciliary veins, episcleral and muscular veins drain into superior and inferior ophthalmic veins.

EYELIDS AND LACRIMAL APPARATUS

The **accessory structures** of the eye are the eyelids and lacrimal apparatus, whose function is to protect and lubricate the eye.

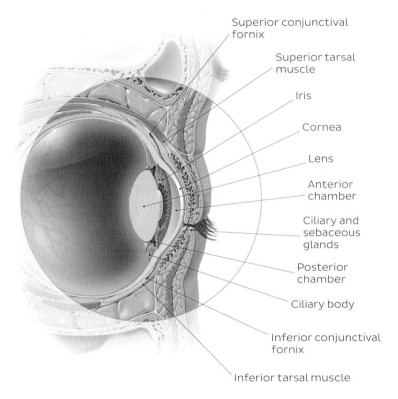

Superior conjunctival fornix

Superior tarsal muscle

Iris

Cornea

Lens

Anterior chamber

Ciliary and sebaceous glands

Posterior chamber

Ciliary body

Inferior conjunctival fornix

Inferior tarsal muscle

FIGURE 8.58. **Eyelids and conjunctiva (sagittal section).** Directly adjacent to the cornea is the **bulbar conjunctiva**, a mucous membrane which lines the anterior surface of the eyeball and continues along the inner surface of the eyelids as the palpebral conjunctiva.

Also depicted in the image are the numerous layers composing the eyelid: Outermost the skin and eye-lashes (cilia), followed by a layer of subcutaneous tissue, skeletal muscle, tarsal plate and innermost, the palpebral conjunctiva. The skeletal muscle within the eyelid is mainly fibers of the palpebral portion of the **orbicularis oculi muscle**, which surrounds the eye and acts as a type of sphincter, as it closes the eyes upon contraction. The **tarsal plate** is a plate of dense connective tissue, responsible for the crescent-shaped form of the eyelid, conforming to the convex anterior surface of the eyeball.

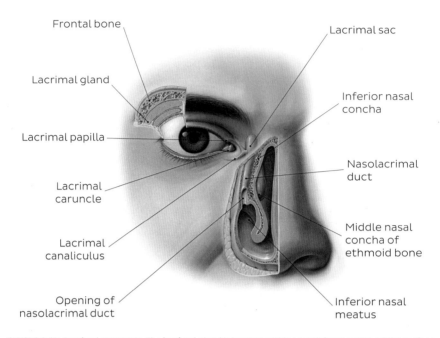

Frontal bone

Lacrimal gland

Lacrimal papilla

Lacrimal caruncle

Lacrimal canaliculus

Opening of nasolacrimal duct

Lacrimal sac

Inferior nasal concha

Nasolacrimal duct

Middle nasal concha of ethmoid bone

Inferior nasal meatus

FIGURE 8.59. **Lacrimal apparatus.** The **lacrimal gland** is located within a small fossa on the orbital surface of the frontal bone and is separated into a superior orbital part and an inferior palpebral part by the aponeurosis of the levator palpebrae superioris muscle. It produces **lacrimal fluid**, which is the aqueous component of the tear film and reaches the eye through 6–12 excretory ducts that open up into the superolateral aspect of the conjunctival sac between the eyelids and eyeball. The fluid then moves from lateral to medial across the eyeball, facilitated by the blinking of the eyelids, and collects in the lacrimal lake in the medial angle of the eye. This accumulation of fluid is drained by the **lacrimal papillae**, which conduct the fluid through the **lacrimal canaliculi** into the **lacrimal sac**, which continues inferiorly as the **nasolacrimal duct** opening on the lateral wall of the **inferior nasal meatus**.

Key points about the eyelids	
Function	Shield eyes from dust and other foreign particles; protect eyes from injury and excessive light; maintain a moist surface on the cornea
Layers	From superficial to deep: skin and eyelashes (cilia), subcutaneous tissue, skeletal muscle (orbicularis oculi muscle/levator palpebrae superioris), tarsal plate, palpebral conjunctiva
Secretions of the eyelid	Ciliary glands (of Moll): secrete a lipid-based compound, prevents evaporation of tear film
	Sebaceous glands (of Zeis): secrete sebum for hair follicles of the eyelashes (cilia)
	Tarsal glands (Meibomian glands): secrete a sebaceous substance (meibum), for an oily layer across the anterior eyeball to prevent evaporation of tear film

Key points about the lacrimal apparatus	
Function	Production, movement and drainage of lacrimal fluid
Components	Production of lacrimal fluid: lacrimal gland
	Excretion: 6–12 excretory ducts of lacrimal gland
	Drainage: through lacrimal caruncle, lacrimal papilla, lacrimal canaliculus, lacrimal sac, nasolacrimal duct → inferior nasal meatus

NASAL CAVITY

The nasal cavities are spaces within the anterior aspect of the skull, located directly behind the external nose. The left and right cavities are separated in the midline by a central nasal septum (medial wall) and both chambers are also bounded by a roof, floor and lateral wall.

Each cavity has **three regions**: Vestibule region, respiratory region and the olfactory region. The **vestibule** is located within the nares. It is lined by skin and houses hair follicles. The **olfactory region** is the most superior part of the nasal cavity, it is lined by olfactory epithelium and contains olfactory receptors. The remaining nasal cavity forms the large **respiratory region**. This area is lined by **respiratory epithelium** with ciliated and mucous cells and contains the nasal conchae and meatuses.

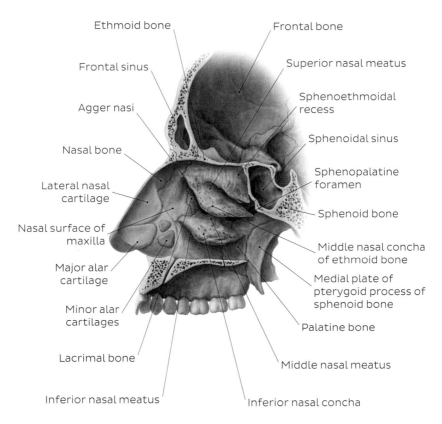

Ethmoid bone — **Frontal bone**
Frontal sinus — **Superior nasal meatus**
Agger nasi — **Sphenoethmoidal recess**
Nasal bone — **Sphenoidal sinus**
Lateral nasal cartilage — **Sphenopalatine foramen**
Nasal surface of maxilla — **Sphenoid bone**
Major alar cartilage — **Middle nasal concha of ethmoid bone**
Minor alar cartilages — **Medial plate of pterygoid process of sphenoid bone**
Lacrimal bone — **Palatine bone**
Inferior nasal meatus — **Middle nasal meatus**
Inferior nasal concha

FIGURE 8.60. **Lateral wall of the nasal cavity.** The anterior apertures to the nasal cavity are the **nostrils** (nares), while posteriorly the nasal cavity opens into the nasopharynx via the **choanae**. The roof houses the **cribriform plate**, which allows the passage of olfactory fibers conveying the sense of smell. The hard palate is the **floor**, separating the nasal from the oral cavity. The **medial wall** is formed anteriorly by cartilage and posteriorly by the very thin vomer bone and the perpendicular plate of the ethmoid bone. Both are covered by a thin, mucosal lining.

The **lateral wall** of each nasal cavity exhibits three curved bony shelves. These are the superior, middle and inferior **conchae**. The conchae project medially into the nasal cavity forming four air channels through which inhaled air can flow, increasing the surface area between the lateral wall and the passing air. From inferior to superior the four air channels are the **inferior nasal meatus**, **middle nasal meatus**, **superior nasal meatus** and the **sphenoethmoidal recess**.

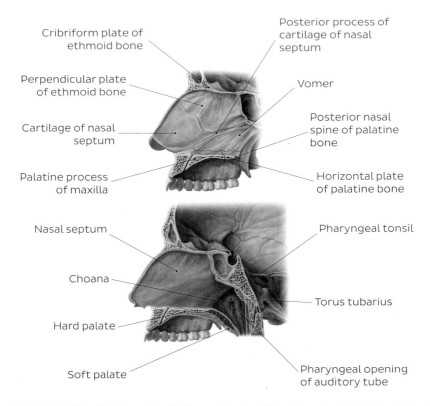

Cribriform plate of ethmoid bone

Posterior process of cartilage of nasal septum

Perpendicular plate of ethmoid bone

Vomer

Cartilage of nasal septum

Posterior nasal spine of palatine bone

Palatine process of maxilla

Horizontal plate of palatine bone

Nasal septum

Pharyngeal tonsil

Choana

Torus tubarius

Hard palate

Soft palate

Pharyngeal opening of auditory tube

FIGURE 8.61. **Medial wall of the nasal cavity.** The **nasal septum** divides the nasal cavity into the right and left chambers. This septum has both bony and cartilaginous parts, composed mainly by the perpendicular plate of the ethmoid, the vomer and the septal cartilage. The septum is smooth and mostly featureless, and like the rest of the nasal cavity, it is covered with nasal mucosa.

Key points about the nasal cavity	
Skeletal framework	Ethmoid bone, sphenoid bone, frontal bone, vomer, nasal bone (2), maxilla (2), palatine bone (2), lacrimal bone (2) and inferior nasal concha bone (2)
Boundaries	Roof – cribriform plate
	Floor – hard palate
	Medial wall – nasal septum
	Lateral wall – houses the conchae and meatuses
Apertures	Anterior – nostrils
	Posterior – nasopharynx (choana)
	Superior – cribriform plate
	Inferior – Incisive canal
	Posterosuperior – sphenopalatine foramen

NEUROVASCULATURE OF THE NASAL CAVITY

The nasal cavity has a rich neurovascular supply, provided by the **nasal arteries**, **veins** and **nerves**. Nasal arteries warm and humidify inhaled air, preparing the air to travel down into our lungs. Nasal veins drain the deoxygenated blood. Nasal nerves carry olfactory information and general sensation, as well as parasympathetic (secretomotor) signals to and from the brain allowing for the sense of smell and taste.

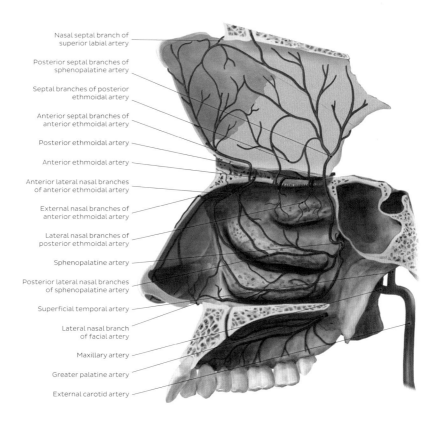

Nasal septal branch of superior labial artery

Posterior septal branches of sphenopalatine artery

Septal branches of posterior ethmoidal artery

Anterior septal branches of anterior ethmoidal artery

Posterior ethmoidal artery

Anterior ethmoidal artery

Anterior lateral nasal branches of anterior ethmoidal artery

External nasal branches of anterior ethmoidal artery

Lateral nasal branches of posterior ethmoidal artery

Sphenopalatine artery

Posterior lateral nasal branches of sphenopalatine artery

Superficial temporal artery

Lateral nasal branch of facial artery

Maxillary artery

Greater palatine artery

External carotid artery

FIGURE 8.62. **Arteries of the nasal cavity.** The lateral wall and nasal septum of the nasal cavity receive arterial supply from five main arteries: The anterior and posterior ethmoidal arteries (ophthalmic artery), the sphenopalatine and greater palatine arteries (maxillary artery) and the septal branch of the superior labial artery (facial artery). The **anterior** and **posterior ethmoidal** and **sphenopalatine arteries** divide into lateral and septal branches as they enter the nasal cavity, while the **greater palatine artery** enters the nasal cavity via the incisive canal of the hard palate. The **septal branch of the superior labial artery** does not give off any named branches and terminates by anastomosing with the **anterior septal branches of the anterior ethmoidal artery**. These arteries collectively supply the ethmoidal and frontal sinuses, the roof of the nasal cavity as well as the mucosa of the nasal conchae, the nasal meatuses and the nasal septum. All 5 arteries anastomose in an arterial plexus located in the anterior nasal septum termed the **Kiesselbach area**. This region is a common site for nose bleeds (epistaxis).

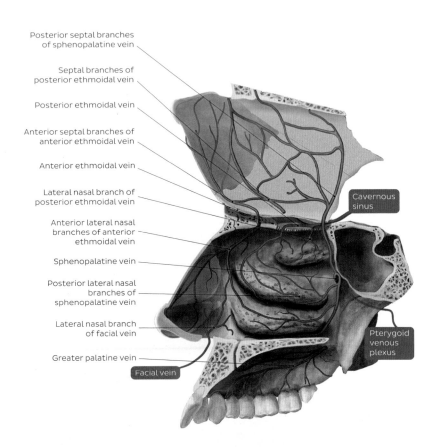

Posterior septal branches
of sphenopalatine vein

Septal branches of
posterior ethmoidal vein

Posterior ethmoidal vein

Anterior septal branches of
anterior ethmoidal vein

Anterior ethmoidal vein

Lateral nasal branch of
posterior ethmoidal vein

Anterior lateral nasal
branches of anterior
ethmoidal vein

Sphenopalatine vein

Posterior lateral nasal
branches of
sphenopalatine vein

Lateral nasal branch
of facial vein

Greater palatine vein

Facial vein

Cavernous
sinus

Pterygoid
venous
plexus

FIGURE 8.63. Veins of the nasal cavity. The nasal veins (sphenopalatine, facial, and ophthalmic veins) follow the pathways of the arteries forming a rich venous plexus within the mucosa of the nasal cavity, particularly at the posterior end of the inferior nasal meatus (Woodruff's plexus). Veins of the nasal cavity have three main drainage points: The **facial vein**, **cavernous sinus** and **pterygoid venous plexus**. The **sphenopalatine vein** and its associated tributaries generally travel through the sphenopalatine foramen to drain into the pterygoid venous plexus. The **greater palatine vein** drains the hard palate and gingiva and enters the infratemporal fossa to also drain into the pterygoid venous plexus. The **ethmoidal veins** drain the roof and upper septal and lateral walls of the nasal cavity, ethmoidal air sinuses, dorsum of the nose and dura mater. The **posterior ethmoidal vein** and its associated tributaries empty into the cavernous sinus while the **anterior ethmoidal vein** and its tributaries drain to the facial or superior ophthalmic vein.

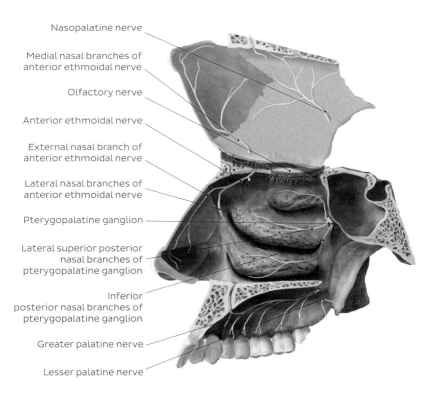

Nasopalatine nerve

Medial nasal branches of anterior ethmoidal nerve

Olfactory nerve

Anterior ethmoidal nerve

External nasal branch of anterior ethmoidal nerve

Lateral nasal branches of anterior ethmoidal nerve

Pterygopalatine ganglion

Lateral superior posterior nasal branches of pterygopalatine ganglion

Inferior posterior nasal branches of pterygopalatine ganglion

Greater palatine nerve

Lesser palatine nerve

FIGURE 8.64. **Nerves of the nasal cavity.** The nasal cavity is innervated by 3 nerves

1. Cranial nerve I – Olfactory nerve
2. Cranial nerve V – Trigeminal nerve
3. Cranial nerve VII – Facial nerve

The **olfactory nerve** carries information of smell to the brain. The **trigeminal nerve** supplies the nasal cavity with sensation, where CN V$_1$ (**ophthalmic nerve**) innervates the anterior nasal cavity and CN V$_2$ (**maxillary nerve**) the posterior cavity. The **facial nerve** carries parasympathetic supply to nasal mucous glands.

Lateral wall of the nasal cavity

Medial wall of the nasal cavity

Kiesselbach's plexus

Olfactory pathway

EXTERNAL EAR

The external ear consists of the **auricle** and the **external acoustic meatus**. It is separated from the middle ear by the **tympanic membrane** (eardrum).

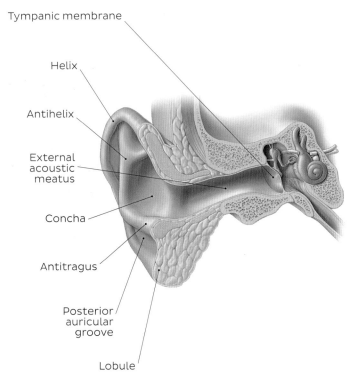

Tympanic membrane

Helix

Antihelix

External acoustic meatus

Concha

Antitragus

Posterior auricular groove

Lobule

FIGURE 8.65. **External ear (coronal section).** The **auricle** is an irregularly shaped cartilaginous structure covered by a thin layer of skin. It is continuous with the **external acoustic meatus**, a tubular component of the external ear. The lateral one-third of the meatus is **cartilaginous**, while its medial two-thirds are **osseous** (temporal bone). The external acoustic meatus terminates with the **tympanic membrane** (eardrum) which is connected to the ossicles of the middle ear.

HEAD AND NECK

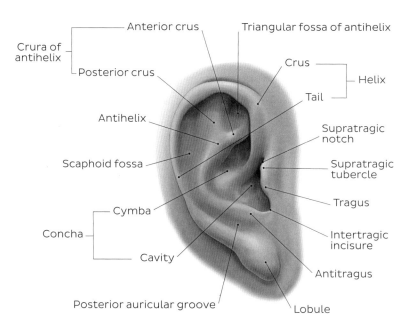

Crura of antihelix — Anterior crus
Posterior crus
Triangular fossa of antihelix
Crus
Helix
Tail
Antihelix
Supratragic notch
Scaphoid fossa
Supratragic tubercle
Cymba
Tragus
Concha
Cavity
Intertragic incisure
Antitragus
Posterior auricular groove
Lobule

FIGURE 8.66. **Auricle (lateral view).** The auricle has several depressions and elevations that comprise its unique shape. The **tragus** is one of several cartilaginous flaps in the external ear and provides a lateral border to the distal end of the external acoustic meatus. The **antitragus** is located posteroinferior to the tragus, from which it is separated by the **intertragic incisure**. The **helix** forms the outer concave border of the ear and may present a small congenital protuberance called the **auricular tubercle** (of Darwin (not shown)). Internal to the helix is another raised cartilaginous structure called the **antihelix** which presents paired, fork-like crura at its superior extremity. It is separated from the helix by the scaphoid fossa. Finally, the inferior most structure of the auricle is the soft, fibrofatty structure known as the **lobule**.

Key points about the external ear	
Parts	Auricle, external acoustic meatus, tympanic membrane
Muscles	**Extrinsic:** auricularis superior, auricularis anterior, auricularis posterior
	Intrinsic: tragicus, antitragicus, obliquus auriculae, transversus auriculae, helicis major, helicis minor
Blood supply	Posterior auricular artery;
	Anterior auricular branches of superficial temporal artery;
	Small branches of occipital artery, deep auricular artery (of maxillary artery), and inferior tympanic artery (of ascending pharyngeal artery)
Innervation	Great auricular nerve;
	Auriculotemporal nerve (branch of mandibular nerve [CN V$_3$])
Function	Conduction of sound waves to the middle ear

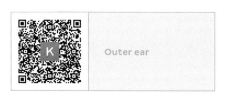

Outer ear

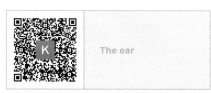

The ear

MIDDLE EAR

The middle ear consists of an air-filled chamber within the temporal bone known as the **tympanic cavity**, located between the external and internal parts of the ear. It is often divided into two main parts: The **inferior tympanic cavity proper (atrium)** and the **superior epitympanic recess (attic)**.

The middle ear is bounded laterally by the tympanic membrane and medially by the lateral wall of the internal ear. The roof of the cavity is formed by a thin plate of bone, the tegmen tympani, while the floor is similarly thin, overlying the internal jugular vein.

The tympanic cavity is directly connected to neighboring anatomical structures and spaces. Anteromedially, it is directly connected with the auditory tube (Eustachian tube) which facilitates equalization of air pressure within the tympanic cavity with ambient pressure. Posteriorly, the tympanic cavity communicates with the mastoid cell of the temporal bone via the mastoid antrum. The result of these direct connections is a continuous mucous membrane between the tympanic cavity, auditory tube, mastoid cells and antrum.

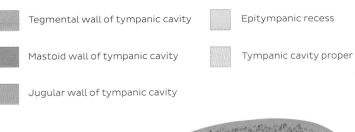

- Tegmental wall of tympanic cavity
- Mastoid wall of tympanic cavity
- Jugular wall of tympanic cavity
- Epitympanic recess
- Tympanic cavity proper

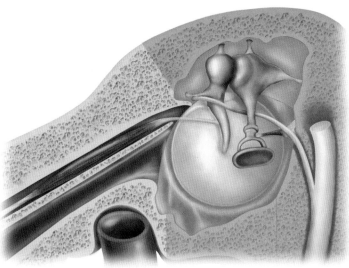

FIGURE 8.67. **Parts and walls of tympanic cavity (medial view).** The tympanic cavity has two main parts: The tympanic cavity proper and the epitympanic recess. The **tympanic cavity proper** is located medially to the tympanic membrane, while the **epitympanic recess** lies above the level of the tympanic membrane, next to the mastoid air cells.

HEAD AND NECK

The tympanic cavity is shaped like a cube, containing **6 walls**: Membranous, tegmental, jugular, mastoid, labyrinthine and carotid wall, with the latter 2 not shown in this section. The **membranous (lateral) wall** is formed by the tympanic membrane and the squamous part of temporal bone. The **labyrinthine (medial) wall** separates the tympanic cavity from the labyrinth. The **tegmental wall (roof)** is a thin plate of bone that separates the tympanic cavity from the cranial cavity, while the **jugular wall (floor)** separates it from the jugular vein and the carotid artery below. The **carotid (anterior) wall** corresponds to the carotid canal and contains the tympanic opening of the auditory tube, while the **mastoid (posterior) wall** partly separates the tympanic cavity from the mastoid antrum.

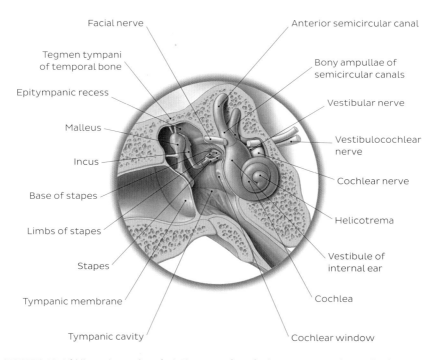

Facial nerve

Tegmen tympani
of temporal bone

Epitympanic recess

Malleus

Incus

Base of stapes

Limbs of stapes

Stapes

Tympanic membrane

Tympanic cavity

Anterior semicircular canal

Bony ampullae of
semicircular canals

Vestibular nerve

Vestibulocochlear
nerve

Cochlear nerve

Helicotrema

Vestibule of
internal ear

Cochlea

Cochlear window

FIGURE 8.68. Middle ear (coronal section). The **tympanic cavity** is a narrow space located in the petrous part of the temporal bone. It contains three **auditory ossicles** (malleus, incus and stapes) which are suspended via small **ossicular ligaments** and regulate the transmission of sound from the external environment to the internal ear. The **jugular wall/floor** of the tympanic cavity features the pharyngeal opening of the auditory tube, a part osseous-part cartilaginous conduit which links the tympanic cavity with the nasopharynx.

Key points about the middle ear	
Parts	Tympanic cavity (proper), epitympanic recess
Walls	Tegmental wall (roof)
	Jugular wall (floor)
	Membranous (lateral) wall (tympanic membrane)
	Labyrinthine (medial) wall
	Mastoid (posterior) wall
	Carotid (anterior) wall
Auditory ossicles	Malleus, incus, stapes
Muscles	Tensor tympani muscle, stapedius muscle
Arterial supply	Anterior tympanic artery (of maxillary artery), deep auricular artery (of maxillary artery), stylomastoid artery (of occipital artery)

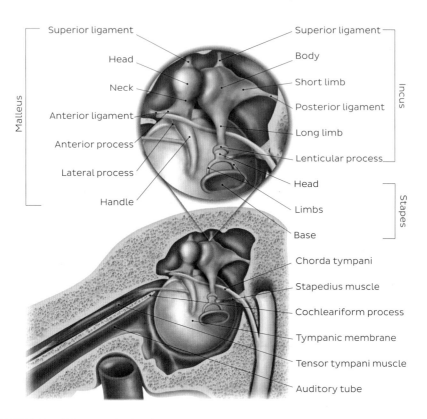

FIGURE 8.69. **Middle ear (sagittal section).** This sagittal section (medial view) of the middle ear provides a better view of the three auditory ossicles, their parts and their ligaments. The **malleus** consists of a head, neck, anterior and lateral processes and handle. It is suspended via three **ligaments**: The superior, anterior and lateral ligaments of malleus (the former of which is not seen on this view).

The **incus** consists of a body, short and long limbs, and lenticular process. It is suspended by two **ligaments**: The superior and posterior ligaments of incus.

The **stapes** consists of a head, anterior and posterior limbs, and base; it is suspended via the **anular ligament of stapes** (not shown). In addition, the **tensor tympani muscle** is clearly seen on this view, running through the semicanal for the tensor tympani muscle of the temporal bone across the cochleariform process which acts as a pulley for this muscle. This view also provides a visual of the stapedius muscle, which attaches on the neck of the stapes.

Key points about the middle ear	
Innervation	Tympanic plexus (glossopharyngeal nerve [CN IX]), nerve to stapedius (facial nerve [CN VII]), nerve to tensor tympani (of mandibular nerve [CN V$_3$]), caroticotympanic nerves
Function	Conduction of sound waves to the inner ear

Auditory ossicles

Middle ear

INTERNAL EAR

The **internal ear** is located in the petrous part of the temporal bone, between the tympanic cavity (middle ear) laterally and the internal acoustic meatus medially. It is formed by a number of bony cavities (**bony labyrinth**), which contain several membranous ducts and sacs (**membranous labyrinth**).

The cavities forming the **bony labyrinth** are the vestibule, cochlea, and three semicircular canals. These cavities are filled with a clear fluid, called perilymph. The **membranous labyrinth** lies suspended within the bony labyrinth, and is also filled with a fluid, the endolymph. It consists of three semicircular ducts (one inside each semicircular canal), the cochlear duct (inside the cochlea) and two sacs found in the vestibule, the saccule and the utricle.

The internal ear has two main **functions**, acting as a transducer transforming the mechanical energy of **sound waves** into neuronal impulses (cochlear part of the internal ear), and also playing an important role in the maintenance of **balance** (vestibular part of the internal ear and semicircular canals).

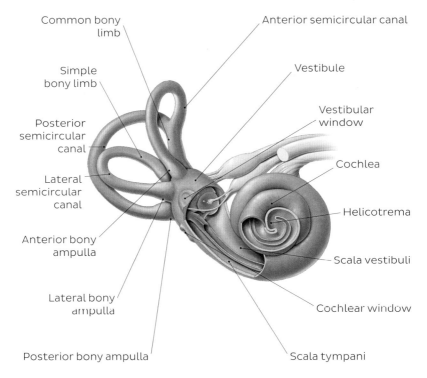

Common bony limb · Anterior semicircular canal · Simple bony limb · Vestibule · Vestibular window · Posterior semicircular canal · Lateral semicircular canal · Cochlea · Helicotrema · Anterior bony ampulla · Scala vestibuli · Lateral bony ampulla · Cochlear window · Posterior bony ampulla · Scala tympani

FIGURE 8.70. **Bony labyrinth.** The bony labyrinth is located within the petrous part of the temporal bone. It consists of three continuous parts: Vestibule, cochlea and semicircular canals.

The **vestibule** is a central bony cavity which communicates with the middle ear through the vestibular window on its lateral wall.

Posterosuperiorly, the vestibule is continued by the three **semicircular bony canals**, each placed in a specific anatomical plane. The **anterior canal** lies in the sagittal plane, the **posterior** is in the lateral plane, while the **lateral canal** lies in the transverse plane. The canals arise from the vestibule via bony **ampullae** (anterior, posterior, lateral). They curve through their respective planes, diving back into the bony vestibule. The lateral canal does so directly via the **simple bony limb**, while the anterior and posterior canals merge forming the **common bony limb** which then joins the vestibule.

The **cochlea** is a snail-like structure that spirals from the anterior part of the vestibule. The cochlea is essentially a bony canal that spirals around its axis two and a half times. The central portion of the cochlea, i.e. the axis, around which it spirals, is called the **modiolus**. Along the entire length of the cochlea is a thin bony lamina which divides the cochlea into two parts: **Scala vestibuli** and **scala tympani**. These sub-canals are entirely separate except at the apex of the cochlea, where they communicate through a narrow slit called the helicotrema.

The whole bony labyrinth is filled with **perilymph**.

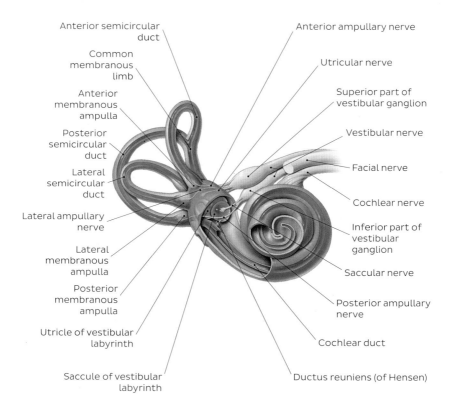

Anterior semicircular duct
Common membranous limb
Anterior membranous ampulla
Posterior semicircular duct
Lateral semicircular duct
Lateral ampullary nerve
Lateral membranous ampulla
Posterior membranous ampulla
Utricle of vestibular labyrinth
Saccule of vestibular labyrinth

Anterior ampullary nerve
Utricular nerve
Superior part of vestibular ganglion
Vestibular nerve
Facial nerve
Cochlear nerve
Inferior part of vestibular ganglion
Saccular nerve
Posterior ampullary nerve
Cochlear duct
Ductus reuniens (of Hensen)

FIGURE 8.71. **Membranous labyrinth.** The membranous labyrinth is suspended within the perilymph of the bony labyrinth thus mirroring its overall structure. The central part of the membranous labyrinth is located within the bony vestibule. It consists of two sacs: Utricle and saccule, which communicate via a small duct called the ductus reuniens. The **utricle** lies in the posterior part of the vestibule, while the **saccule** lies anteriorly. The three **membranous semicircular ducts** branch from the utricle and pass through the semicircular canals. Similar to their bony counterparts, the canals originate with membranous **ampullae** (anterior, posterior, lateral). The anterior and posterior duct unite as well, forming the **common membranous limb**.

The bony cochlea houses the membranous **cochlear duct** which follows its spiral course.

The whole membranous labyrinth is filled with **endolymph**. Movement of endolymph stimulates the receptor cells within the walls of the labyrinth, producing neuronal stimuli related to balance and hearing. These stimuli are conveyed via the **vestibulocochlear nerve**, whose components can be seen innervating different parts of the labyrinth. Essentially, the **vestibular nerve** innervates the utricle, saccule and semicircular ducts, via its branches, conveying the information about **balance**. Branches of the **cochlear nerve** innervate the spiral organ of Corti that is located in the cochlea, providing information about **hearing**.

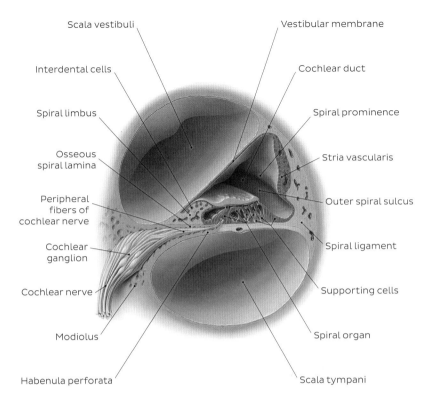

Scala vestibuli

Vestibular membrane

Interdental cells

Cochlear duct

Spiral limbus

Spiral prominence

Osseous spiral lamina

Stria vascularis

Peripheral fibers of cochlear nerve

Outer spiral sulcus

Cochlear ganglion

Spiral ligament

Cochlear nerve

Supporting cells

Modiolus

Spiral organ

Habenula perforata

Scala tympani

FIGURE 8.72. Cochlea (cross section). The cochlea is the structure of the internal ear responsible for **hearing**. Its structure resembles a snail shell situated in the bony labyrinth of the temporal bone. The 'shell' of the cochlea is wrapped two and a half times around its axis, known as the **modiolus**. The cross section of the cochlea reveals its internal structure which is characterized by the cavity of the cochlea (spiral canal) and a triangular membranous duct, called the cochlear duct (also known as the scala media).

The **scala media** is filled with endolymph. In addition to the scala media, there are two more canals that run parallel to one another, the scala vestibuli and scala tympani. In contrast to the scala media, the **scala vestibuli** and **scala tympani** are filled with perilymph. Sound vibrations transmitted from the middle ear through the vestibular window result in mechanical movements of the fluids inside the cochlea which moves the **basilar membrane**. Movements of the basilar membrane in turn cause movements of the structures within the cochlear duct. These movements are converted to electrical impulses in the receptor part of the cochlea known as the spiral organ (of Corti).

Key points about the internal ear	
Parts	**Bony labyrinth**: vestibule, semicircular canals, cochlea
	Membranous labyrinth: utricle, saccule, semicircular ducts, cochlear duct
Functions	**Utricle and saccule**: information about the position of the head (via vestibular nerve)
	Semicircular ducts: information about movements of the head (via vestibular nerve)
	Cochlear duct: hearing information (via cochlear nerve)

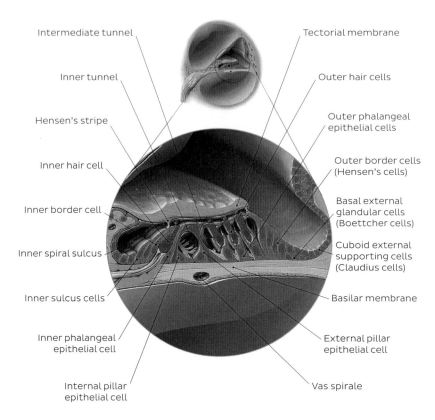

Intermediate tunnel

Inner tunnel

Hensen's stripe

Inner hair cell

Inner border cell

Inner spiral sulcus

Inner sulcus cells

Inner phalangeal epithelial cell

Internal pillar epithelial cell

Tectorial membrane

Outer hair cells

Outer phalangeal epithelial cells

Outer border cells (Hensen's cells)

Basal external glandular cells (Boettcher cells)

Cuboid external supporting cells (Claudius cells)

Basilar membrane

External pillar epithelial cell

Vas spirale

FIGURE 8.73. Cochlear duct/spiral organ (cross section). The **spiral organ (of Corti)** is the receptor organ for hearing that produces electrical impulses in response to auditory stimuli. It is located in the cochlear duct of the cochlear canal sitting on top of the basilar membrane.

The spiral organ (of Corti) contains a number of receptor cells known as **hair cells**. More specifically, it contains three rows of outer hair cells and one row of inner hair cells. Hair cells are so named because they contain hair-like projections on the apical part of their cell membrane, known as **stereocilia**, which are embedded in a gel-like structure called the tectorial membrane. As perilymph moves in response to sound waves, it shifts the basilar membrane respectively to the tectorial membrane. These shifts between the tectorial and basilar membranes bend the stereocilia, causing the hair cells to depolarize and release neurotransmitters (glutamate) that transmits the sound information to the cochlear nerve.

Inner ear

Vestibular system

Auditory pathway

HEAD AND NECK

OVERVIEW OF THE ORAL CAVITY

The **oral cavity** is the initial part of the digestive system that contains the structures necessary for mastication and speech; teeth, tongue and salivary glands. It allows food to be tasted and broken down to form the food bolus, which is pushed back into the pharynx to initiate the process of deglutition (swallowing). Moreover, the oral cavity also has a role in the process of articulation, which is the modification of sounds to facilitate communication; it can also be an alternative route for the inhalation of air into the respiratory system.

The oral cavity is divided in two regions: Oral vestibule and oral cavity proper.

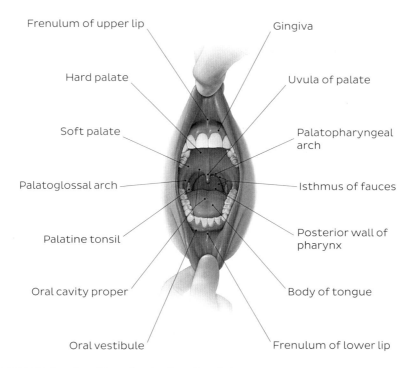

Frenulum of upper lip

Gingiva

Hard palate

Uvula of palate

Soft palate

Palatopharyngeal arch

Palatoglossal arch

Isthmus of fauces

Palatine tonsil

Posterior wall of pharynx

Oral cavity proper

Body of tongue

Oral vestibule

Frenulum of lower lip

FIGURE 8.74. **Overview of the oral cavity.** The **oral vestibule** contains the lingual/buccal gingiva which are firmly attached to the maxilla and mandible, as well as the median mucosal folds known as the superior and inferior labial frenula. The space enclosed by the teeth is the **oral cavity proper**, whose roof is formed by the hard and soft palates. The **uvula** can be seen hanging from the posterior part of the soft palate.

The **floor** of that cavity is composed of the geniohyoid and mylohyoid muscles (not shown). Its **lateral walls** are formed by the dental arches. Posteriorly, the oral cavity proper opens into the **isthmus of fauces** (oropharyngeal isthmus), a transitional space located between the oral cavity and oropharynx, bounded anteriorly by the palatoglossal arches and posteriorly by the palatopharyngeal arches. The space between these arches is called **tonsillar fossa** (sinus) and contains the palatine tonsils.

Oral cavity

Tongue

SURFACE OF THE TONGUE

The tongue consists of a body, apex and root containing the lingual papillae and tonsils.

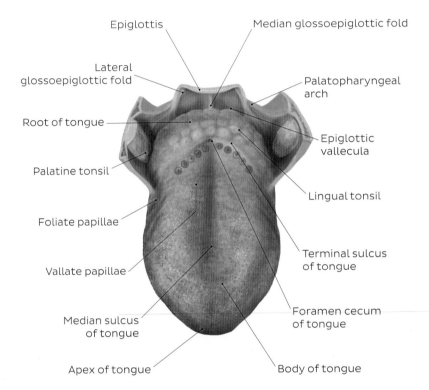

FIGURE 8.75. **Superior view of the surface of the tongue.** The **apex** of the tongue lies most anteriorly. The **body** of the tongue is divided into two hemispheres by the median sulcus of the tongue and contains numerous lingual papillae. It has a rough dorsal (superior) and a smooth ventral (inferior) surface. The **root** of the tongue with the lingual tonsils is located posteriorly. Just anterior to it lies the **foramen cecum**, an embryological remnant of the thyroglossal duct. The epiglottis is located posteriorly to the root of the tongue and the palatine tonsils laterally.

The **lingual papillae** are located on the presulcal part of the tongue, just anterior to the **terminal sulcus**. The **vallate papillae** run parallel to the terminal sulcus, whereas the **foliate papillae** are located on the posterolateral end of the body of the tongue on each side. The **filiform papillae** are the most numerous lingual papillae and cover most of the presulcal area of the dorsum of the tongue. Their main function is to increase the friction between the food and the tongue. The **fungiform papillae** are larger than the filiform papillae and rounder in shape. They are mostly found at the tip and side of the tongue and contain taste buds on their upper surface.

The **taste sensation** is transmitted to the brainstem via three nerves: The facial nerve (chorda tympani) innervating the anterior ⅔ of tongue and soft palate, the glossopharyngeal nerve innervating the posterior ⅓ of the tongue and the vagus nerve innervating the epiglottis.

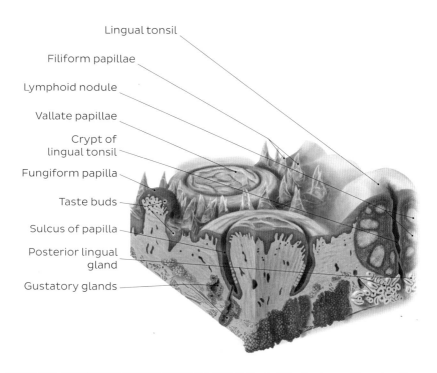

Lingual tonsil

Filiform papillae

Lymphoid nodule

Vallate papillae

Crypt of
lingual tonsil

Fungiform papilla

Taste buds

Sulcus of papilla

Posterior lingual
gland

Gustatory glands

FIGURE 8.76. **Overview of the lingual papillae.** The distinct shapes of the four types of lingual papillae can be seen. The vallate papillae are separated from their walls by the sulcus of papilla. In addition to this, the gustatory glands, also known as von Ebner's glands, are located deep to the vallate papillae. The posterior lingual glands are located at the root of the tongue. Above the posterior lingual glands, the lingual tonsil is illustrated.

Key points of the lingual papillae	
Filiform papillae	Stretched, conical, gray-white papillae
	Covered with keratinized squamous epithelium
	Provide friction to allow movement of the food bolus during chewing
	Do not possess taste buds
Fungiform papillae	Highly vascular, mushroom-shaped papillae
	Scattered across the entire dorsal surface of the tongue
	Contain few taste buds on the apical aspect
Foliate papillae	Bilaterally paired, parallel, "leaf-like" ridges of mucosa
	On the posterolateral margin of the tongue, near the terminal sulcus
	Non-keratinized mucosa
	Contain numerous taste buds
Vallate papillae	Usually between 8–12 cylindrical papillae
	Anterior and parallel to the terminal sulcus of the tongue

Anatomy of taste

MUSCLES OF THE TONGUE

The tongue consists of two major muscle groups: Extrinsic and intrinsic. The **extrinsic muscles** originate outside of the tongue and mainly function to move the tongue as a whole (i.e. gross movement). They are the genioglossus, hyoglossus, styloglossus and palatoglossus. The **intrinsic muscles** are contained within the tongue itself and alter its size and shape to produce fine movements for talking and swallowing. They are the superior and inferior longitudinal muscles, vertical and transverse muscles of the tongue.

All of the lingual muscles innervated by the **hypoglossal nerve (CN XII)**, except for the palatoglossus muscle, which receives its innervation from the **vagus nerve (CN X)** via the pharyngeal plexus.

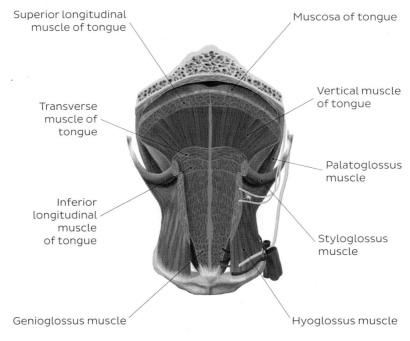

Superior longitudinal muscle of tongue

Muscosa of tongue

Transverse muscle of tongue

Vertical muscle of tongue

Palatoglossus muscle

Inferior longitudinal muscle of tongue

Styloglossus muscle

Genioglossus muscle

Hyoglossus muscle

FIGURE 8.77. **Muscles of the tongue (coronal section).** The tongue is composed of 8 paired muscles, which are separated left from right by a **median lingual septum**. The intrinsic muscles (superior longitudinal muscle, inferior longitudinal muscle, vertical muscle and transverse muscle) are confined within the core of the tongue. They are flanked on either side by the styloglossus, hyoglossus and palatoglossus muscles which enter the side of the tongue, decussating with each other as well as the inferior longitudinal muscle. The genioglossus muscle is located medially on either side of the lingual septum. The **hypoglossal nerve (CN XII)**, which innervates most of the muscles of the tongue, is also shown in this image.

Palatoglossus muscle

Superior longitudinal
muscle of tongue

Styloglossus muscle

Vertical muscle of tongue

Transverse muscle
of tongue

Inferior longitudinal
muscle of tongue

Hyoglossus muscle

Genioglossus muscle

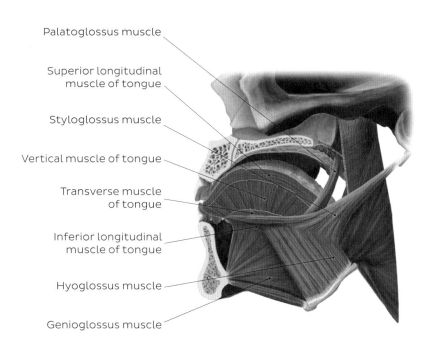

FIGURE 8.78. **Muscles of the tongue (sagittal section).** The attachment points of the **extrinsic muscles** are visible in this image. The **genioglossus** muscle originates from the superior mental spine of the mandible; its triangular shape inserts along the entire length of the tongue as well as the body of the hyoid bone. The **styloglossus** muscle originates from the styloid process of the temporal bone; its longitudinal fibers blend with the inferior longitudinal muscle while its oblique fibers decussate with those of the **hyoglossus** muscle which extends from body and greater horn of the hyoid bone. Finally, the **palatoglossus** muscle can be identified arising from tissues of the soft palate extending towards the tongue, forming the wall of the palatoglossal arch.

Extrinsic tongue muscles	Origin	Insertion	Innervation	Function
Genioglossus	Superior mental spine of mandible	Entire length of dorsum of tongue/Lingual aponeurosis, Body of hyoid bone		Bilateral contraction – Depresses and protrudes tongue; Unilateral contraction – Deviates tongue contralaterally
Hyoglossus	Body and greater horn of hyoid bone	Inferior/Ventral parts of lateral tongue	Hypoglossal nerve (CN XII)	Depresses and retracts tongue
Styloglossus	Anterolateral aspect of styloid process (of temporal bone), Stylomandibular ligament	**Longitudinal part**: blends with inferior longitudinal muscle **Oblique part**: blends with hyoglossus muscle		Retracts and elevates lateral aspects of tongue
Palatoglossus	Palatine aponeurosis of soft palate	Lateral margins of tongue, Blends with intrinsic muscles of tongue	Vagus nerve (CN X) (via branches of pharyngeal plexus)	Elevates root of tongue, Constricts isthmus of fauces

Intrinsic tongue muscles	Origin	Insertion	Innervation	Function
Superior longitudinal muscle	Submucosa of posterior tongue, Lingual septum	Apex/Anterolateral margins of tongue	Hypoglossal nerve (CN XII)	Retracts and broadens tongue, Elevates apex of tongue
Inferior longitudinal muscle	Root of tongue, Body of hyoid bone	Apex of tongue		Retracts and broadens tongue, Lowers apex of tongue
Transverse muscle	Lingual septum	Lateral margin of tongue		Narrows and elongates tongue
Vertical muscle	Root of tongue, Genioglossus muscle	Lingual aponeurosis		Broadens and elongates tongue

Muscles and taste sensation of the tongue

HEAD AND NECK

NEUROVASCULATURE OF THE TONGUE

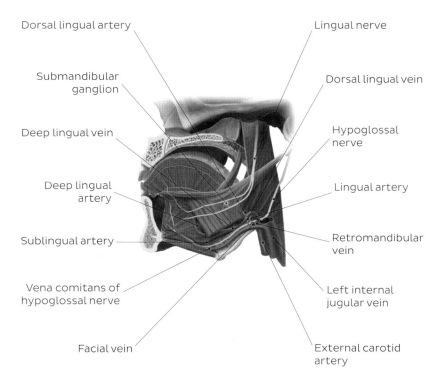

Dorsal lingual artery

Lingual nerve

Submandibular ganglion

Dorsal lingual vein

Deep lingual vein

Hypoglossal nerve

Deep lingual artery

Lingual artery

Sublingual artery

Retromandibular vein

Vena comitans of hypoglossal nerve

Left internal jugular vein

Facial vein

External carotid artery

FIGURE 8.79. **Nervous and vascular supply of the tongue.** Sagittal section of the lower face showing the tongue and its neurovascular supply. The image shows the **lingual nerve**, a branch of the mandibular nerve (CN V$_3$), and the submandibular ganglion, a parasympathetic ganglion associated with the chorda tympani. **Chorda tympani** is a branch of the facial nerve (CN VII) that carries special sensory innervation to the tongue and parasympathetic innervation to the submandibular and sublingual glands. The **hypoglossal nerve (CN XII)** carries motor innervation to all the intrinsic muscles of the tongue. The **lingual artery** originates from the external carotid artery and gives off 3 main branches: The dorsal lingual, deep lingual and sublingual arteries, which supply the root of the tongue, the body of tongue and the floor of the oral cavity and sublingual glands, respectively. Lastly, the veins that drain the tongue into the **internal jugular vein** are visible.

Key points about the neurovasculature of the tongue	
Innervation	Motor innervation: hypoglossal nerve (CN XII) innervates all except palatoglossus muscle (pharyngeal plexus from vagus nerve, CN X)
	Sensory and parasympathetic innervation: • Anterior ¾: lingual nerve for general sensory (branch of mandibular nerve V$_3$) and chorda tympani nerve for special sensory (branch of facial nerve, CN VII) • Posterior ⅓ and vallate papillae: glossopharyngeal nerve (CN IX)
Arterial supply	Lingual artery and its branches: • Dorsal lingual artery: supplies the root of tongue • Deep lingual artery: supplies the body of tongue • Sublingual artery: supplies the floor of the oral cavity and sublingual glands
Venous drainage	Dorsal lingual vein: drains the root of tongue → lingual vein → internal jugular vein (IJV)
	Deep lingual vein: drains the body of tongue → lingual vein → IJV
	Sublingual veins: drain the floor of oral cavity and sublingual glands to vena comitans of hypoglossal nerve → lingual vein → IJV

Nerve and blood
supply of the tongue

SALIVARY GLANDS

The salivary glands are exocrine tubuloacinar structures whose excretory ducts open into the oral cavity. The main function of these glands is to secrete saliva, a seromucous liquid that has several major functions within the oral cavity including lubrication, digestion, physicochemical/immune defense and taste transmission. The total daily output of **saliva** in an adult is about 1.5 liters. The **major salivary glands** are the paired parotid, submandibular and sublingual glands. Additionally, there are as many as 600 **minor salivary glands** scattered throughout the oral cavity.

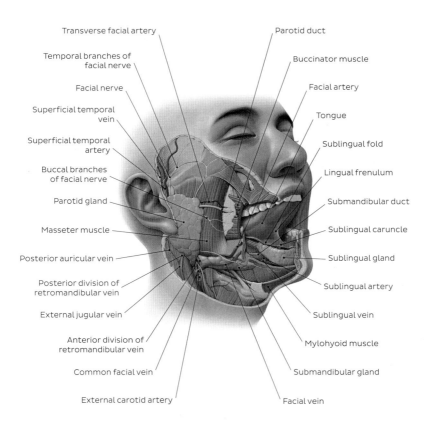

FIGURE 8.80. **Salivary glands (overview).** The **parotid gland** is the largest of the major salivary glands, located superficially in the front of the ear (preauricular region). It is shaped like an inverted pyramid and

enclosed in a fibrous capsule. A number of important neurovascular structures traverse the parotid gland including the **external carotid artery**, **retromandibular** vein **and facial nerve**. The secreted content of the parotid gland gets released through the **parotid duct** (Stensen's duct) whose orifice can be seen on the buccal wall at the level of the maxillary second molar.

The **submandibular gland** is the second largest salivary gland, located inferior and deep to the ramus of the mandible in the submandibular triangle of the neck (a.k.a. digastric triangle). This gland produces the largest amount of saliva that gets excreted through the **submandibular duct** (of Wharton) which opens at the sublingual papilla under the tongue.

The **sublingual gland** is an almond-shaped gland and is the smallest of the major salivary glands. It lies on the mylohyoid muscle and is covered by the mucosa of the floor of the mouth, which is raised as a sublingual fold. It has several ductal openings that run along the sublingual folds: A **major sublingual duct** (of Bartholin) and as many as 20 **minor sublingual ducts** (of Rivinius).

Salivary glands	Location	Type	Excretory duct	Blood supply	Innervation
Parotid	Preauricular region	Serous gland	Parotid duct (of Stensen)	Superficial temporal artery, maxillary artery, transverse facial artery	Auriculotemporal nerve (V_3), glossopharyngeal nerve (CN IX), external carotid plexus
Submandibular	Submandibular triangle	Mixed gland	Submandibular duct (of Wharton)	Sublingual artery, submental artery	Chorda tympani (CN VII)
Sublingual	Beneath the sublingual fold	Mucous gland	Major sublingual duct (of Bartholin), minor sublingual ducts (of Rivinius)	Sublingual artery, submental artery	Chorda tympani (CN VII)

Submandibular gland

Parotid gland

Sublingual gland

HEAD AND NECK

TYPES OF TEETH

The teeth are organized in two arches, a **maxillary** or superior arch and a **mandibular** or inferior arch, each of which is divided into two quadrants.

Each quadrant on the permanent dentition is made up of eight teeth (one central incisor, one lateral incisor, one canine, two premolars and three molars). The morphology and anatomical characteristics of each of these are specific to each tooth since they have different functions.

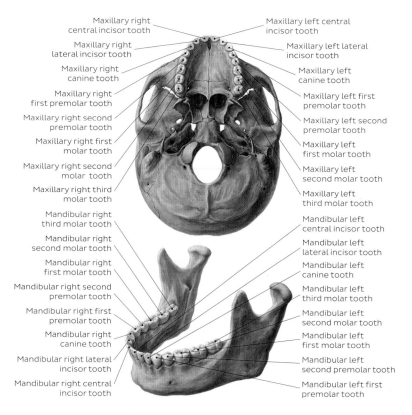

Maxillary right central incisor tooth
Maxillary right lateral incisor tooth
Maxillary right canine tooth
Maxillary right first premolar tooth
Maxillary right second premolar tooth
Maxillary right first molar tooth
Maxillary right second molar tooth
Maxillary right third molar tooth
Mandibular right third molar tooth
Mandibular right second molar tooth
Mandibular right first molar tooth
Mandibular right second premolar tooth
Mandibular right first premolar tooth
Mandibular right canine tooth
Mandibular right lateral incisor tooth
Mandibular right central incisor tooth

Maxillary left central incisor tooth
Maxillary left lateral incisor tooth
Maxillary left canine tooth
Maxillary left first premolar tooth
Maxillary left second premolar tooth
Maxillary left first molar tooth
Maxillary left second molar tooth
Maxillary left third molar tooth
Mandibular left central incisor tooth
Mandibular left lateral incisor tooth
Mandibular left canine tooth
Mandibular left third molar tooth
Mandibular left second molar tooth
Mandibular left first molar tooth
Mandibular left second premolar tooth
Mandibular left first premolar tooth

FIGURE 8.81. **Teeth in situ.** Overview of the permanent dentition with all 32 teeth: 16 maxillary/superior teeth and 16 mandibular/inferior teeth.

HEAD AND NECK

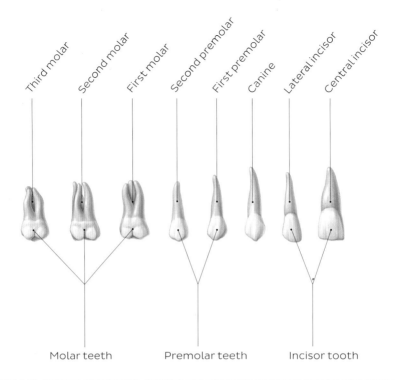

Third molar
Second molar
First molar
Second premolar
First premolar
Canine
Lateral incisor
Central incisor

Molar teeth   Premolar teeth   Incisor tooth

FIGURE 8.82. **Anatomy of each tooth.** Dentition of maxillary left quadrant in isolation with crowns and roots visible. Each tooth has a **clinical crown**, which is the portion of the tooth seen in the oral cavity. **Cusps** are prominent landmarks on the crown presenting as eminences or projections that help teeth with their functions. Canine teeth only have a single predominant cusp, while premolars have 2 cusps except for the mandibular second premolar which generally has 3 cusps. The mandibular first molar has 5 cusps whereas the maxillary first molar has 4 cusps with a small accessory cusp (of Carabelli) sometimes described as a fifth cusp. Both the maxillary and mandibular second molars have 4 cusps.

The number of **roots** for each tooth is similarly variable; the central and lateral incisors, canines and premolars all have a single root with the exception of the maxillary first premolar which generally has 2 roots. The maxillary first and second molars have 3 roots and the mandibular first and second molars have 2 roots. Regarding third molars or wisdom teeth, the number of cusps and roots is subject to a deal of interindividual variation, however generally varies between 3–4 cusps in the maxillary third molars and 4–5 cusps in the mandibular third molars. Regarding roots the maxillary third molar varies between 1–3 roots while the mandibular third molar can vary between 1–2 roots.

	Teeth	Number	Function	Roots	Cusps
	Incisor	8	Cut and bite	1	None
	Canine	4	Tear	1	1
	Premolar	8	Tear and grind	1	2
Molar	Maxillary	6	Crush and grind	3	First: 4 / Second: 4 / Third: variable
	Mandibular			2	First: 5 / Second: 4 / Third: variable

Teeth

Ace your exam
with these teeth
diagrams and tooth
identification quizzes

ANATOMY OF THE TOOTH

Each tooth is made up of a crown and root(s). The **crown** can be defined either as a clinical crown, which is the portion exposed to the oral cavity, or as an anatomical crown, going from the cementoenamel junction to the cusps or the incisal edge of the tooth. Below it, the part of the tooth attached to the surrounding alveolar bone of the maxilla or mandible, is known as the **root**. The alveolar processes of the maxilla and mandible contain sockets known as **dental alveoli**. Each dental alveolus houses a tooth, and is bound to it by a specific fibrous joint known as gomphosis or dentoalveolar syndesmosis (a.k.a. peg and socket joint). The root of the tooth is held in place by the **peridodontium**, which is composed of the periodontal ligament, cementum and gingiva (gum).

Each tooth is composed of a variety of tissues. **Enamel** is a hard calcareous substance which covers the anatomical crown of the tooth; it is the hardest tissue in the human body. **Dentin** is covered by the enamel in the crown and the cementum in the roots. **Dental pulp** is the innermost portion of the tooth, containing nerves, blood vessels and connective tissue. It's found in the pulp cavity of the crown as well as within the root canal(s).

HEAD AND NECK

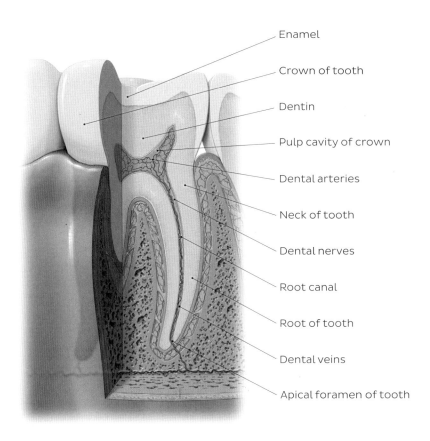

Enamel

Crown of tooth

Dentin

Pulp cavity of crown

Dental arteries

Neck of tooth

Dental nerves

Root canal

Root of tooth

Dental veins

Apical foramen of tooth

FIGURE 8.83. **Tooth: Parts and landmarks.** Section of a molar tooth. The **enamel** consists of a highly mineralized and resistant layer which functions as a hard chewing surface and as a barrier which protects the tooth from possible physical, thermal and chemical damage. **Dentin** provides support to the enamel, while the dental pulp is responsible for nourishing surrounding tissue and perceiving pain or discomfort in cases of drastic temperature changes, pressure, trauma and possible infections. Important landmarks found in every tooth are the **cementoenamel junction** 'CEJ' (the point at the neck of the tooth where the cementum and the enamel border each other), and the **dentinoenamel junction** 'DEJ' (point where the enamel and dentin meet).

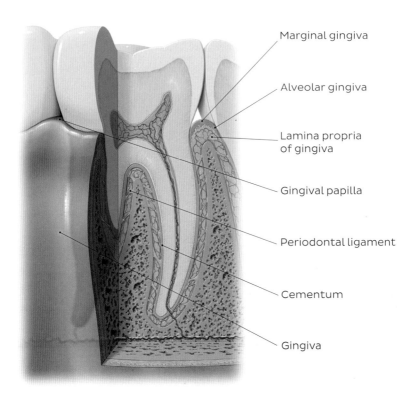

Marginal gingiva

Alveolar gingiva

Lamina propria of gingiva

Gingival papilla

Periodontal ligament

Cementum

Gingiva

FIGURE 8.84. Tooth: Supporting structures. Teeth are held in place by the **periodontium** composed of a variety of supporting structures such as the gum or gingiva, periodontal ligament, cementum and alveolar bone. Integrity of these structures is important since without them, teeth can become loose and eventually detach completely. The **gingiva** is the external portion of the periodontium surrounding each tooth. It is divided into an alveolar/fixed gingiva (going from the mucogingival junction until the level of the cementoenamel junction 'CEJ' or more specifically, the free gingival groove) and a marginal/free gingiva (from the free gingival groove until the gingival margin surrounding the tooth).

Anatomy of the tooth

Gingiva

HEAD AND NECK

PHARYNGEAL MUCOSA

The pharynx, commonly known as the throat, is a muscular tube extending from the nasal and oral cavities until the larynx and the esophagus: A place of passage for air, food and liquids.

Based on its anterior relations, the pharynx is divided into three mains sections: The **nasopharynx**, posterior to the nasal cavity; the **oropharynx**, posterior to the oral cavity; and the **laryngopharynx** posterior to the larynx. The pharyngeal wall is formed essentially by muscles and fascia and is covered internally by a mucous membrane.

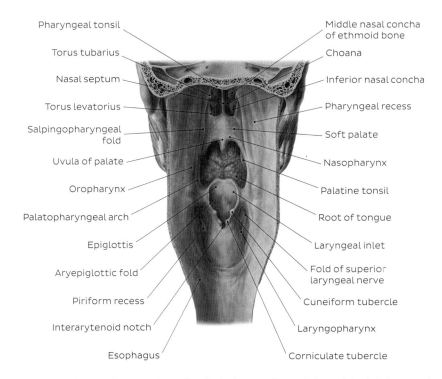

Pharyngeal tonsil — Middle nasal concha of ethmoid bone
Torus tubarius — Choana
Nasal septum — Inferior nasal concha
Torus levatorius — Pharyngeal recess
Salpingopharyngeal fold — Soft palate
Uvula of palate — Nasopharynx
Oropharynx — Palatine tonsil
Palatopharyngeal arch — Root of tongue
Epiglottis — Laryngeal inlet
Aryepiglottic fold — Fold of superior laryngeal nerve
Piriform recess — Cuneiform tubercle
Interarytenoid notch — Laryngopharynx
Esophagus — Corniculate tubercle

FIGURE 8.85. **Pharyngeal mucosa (posterior view).** The **nasopharynx** is located behind the posterior aperture of the nasal cavity (choanae), above the level of the soft palate and below the base of the skull. It is continuous inferiorly with the **oropharynx** which is located between the level of the soft palate and upper margin of the epiglottis. The oropharynx communicates anteriorly with the oral cavity and is continuous inferiorly with the **laryngopharynx**, which is the inferior most part of the pharynx. It extends from the superior margin of the epiglottis to the top of the esophagus. The laryngopharynx communicates anteriorly with the larynx through the **laryngeal inlet**.

The pharynx

MUSCLES OF THE PHARYNX

The functions of the pharynx are accomplished by several muscles, divided into two groups based on the orientation of their fibers. The **constrictor muscles** are formed by a series of overlapping circularly oriented fibers while the longitudinal/elevator muscles have fibers that are oriented vertically.

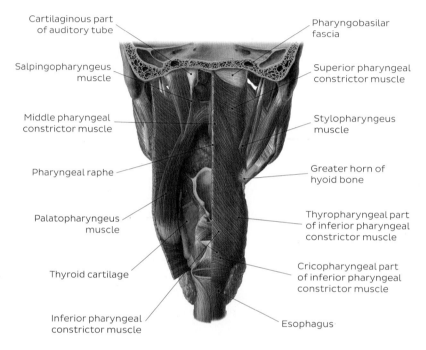

Cartilaginous part of auditory tube

Salpingopharyngeus muscle

Middle pharyngeal constrictor muscle

Pharyngeal raphe

Palatopharyngeus muscle

Thyroid cartilage

Inferior pharyngeal constrictor muscle

Pharyngobasilar fascia

Superior pharyngeal constrictor muscle

Stylopharyngeus muscle

Greater horn of hyoid bone

Thyropharyngeal part of inferior pharyngeal constrictor muscle

Cricopharyngeal part of inferior pharyngeal constrictor muscle

Esophagus

FIGURE 8.86. Pharyngeal muscles (posterior view). The **constrictor muscles** on either side of the pharynx form the main components of the pharyngeal wall and are named according to their position: Superior, middle, and inferior. The inferior constrictor muscle is further divided into thyropharyngeal and cricopharyngeal parts. Posteriorly, these muscles come together in the midline at the **pharyngeal raphe**. The muscular sleeve formed by these muscles has a strong internal lining known as the **pharyngobasilar fascia** which is particularly evident superior to the level of the superior constrictor; here the pharyngeal wall is formed almost completely of fascia.

The **longitudinal/elevator muscles** of the pharynx are located deep to their circular counterparts and include the stylopharyngeus, salpingopharyngeus and palatopharyngeus muscles, which originate from the styloid process of temporal bone, auditory tube and soft palate, respectively.

Pharyngeal constrictors	Origin	Insertion	Innervation	Function
Superior pharyngeal constrictor	Pterygoid hamulus, Pterygomandibular raphe, Posterior end of mylohyoid line of mandible	Pharyngeal tubercle on basilar part of occipital bone	Branches of pharyngeal plexus (CN X)	Constricts wall of pharynx during swallowing
Middle pharyngeal constrictor	Stylohyoid ligament, Greater and lesser horn of hyoid bone	Median pharyngeal raphe, Blends with superior and inferior pharyngeal constrictors		
Inferior pharyngeal constrictor	**Thyropharyngeal part**: oblique line of thyroid cartilage	**Thyropharyngeal part**: median pharyngeal raphe	**Both parts**: branches of pharyngeal plexus (CN X)	
	Cricopharyngeal part: cricoid cartilage	**Cricopharyngeal part**: blends inferiorly with circular esophageal fibres	**Cricopharyngeal part**: also receives branches of external and/or recurrent laryngeal branches of vagus nerve (CN X)	

Longitudinal pharyngeal muscles	Origin	Insertion	Innervation	Function
Stylopharyngeus	Medial base of styloid process of temporal bone	Blends with pharyngeal constrictors, Lateral glossoepiglottic fold, Posterior border of thyroid cartilage	Glossopharyngeal nerve (CN IX)	Elevates pharynx and larynx
Salpingopharyngeus	Inferior/ cartilaginous part of auditory (Eustachian) tube	Blends with palatopharyngeus muscle	Branches of pharyngeal plexus (CN X)	Elevates pharynx, Opens auditory tube during swallowing
Palatopharyngeus	Posterior border of hard palate, Palatine aponeurosis	Posterior border of thyroid cartilage, Blends with contralateral palatopharyngeus muscle		Elevates pharynx superiorly, anteriorly and medially (shortening it to swallow)

Muscles and walls of the pharynx

Pharynx

HEAD AND NECK

BLOOD VESSELS OF THE PHARYNX

The pharynx has a very rich blood supply. Its upper parts are supplied by branches of the **external carotid artery**, while the lower parts are supplied by branches from the **subclavian artery**. The venous drainage of this region is done through a network of **pharyngeal veins** that form a venous plexus.

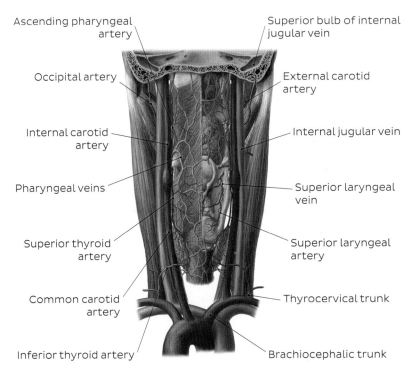

Ascending pharyngeal artery

Occipital artery

Internal carotid artery

Pharyngeal veins

Superior thyroid artery

Common carotid artery

Inferior thyroid artery

Superior bulb of internal jugular vein

External carotid artery

Internal jugular vein

Superior laryngeal vein

Superior laryngeal artery

Thyrocervical trunk

Brachiocephalic trunk

FIGURE 8.87. **Overview of the blood vessels of the pharynx.** In this posterior perspective, important blood vessels of the head and neck can be seen on either side of the pharynx. The **external carotid artery** gives off several branches, some of them responsible for supplying the upper part of the pharynx. The **ascending pharyngeal artery** arises from the external carotid artery close to the carotid bifurcation and ascends superiorly along the pharynx, giving off branches that supply various structures located in the upper part of the pharynx.

The lower part of the pharynx is supplied by pharyngeal branches of the **inferior thyroid artery**, which originates from the thyrocervical trunk of the subclavian artery. The **pharyngeal veins** form a venous plexus which drains inferiorly into the internal jugular veins.

Key points about the blood vessels of the pharynx	
Upper pharynx	Supplied by branches of external carotid artery: • Ascending pharyngeal artery • Ascending palatine and tonsillar branches of the facial artery • Branches of lingual artery • Branches of maxillary artery
Lower pharynx	Supplied by branches of subclavian artery: • Pharyngeal branches of inferior thyroid artery (from thyrocervical trunk)

NERVES OF THE PHARYNX

Nearly all of the innervation of the pharynx, either motor or sensory, is derived from the **pharyngeal plexus**, located in the outer fascia of the pharyngeal wall. This plexus is formed mainly through the branches of the vagus (CN X) and glossopharyngeal (CN IX) nerves with contributions from the superior cervical sympathetic ganglion.

Other important nerves located in the parapharyngeal space are the accessory (CN XI) and the hypoglossal (CN XII) nerve, as well as all nerves of the cervical sympathetic trunk. These nervous structures are not directly involved in the nerve supply of the pharynx but are closely related to this organ.

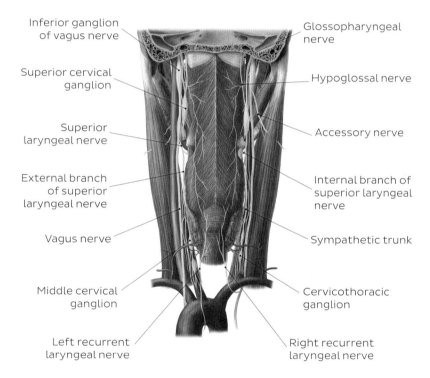

Inferior ganglion of vagus nerve

Superior cervical ganglion

Superior laryngeal nerve

External branch of superior laryngeal nerve

Vagus nerve

Middle cervical ganglion

Left recurrent laryngeal nerve

Glossopharyngeal nerve

Hypoglossal nerve

Accessory nerve

Internal branch of superior laryngeal nerve

Sympathetic trunk

Cervicothoracic ganglion

Right recurrent laryngeal nerve

FIGURE 8.88. **Overview of the nerves of the pharynx.** In this posterior view we can see the nerves that supply the pharynx and other important nervous structures of the parapharyngeal space. The **pharyngeal plexus** is mainly composed of pharyngeal branches of the glossopharyngeal and vagus nerves and lies on the external surface of the pharynx.

On the right side of the image, superiorly, the **glossopharyngeal nerve (CN IX)** is seen after leaving the skull through the jugular foramen. The **vagus nerve (CN X)** also leaves the skull through this foramen and has two sensory ganglia in this location (in this image the inferior ganglion is visible). The **superior laryngeal nerve** arises from the inferior ganglion of the vagus nerve and descends against the lateral wall of the pharynx. It divides into the external and internal branches. The **recurrent laryngeal nerve** is also a branch of the vagus nerve that supplies the larynx. The right and left nerves are not symmetrical, with the left nerve looping under the aortic arch, and the right nerve looping under the right subclavian artery then traveling upwards.

The **accessory nerve (CN XI)** also passes through the jugular foramen and courses through the neck; it pierces the sternocleidomastoid muscle which it innervates. The **hypoglossal nerve (CN XII)** leaves the skull, travels down the neck and ends at the base and underside of the tongue, being responsible for its nerve supply. The **cervical sympathetic trunk** lies behind the carotid sheath (a condensation of deep fascia of the neck in which is embedded the common and internal carotid arteries, internal jugular vein, and the vagus nerve). This trunk contains three interconnected ganglia: The superior, middle and inferior (stellate or cervicothoracic).

Key points about the nerves of the pharynx	
Pharyngeal plexus (composition)	1. Pharyngeal branches of the glossopharyngeal nerve (CN IX) 2. Pharyngeal branch of the vagus nerve (CN X) 3. Branches from the external laryngeal nerve from the superior laryngeal branch of the vagus nerve (CN X) 4. Contributions from the superior cervical sympathetic ganglion
Sensory innervation	**Nasopharynx**: pharyngeal branch of the maxillary nerve (CN V$_2$) **Oropharynx**: glossopharyngeal nerve (CN IX) via the pharyngeal plexus **Laryngopharynx**: vagus nerve (CN X) via the internal branch of the superior laryngeal nerve
Motor innervation	All pharyngeal muscles: pharyngeal branch of the vagus nerve (CN X) (except for the stylopharyngeus muscle which is innervated by a branch of the glossopharyngeal nerve)

HYOID BONE

The **hyoid bone** is a small U-shaped bone located in the anterior neck between the epiglottis and the thyroid cartilage. It does not articulate directly with other bones but instead is connected to adjacent bones via muscles and ligaments. The hyoid bone serves as an attachment site for the muscles of the floor of the mouth, tongue, larynx, epiglottis, and pharynx.

Together with these muscles, the hyoid bone assists in movements, such as opening the jaw, articulating, swallowing, and coughing.

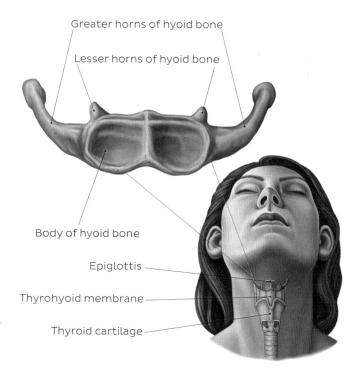

Greater horns of hyoid bone

Lesser horns of hyoid bone

Body of hyoid bone

Epiglottis

Thyrohyoid membrane

Thyroid cartilage

FIGURE 8.89. **Hyoid bone.** Anterior view of the neck region with the larynx and the trachea visible. The magnified illustration depicts the structure and bony landmarks of the hyoid bone. It consists of three parts: A rectangular **body** with two **lesser** and two **greater horns** protruding from it. The illustration below shows the *in situ* position of the hyoid bone, anterior to the epiglottis and superior to the thyroid cartilage of the larynx. The hyoid bone is connected to the thyroid cartilage via the **thyrohyoid membrane**. The stylohyoid ligament and stylohyoid muscle (not depicted) connect the hyoid bone to the styloid process of the temporal bone (not shown).

Hyoid bone

MUSCLES OF THE ANTERIOR NECK

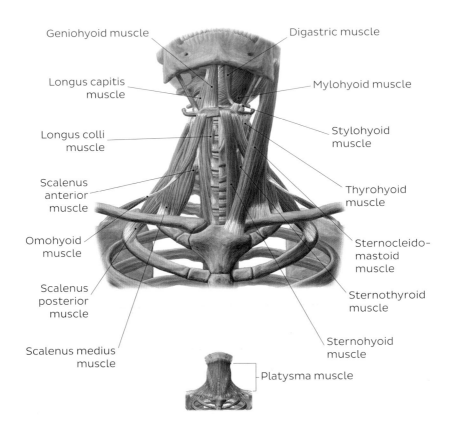

Geniohyoid muscle

Longus capitis muscle

Longus colli muscle

Scalenus anterior muscle

Omohyoid muscle

Scalenus posterior muscle

Scalenus medius muscle

Digastric muscle

Mylohyoid muscle

Stylohyoid muscle

Thyrohyoid muscle

Sternocleido-mastoid muscle

Sternothyroid muscle

Sternohyoid muscle

Platysma muscle

FIGURE 8.90. Muscles of the anterior neck (anterior view). The lower image shows the **platysma**. This sheet-like muscle lies most superficially within the subcutaneous tissue and covers all of the anterior aspect of the neck. The upper image shows all other anterior neck muscles that are situated deep to the platysma.

The **sternocleidomastoid** is a two-headed muscle and can be prominently seen and palpated along the lateral sides of the neck creating a 'V-shape'. The **suprahyoid** (digastric, mylohyoid, geniohyoid and stylohyoid) and **infrahyoid** (sternohyoid, omohyoid, sternothyroid and thyrohyoid muscle) muscles position the hyoid bone, thus playing an active role in swallowing and the movement of the larynx. The **scalene muscles** (scalenus anterior, middle and posterior) attach to the upper two ribs, making them accessory muscles of respiration. The **prevertebral muscles** (rectus capitis anterior, rectus capitis lateralis, longus capitis and longus colli) are located along the length of the anterior cervical spine and are surrounded by the prevertebral fascia of the neck. These muscles help with flexion of the head to varying degrees.

Anterior neck muscles		Origin	Insertion	Innervation	Function
	Platysma	Skin/Fascia of infra- and supraclavicular regions	Lower border of mandible, Skin of buccal/cheek region, Lower lip, Modiolus, Orbicularis oris muscle	Cervical branch of facial nerve (CN VII)	Depresses mandible and angle of mouth, Tenses skin of lower face and anterior neck
Superficial muscles	**Sternocleidomastoid**	**Sternal head**: superoanterior surface of manubrium of sternum **Clavicular head**: superior surface of medial third of clavicle	Lateral surface of mastoid process of temporal bone, Lateral half of superior nuchal line of occipital bone	**Motor**: accessory nerve (CN XI), **Sensory**: anterior rami of spinal nerves C2–C3	**Bilateral contraction** – Atlantooccipital joint/Superior cervical spine: head/Neck extension; inferior cervical vertebrae: neck flexion; **Sternoclavicular joint**: elevation of clavicle and manubrium of sternum **Unilateral contraction** – Cervical spine: neck ipsilateral flexion, neck contralateral rotation
Scalene muscles	**Scalenus anterior**	Anterior tubercle of transverse processes of vertebrae C3–C6	Scalene tubercle and superior border of rib 1 (anterior to subclavian groove)	Anterior rami of spinal nerves C4–C6	**Bilateral contraction** – Neck flexion **Unilateral contraction** – Neck lateral flexion (ipsilateral), Neck rotation (contralateral), Elevates rib 1
	Scalenus medius	Transverse processes of C1/C2 → C7 (posterior tubercles of transverse proc. in C3–C7)	Superior border of rib 1 (posterior to subclavian groove)	Anterior rami of spinal nerves C3–C8	Neck lateral flexion, Elevates rib 1
	Scalenus posterior	Posterior tubercles of transverse processes of vertebrae C4–C6/C5–C7	External surface of rib 2	Anterior rami of spinal nerves C6–C8	Neck lateral flexion, Elevates rib 2

Anterior neck muscles		Origin	Insertion	Innervation	Function
	Digastric	**Anterior belly**: digastric fossa of mandible **Posterior belly**: mastoid notch of temporal bone	Intermediate digastric tendon (Body of hyoid bone)	**Anterior belly**: nerve to mylohyoid (of inferior alveolar nerve) (CN V₃) **Posterior belly**: digastric branch of facial nerve (CN VII)	Depresses mandible, Elevates hyoid bone during swallowing and speaking
Suprahyoid muscles	Mylohyoid	Mylohyoid line of mandible	Mylohyoid raphe, Body of hyoid bone	Nerve to mylohyoid (of inferior alveolar nerve (CN V₃))	Forms floor of oral cavity, Elevates hyoid bone and floor of mouth, Depresses mandible
	Geniohyoid	Inferior mental spine (Inferior genial tubercle)	Body of hyoid bone	Anterior ramus of spinal nerve C1 (via hypoglossal nerve [CN XII])	Elevates and draws hyoid bone anteriorly
	Stylohyoid	Styloid process of temporal bone		Stylohyoid branch of facial nerve (CN VII)	Elevates and draws hyoid bone posteriorly
	Sternothyroid	Posterior surface of manubrium of sternum, Costal cartilage of rib 1	Oblique line of thyroid cartilage		Depresses larynx
	Sternohyoid	Manubrium of sternum, Medial end of clavicle	Inferior border of body of hyoid bone	Anterior rami of spinal nerves C1-C3 (via ansa cervicalis)	Depresses hyoid bone (from elevated position)
Infrahyoid muscles	Omohyoid	**Inferior belly**: superior border of scapula (near suprascapular notch) **Superior belly**: intermediate tendon of omohyoid muscle	**Inferior belly**: intermediate tendon of omohyoid muscle **Superior belly**: body of hyoid bone		Depresses and draws hyoid bone posteriorly
	Thyrohyoid	Oblique line of thyroid cartilage	Inferior border of body and greater horn of hyoid bone	Anterior ramus of spinal nerve C1 (via hypoglossal nerve [CN XII])	Depresses hyoid bone, Elevates larynx

HEAD AND NECK

Prevertebral muscles				
Rectus capitis anterior	Anterior surface of lateral mass and transverse process of atlas	Inferior surface of basilar part of occipital bone	Anterior rami of spinal nerves C1, C2	**Atlantooccipital joint:** head flexion
Rectus capitis lateralis	Superior surface of transverse process of atlas	Inferior surface of jugular process of occipital bone		**Unilateral contraction –** **Atlantooccipital joint:** head lateral flexion (ipsilateral), stabilizes joint
Longus capitis	Anterior tubercles of transverse processes of C3–C6	Basilar part of occipital bone	Anterior rami of spinal nerves C1–C3	**Bilateral contraction** – Head flexion; **Ipsilateral contraction** – Head rotation (ipsilateral)
Longus colli	**Superior part:** anterior tubercles of transverse processes of vertebrae C3–C5; **Intermediate part:** anterior surface of bodies of vertebrae C5–T3; **Inferior part:** anterior surface of bodies of vertebrae T1–T3	**Superior part:** anterior tubercle of vertebra C1; **Intermediate part:** anterior surface of bodies of vertebrae C2–C4; **Inferior part:** anterior tubercles of transverse processes of vertebrae C5–C6	Anterior rami of spinal nerves C2–C6	**Bilateral contraction** – Neck flexion, Neck lateral flexion (ipsilateral); **Unilateral contraction** – Neck contralateral rotation

Muscles of the neck

LARYNX

The **larynx** houses and protects the vocal cords, as well as the entrance to the trachea, preventing food particles or fluids from entering the lungs during swallowing.

The larynx lies anterior to the esophagus at the level of the third to the sixth cervical vertebrae and is continuous with the laryngopharynx above and trachea below. It consists of a complex cartilaginous skeleton connected by membranes, ligaments and associated muscles. The muscles are grouped into **extrinsic muscles**, suspending the larynx to its neighboring structures and moving it as a whole, and **intrinsic muscles**, which move the vocal cords in order to produce speech sounds (phonation).

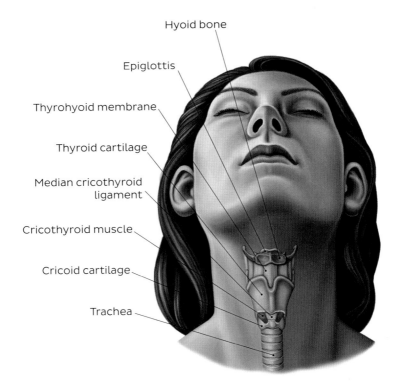

Hyoid bone

Epiglottis

Thyrohyoid membrane

Thyroid cartilage

Median cricothyroid ligament

Cricothyroid muscle

Cricoid cartilage

Trachea

FIGURE 8.91. **Larynx *in situ*: Anterior view.** The **thyroid cartilage** is the largest of the laryngeal cartilages and presents broad flat right and left halves of hyaline cartilage which fuse anteriorly in the midline to form the **laryngeal prominence**, commonly called the "Adam's apple". The thyroid cartilage is attached superiorly to the hyoid bone via the thyrohyoid membrane. Directly below the thyroid cartilage lies the **cricoid cartilage**, a ring-shaped hyaline cartilage which is connected to the trachea inferiorly.

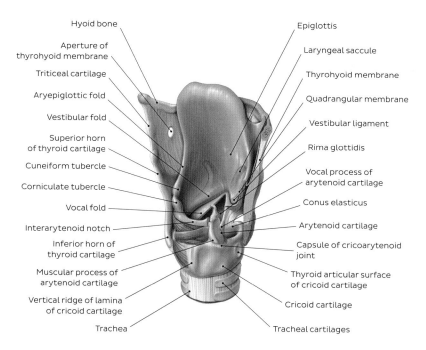

Hyoid bone

Aperture of
thyrohyoid membrane

Triticeal cartilage

Aryepiglottic fold

Vestibular fold

Superior horn
of thyroid cartilage

Cuneiform tubercle

Corniculate tubercle

Vocal fold

Interarytenoid notch

Inferior horn of
thyroid cartilage

Muscular process of
arytenoid cartilage

Vertical ridge of lamina
of cricoid cartilage

Trachea

Epiglottis

Laryngeal saccule

Thyrohyoid membrane

Quadrangular membrane

Vestibular ligament

Rima glottidis

Vocal process of
arytenoid cartilage

Conus elasticus

Arytenoid cartilage

Capsule of cricoarytenoid
joint

Thyroid articular surface
of cricoid cartilage

Cricoid cartilage

Tracheal cartilages

FIGURE 8.92. Structure of the larynx (posterolateral view). The **epiglottis** is a leaf-shaped piece of elastic cartilage attached to the internal surface of the thyroid cartilage. When oral contents are swallowed, it folds over the laryngeal inlet preventing food/fluids from entering the trachea.

A thin layer of connective tissue, the **quadrangular membrane** extends between the lateral borders of the epiglottis and the arytenoid cartilages. Its free lower edge is thickened and forms the **vestibular ligament**. This ligament is enclosed by a fold of mucous membrane to form the **vestibular fold** (false vocal cord) which extends from the thyroid cartilage to the arytenoid cartilage. The **(true) vocal cords** consist of the vocal ligament which is the medial free edge of the conus elasticus or lateral cricothyroid ligament, as well as the vocalis muscle which comes from the medial fibers of the thyroarytenoid muscle and the overlying mucosa which covers it.

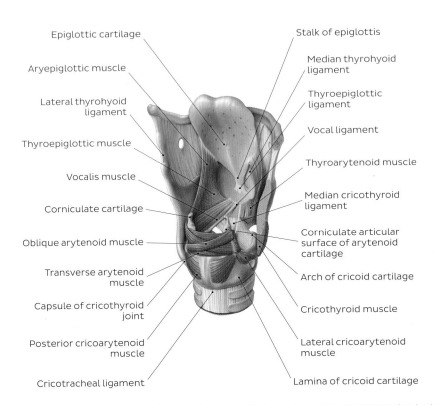

Epiglottic cartilage

Aryepiglottic muscle

Lateral thyrohyoid ligament

Thyroepiglottic muscle

Vocalis muscle

Corniculate cartilage

Oblique arytenoid muscle

Transverse arytenoid muscle

Capsule of cricothyroid joint

Posterior cricoarytenoid muscle

Cricotracheal ligament

Stalk of epiglottis

Median thyrohyoid ligament

Thyroepiglottic ligament

Vocal ligament

Thyroarytenoid muscle

Median cricothyroid ligament

Corniculate articular surface of arytenoid cartilage

Arch of cricoid cartilage

Cricothyroid muscle

Lateral cricoarytenoid muscle

Lamina of cricoid cartilage

FIGURE 8.93. Muscles of the larynx (posterolateral view). The **intrinsic muscles** of the larynx alter both the length and the tension placed upon the vocal cords. They are functionally divided into **adductors** (lateral cricoarytenoid, oblique arytenoid, transverse arytenoid), **abductors** (posterior cricoarytenoid), **sphincters** (transverse arytenoid, aryepiglottic), **tensors** (cricothyroid), and **relaxors** (thyroarytenoid, vocalis). The space between the vocal cords is called **rima glottidis**.

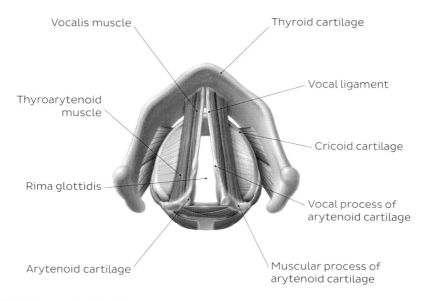

Vocalis muscle

Thyroid cartilage

Vocal ligament

Thyroarytenoid muscle

Cricoid cartilage

Rima glottidis

Vocal process of arytenoid cartilage

Arytenoid cartilage

Muscular process of arytenoid cartilage

FIGURE 8.94. Action of vocalis and thyroarytenoid muscles (superior view). The **thyroarytenoid muscle** is a wide, paired muscle arising from the inner surface of thyroid cartilage, near the midline, as well as the cricothyroid ligament. Its fibers pass posterolaterally to insert into the anterolateral surface of the arytenoid cartilage. The **vocalis muscle** is a small, paired strand-like muscle which sits parallel to the vocal ligament. It originates at the lateral surface of the vocal process of arytenoid cartilage, runs anteromedially across the laryngeal inlet and attaches to the anterior part of the ipsilateral vocal ligament near the thyroid cartilage.

The thyroarytenoid and vocalis muscles both draw the arytenoid cartilages anteriorly allowing the vocal ligaments to shorten, thicken and relax. This means they play a crucial part in controlling and changing the tonal quality of the voice. Concurrently, both muscles rotate the arytenoid cartilages medially which helps in closing the rima glottidis. The narrow/wedge-shaped appearance of the **rima glottidis** in this image represents that seen during normal respirations ('resting' position).

HEAD AND NECK

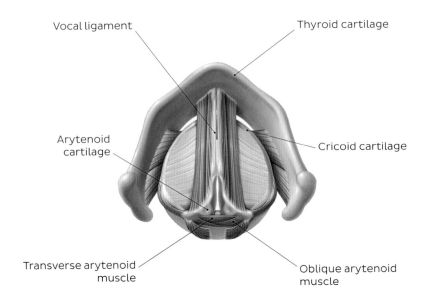

Vocal ligament

Thyroid cartilage

Arytenoid
cartilage

Cricoid cartilage

Transverse arytenoid
muscle

Oblique arytenoid
muscle

FIGURE 8.95. **Action of transverse and oblique arytenoid muscles (superior view).** The **transverse arytenoid muscle** is the only unpaired intrinsic muscle of the larynx and runs horizontally between the arytenoid cartilages. The **oblique arytenoid muscle** is a paired muscle and originates from the muscular process of the arytenoid cartilage. It extends obliquely towards its superiorly located insertion on the contralateral arytenoid cartilage. Along its path, the oblique arytenoid muscle crosses its counterpart from the opposite side, forming the letter "X".

Upon contraction, the transverse and oblique arytenoid muscles **adduct** the vocal folds, closing the posterior portion of the rima glottidis and narrowing the aditus laryngis. The closed/slit-like appearance of the rima glottidis in this image represents that seen during phonation (production of speech sounds).

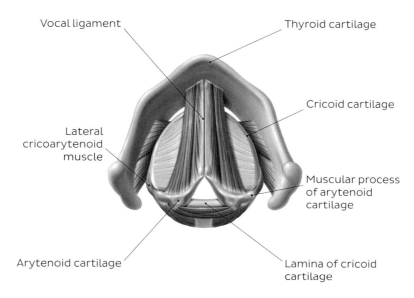

Vocal ligament

Thyroid cartilage

Cricoid cartilage

Lateral cricoarytenoid muscle

Muscular process of arytenoid cartilage

Arytenoid cartilage

Lamina of cricoid cartilage

FIGURE 8.96. **Action of lateral cricoarytenoid muscles (superior view).** The **lateral cricoarytenoid** is a bilateral muscle attaching between the cricoid and arytenoid cartilages. When these muscles contract, they **rotate** the arytenoid cartilages medially which brings the tips of the vocal processes together. This results in **adduction** of the vocal folds and closure of the anterior part of the rima glottidis. The relaxed arytenoid muscles still allow air to pass via the posterior (intercartilaginous) part of the rima glottidis, therefore allowing a toneless sound to be produced i.e., a whisper.

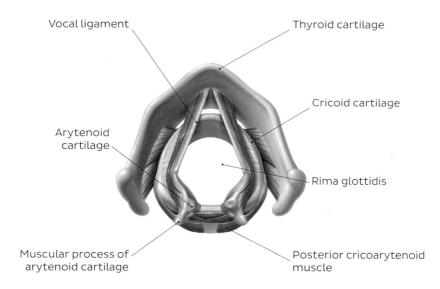

Vocal ligament

Thyroid cartilage

Cricoid cartilage

Arytenoid cartilage

Rima glottidis

Muscular process of arytenoid cartilage

Posterior cricoarytenoid muscle

FIGURE 8.97. **Action of posterior cricoarytenoid muscles (superior view).** The proximal attachment of **posterior cricoarytenoid muscle** is on the posterior surface of the cricoid cartilage and its corresponding insertion point is on the muscular process of the arytenoid cartilage. Contraction of the posterior cricoarytenoid muscle rotates the arytenoid cartilages laterally and pulls them posterolaterally. Therefore, it is the only muscle of the larynx that **abducts** the vocal cords and opens the rima glottidis. This action makes the posterior cricoarytenoid muscle the most important muscle in the larynx in the act of respiration. The open appearance of the rima glottidis in this image represents that seen during forced respiration.

Key points about the larynx	
Spaces	Three parts: vestibule, ventricle, infraglottic cavity
Cartilages	**Unpaired**: epiglottis, cricoid cartilage, thyroid cartilage
	Paired: arytenoid cartilages, corniculate cartilages, cuneiform cartilages, (triticeal cartilages → variable)
	Hyaline: cricoid cartilage, thyroid cartilage
	Elastic: epiglottis, arytenoid cartilages (only vocal process), corniculate cartilages, cuneiform cartilages, (triticeal cartilages)
Ligaments and membranes	**Extrinsic**: thyrohyoid membrane, cricotracheal ligament, hyoepiglottic ligament
	Intrinsic: quadrangular membrane, vestibular fold, thyroepiglottic ligament, median/anterior cricothyroid ligament, conus elasticus, vocal ligaments
Extrinsic muscles	**Depressors**: infrahyoid muscles (sternohyoid muscle, sternothyroid muscle, omohyoid muscle; except thyrohyoid muscle)
	Elevators: thyrohyoid muscle, suprahyoid muscles (digastric muscle, stylohyoid muscle, geniohyoid muscle, mylohyoid muscle, stylopharyngeus muscle)
Intrinsic muscles	**Adductors**: transverse arytenoid muscle, oblique arytenoid muscle, lateral cricoarytenoid muscle
	Abductors: posterior cricoarytenoid muscle
	Sphincters: transverse arytenoid muscle, aryepiglottic muscle
	Tensors: cricothyroid muscle
	Relaxor: thyroarytenoid muscle, vocalis muscle (fine adjustment)
Innervation	**Superior laryngeal nerve**: external branch (external laryngeal nerve) → motor innervation to cricothyroid muscle; internal branch (internal laryngeal nerve) → sensory/secretomotor innervation to laryngeal cavity above vocal cords
	Recurrent laryngeal nerve: anterior laryngeal branch (inferior laryngeal nerve) → motor innervation to all intrinsic muscles (except cricothryoid muscle); posterior laryngeal branch → sensory/secretomotor innervation to laryngeal cavity below vocal cords
Function	Air conduction, airway protection, sound production

Larynx

Cartilages of the larynx

Muscles of the larynx

HEAD AND NECK

THYROID AND PARATHYROID GLANDS

The thyroid and parathyroid glands are endocrine organs, located in the neck, anterior and lateral to the trachea and larynx.

The **thyroid gland** is responsible for producing thyroid hormones regulating metabolism. It consists of two lobes, an isthmus and pyramidal lobe, all of which are supplied by the superior and inferior thyroid arteries. Venous drainage occurs via the superior, middle, and inferior thyroid veins. The thyroid gland receives sympathetic and parasympathetic innervation from the three cervical sympathetic ganglia and branches of the vagus nerve, respectively.

The **parathyroid glands**, located on the back of the thyroid gland, participate in regulating blood calcium levels. Their neurovascular supply is similar to that of the thyroid gland.

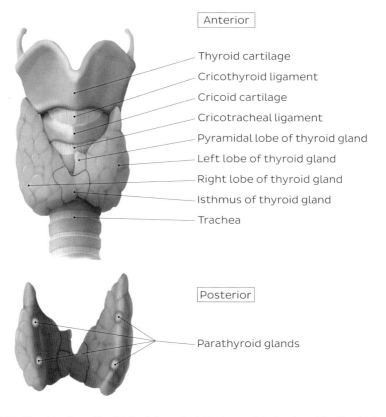

Anterior

- Thyroid cartilage
- Cricothyroid ligament
- Cricoid cartilage
- Cricotracheal ligament
- Pyramidal lobe of thyroid gland
- Left lobe of thyroid gland
- Right lobe of thyroid gland
- Isthmus of thyroid gland
- Trachea

Posterior

- Parathyroid glands

FIGURE 8.98. **Thyroid and parathyroid glands (overview). Top image**: Anterior view of the thyroid gland with thyroid cartilage and the cervical part of the trachea exposed. The butterfly-shaped thyroid gland consists of left and right conical shaped lobes which are connected by a central isthmus. A third pyramidal lobe may be present occasionally. The thyroid gland is located anterior to the trachea and inferior to the thyroid cartilage.

Bottom image: Posterior view of the thyroid gland with the four parathyroid glands exposed. Two pairs of lentil-shaped parathyroid glands are positioned on the back of each lobe of the thyroid gland. According to their location, they are called superior and inferior parathyroid glands.

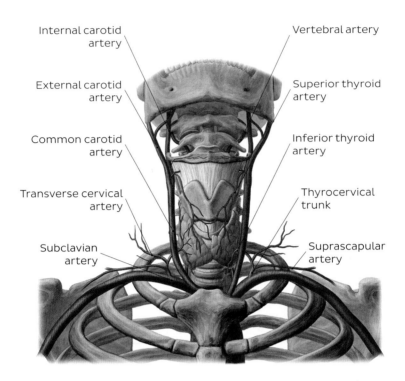

Internal carotid artery

External carotid artery

Common carotid artery

Transverse cervical artery

Subclavian artery

Vertebral artery

Superior thyroid artery

Inferior thyroid artery

Thyrocervical trunk

Suprascapular artery

FIGURE 8.99. **Arterial supply of the thyroid and parathyroid gland.** Anterior view of the neck region with the thyroid gland and its arterial supply. The hyoid bone, thyrohyoid membrane, larynx, and trachea are depicted. The **superior thyroid artery**, a branch of the external carotid artery, supplies the superior portion of the thyroid gland. The inferior portion of the thyroid gland is supplied by the **inferior thyroid artery**, arising from the thyrocervical trunk, a proximal branch of the subclavian artery. The arterial supply of the four parathyroid glands (not depicted) occur via the inferior thyroid artery. In some individuals, an anatomical variant, the **thyroid ima artery**, may be present and contribute to the arterial supply of the thyroid and parathyroid gland.

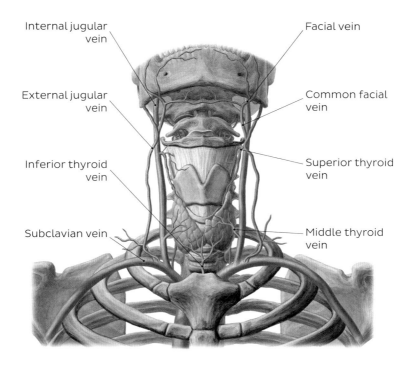

Internal jugular vein

External jugular vein

Inferior thyroid vein

Subclavian vein

Facial vein

Common facial vein

Superior thyroid vein

Middle thyroid vein

FIGURE 8.100. **Venous drainage of the thyroid and parathyroid gland.** Anterior view of the neck region with the thyroid gland and its venous supply. The hyoid bone, thyrohyoid membrane, larynx and trachea are depicted. Venous drainage of the superior aspect of the thyroid gland occurs via the **thyroid venous plexus** and the **superior** and **middle thyroid vein** that empty into the internal jugular vein. The **inferior thyroid vein** drains the inferior aspect of the thyroid gland and empties into the brachiocephalic vein. Venous drainage of the parathyroid glands occurs via the thyroid venous plexus and the thyroid veins.

	Parts	Arterial supply	Venous drainage	Innervation	Functions
Thyroid gland	Left and right lobes, isthmus, pyramidal lobe (variably present)	Superior thyroid artery (from external carotid artery) and inferior thyroid artery (from thyrocervical trunk), thyroid ima artery may be present occasionally	Superior, middle and inferior thyroid veins which form thyroid plexus	Three cervical sympathetic ganglia, external branch of superior laryngeal nerve and recurrent laryngeal nerve	Produces thyroid hormones and regulates metabolism
Parathyroid gland	Four lentil-shaped glands located on back of each lobe of thyroid gland	Inferior thyroid artery	Thyroid plexus	Three cervical sympathetic ganglia	Participate in regulating blood calcium levels

Thyroid gland

Superior thyroid artery

NEUROVASCULATURE OF THE NECK

The neck is a complex thoroughfare for a large number of vessels and nerves which serve to supply, drain and innervate the head, neck, trunk and upper limb.

The main arterial structures of the neck are the **carotid** and **vertebral arteries**. The common carotid artery ascends through the neck bifurcating into the internal and external carotid arteries. The internal carotid artery ascends to provide anterior supply to structures of the cranial cavity while the external carotid artery branches to supply structures of the neck and face. Arising from the subclavian arteries at the root of the neck are the paired vertebral arteries which ascend through the transverse foramina of the upper six cervical verte-brae, to provide posterior supply to the cranial cavity.

The primary venous channels of the neck are the **internal**, **external** and **anterior jugular veins.** Tributaries of these collecting veins largely follow a similar pat-tern to their fellow arteries.

Numerous cranial and peripheral nerves pass through and supply structures of the neck. The **cervical plexus**, located at the superior portion of the neck, gives off several branches to supply cutaneous and muscular innervation to many structures of the neck as well as parts of the face, shoulder region and thorax. The trunks of **brachial plexus** also can be seen passing between the anterior and middle scalene muscles on their way to the axilla and upper limb. **Cranial nerves** of the neck include the glossopharyngeal (CN IX), vagus (CN X), accessory (CN XI) and hypoglossal (CN XII) nerves.

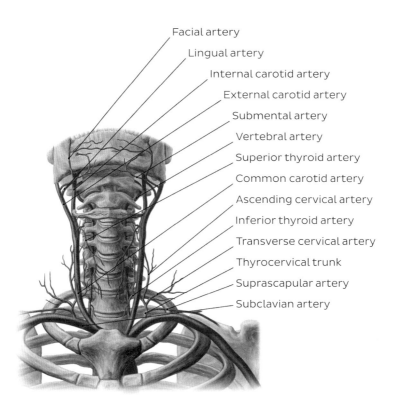

Facial artery

Lingual artery

Internal carotid artery

External carotid artery

Submental artery

Vertebral artery

Superior thyroid artery

Common carotid artery

Ascending cervical artery

Inferior thyroid artery

Transverse cervical artery

Thyrocervical trunk

Suprascapular artery

Subclavian artery

FIGURE 8.101. **Arteries of the neck (anterior view).** Located at the root of the neck are the **subclavian** and **common carotid arteries** which arise from the brachiocephalic trunk on the right and from the arch of the aorta on the left. The **thyrocervical trunk** arises from the first part of the subclavian artery and gives off the inferior thyroid, ascending cervical, transverse cervical and suprascapular arteries. Also arising from the posterosuperior aspect of this part is the **vertebral artery**. Branching from the second part of the subclavian artery is the **costocervical trunk** which gives off a branch, the deep cervical artery at the root of the neck. The **external carotid artery** arises at the level of the hyoid bone, from the bifurcation of the common carotid artery and gives off several branches which include the superior thyroid, lingual artery, ascending pharyngeal, occipital and posterior auricular arteries (not shown).

The rest of the branches of the external carotid artery are located superior to the neck. The internal carotid artery does not give off any cervical branches.

Arteries	Branches/tributaries
Brachiocephalic trunk/arch of aorta	Subclavian arteries, common carotid arteries, thyroid ima artery
Subclavian artery	Vertebral artery, thyrocervical trunk, costocervical trunk
External carotid artery	Superior thyroid artery, ascending pharyngeal artery, lingual artery, facial artery, occipital artery, posterior auricular artery

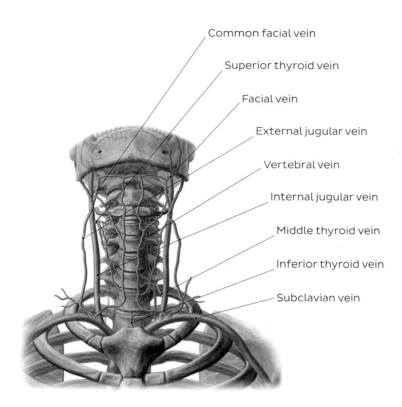

Common facial vein

Superior thyroid vein

Facial vein

External jugular vein

Vertebral vein

Internal jugular vein

Middle thyroid vein

Inferior thyroid vein

Subclavian vein

FIGURE 8.102. **Veins of the neck (anterior view).** The main veins of the neck are the external, internal and anterior jugular veins. The external jugular vein is usually formed by the posterior auricular and posterior division of the retromandibular veins (not shown) and drains into the subclavian vein at the root of the neck. Tributaries of the **external jugular vein** include the anterior jugular, transverse cervical, suprascapular and posterior external jugular veins (not shown). The **internal jugular vein** descends through the neck, joining with the subclavian vein to form the left/right brachiocephalic veins. Unlike its arterial counterpart (the internal carotid artery), the internal jugular vein receives numerous tributaries within the neck, most notably the common facial vein which is received around the level of, or inferior to, the hyoid bone. The **superior** and **middle thyroid veins** drain regions of the thyroid gland and larynx, emptying into the internal jugular vein, while the inferior thyroid vein drains directly into the left brachiocephalic vein. The **vertebral vein** descends within the transverse foramina of the cervical vertebrae and also drains into the brachiocephalic vein.

Veins	Branches/tributaries
External jugular vein	Posterior division of retromandibular vein, posterior auricular vein, anterior jugular vein, suprascapular vein, transverse cervical veins
Internal jugular vein	Common facial vein, superior and inferior bulb of internal jugular vein, pharyngeal venous plexus, superior thyroid vein, lingual vein, middle thyroid vein, sternocleidomastoid vein
Vertebral vein	Occipital vein, anterior vertebral vein, accessory vertebral vein
Subclavian vein	External jugular vein
Brachiocephalic vein	Subclavian vein, internal jugular vein, vertebral vein, deep cervical vein, inferior thyroid vein

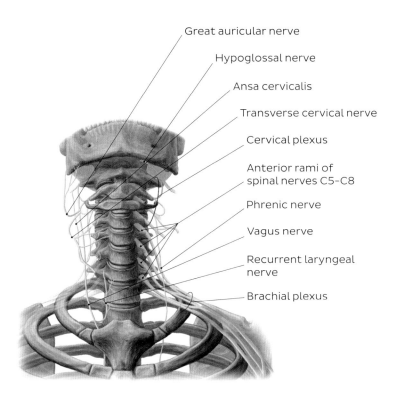

Great auricular nerve

Hypoglossal nerve

Ansa cervicalis

Transverse cervical nerve

Cervical plexus

Anterior rami of
spinal nerves C5-C8

Phrenic nerve

Vagus nerve

Recurrent laryngeal
nerve

Brachial plexus

FIGURE 8.103. **Nerves of the neck (anterior view).** The **cervical plexus** is located at the superior portion of the neck and is formed by the anterior rami of spinal nerves C1-C4. The cervical plexus gives off a number of deep and superficial branches. The **deep branches** include the ansa cervicalis, muscular branches of the cervical plexus and the phrenic nerve, while examples of **superficial branches** include the lesser occipital, great auricular, transverse cervical and supraclavicular nerves (not pictured).

The **glossopharyngeal nerve (CN IX)** descends between the internal carotid artery and internal jugular vein to innervate internal structures of the head and neck, while the **vagus nerve (CN X)** descends towards the thorax, giving off the superior and recurrent laryngeal nerves while doing so. The **accessory nerve** (CN XI; in addition to contributions from spinal nerves C3–4), descends through the posterior aspect of the neck to reach the trapezius muscle of the back. Finally, the **hypoglossal nerve (CN XII)** does not give off any branches within the neck and travels to supply muscles of the tongue.

Nerves	Branches/tributaries
Cervical plexus	**Superficial branches**: lesser occipital nerve, great auricular nerve, transverse cervical nerve, supraclavicular nerves
	Deep branches: ansa cervicalis, phrenic nerve
Brachial plexus (supraclavicular part)	Dorsal scapular nerve, long thoracic nerve, suprascapular nerve, subclavian nerve
Cranial nerves	Glossopharyngeal nerve (CN IX), vagus nerve (CN X), accessory nerve (CN XI), hypoglossal nerve (CN XII)
Autonomic nerves	Sympathetic trunk, superior, middle, inferior cervical ganglia

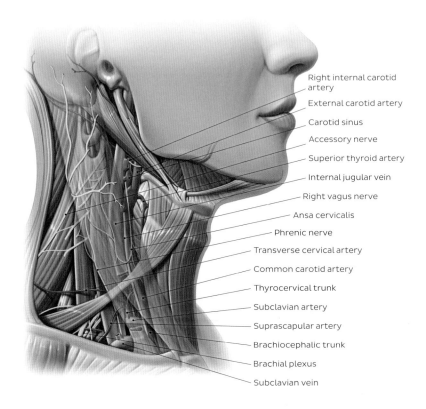

Right internal carotid artery

External carotid artery

Carotid sinus

Accessory nerve

Superior thyroid artery

Internal jugular vein

Right vagus nerve

Ansa cervicalis

Phrenic nerve

Transverse cervical artery

Common carotid artery

Thyrocervical trunk

Subclavian artery

Suprascapular artery

Brachiocephalic trunk

Brachial plexus

Subclavian vein

FIGURE 8.104. Neurovasculature of the neck (lateral view). The anatomical relations between several neurovascular structures of the neck can be appreciated from this lateral perspective. The **carotid arteries** ascend through the neck, just deep to the internal jugular veins. Traveling medial to the internal jugular vein is the **vagus nerve (CN X)**. The **accessory nerve (CN XI)** descends posterolaterally, emerging from behind the posterior border of the sternocleidomastoid muscle, where it receives sensory contributions from spinal nerves C3–4.

Branches of the **cervical plexus**, **ansa cervicalis** and **phrenic nerve** are also located deep to the sterno-cleidomastoid muscle. Passing beneath the intermediate tendon of the omohyoid muscle is the **transverse cervical artery** which branches from the thyrocervical trunk to supply muscles of the neck and back. The **suprascapular artery** also branches from the thyrocervical trunk within the supraclavicular fossa and extends laterally to supply structures of the pectoral girdle. Also located within this region is the supr-aclavicular part of the **brachial plexus** which passes between the anterior and middle scalene muscles (interscalene space).

Neurovasculature
of head neck

HEAD AND NECK

CERVICAL PLEXUS

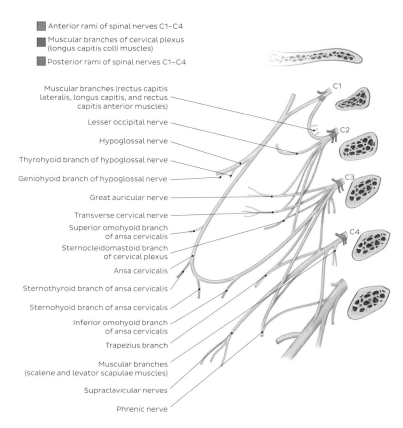

- Anterior rami of spinal nerves C1–C4
- Muscular branches of cervical plexus (longus capitis colli muscles)
- Posterior rami of spinal nerves C1–C4

Muscular branches (rectus capitis lateralis, longus capitis, and rectus capitis anterior muscles)

Lesser occipital nerve

Hypoglossal nerve

Thyrohyoid branch of hypoglossal nerve

Geniohyoid branch of hypoglossal nerve

Great auricular nerve

Transverse cervical nerve

Superior omohyoid branch of ansa cervicalis

Sternocleidomastoid branch of cervical plexus

Ansa cervicalis

Sternothyroid branch of ansa cervicalis

Sternohyoid branch of ansa cervicalis

Inferior omohyoid branch of ansa cervicalis

Trapezius branch

Muscular branches (scalene and levator scapulae muscles)

Supraclavicular nerves

Phrenic nerve

C1
C2
C3
C4

FIGURE 8.105. **Overview of the cervical plexus.** The cervical plexus can be seen as a cluster of nerves originating from the **anterior rami of spinal nerves C1-C4**. A nerve loop known as the **ansa cervicalis** is formed by branches of spinal nerves C1-C3 can be seen in the superior aspect of the illustration. The ansa cervicalis provides motor innervation to all infrahyoid muscles except the thyrohyoid muscle. The **phrenic nerve** originates from C3-C5. It travels into the thoracic cavity and provides motor innervation to the diaphragm and sensory supply to the pericardium and diaphragm. The cervical plexus also provides contributions to the **accessory nerve**, innervating the trapezius muscle. The **superficial/cutaneous branches of the cervical plexus** (lesser occipital, great auricular, transverse cervical and supraclavicular nerves) innervate the skin of the neck, scalp and shoulder.

Key points about the cervical plexus	
Definition	Nervous plexus formed by the anterior rami of the spinal nerves C1-C4.
Deep/muscular branches	**Superior root of ansa cervicalis (C1)**: thyrohyoid muscle
	Inferior root of ansa cervicalis (C2-C3): most of the infrahyoid muscles (omohyoid, sternohyoid and sternothyroid muscles)
	Phrenic nerve (C3-C5): diaphragm (+ sensory innervation of the central tendon of the diaphragm and pericardium)
	Segmental branches: rectus capitis anterior, rectus capitis lateralis, longus colli, longus capitis muscles

Key points about the cervical plexus	
Superficial/ cutaneous branches	**Lesser occipital nerve (C2)**: skin of the neck and scalp posterior to the auricle of the ear
	Great auricular nerve (C2–C3): skin over the parotid gland, posterior to the auricle and the mastoid area
	Transverse cervical nerve (C2–C3): anterior and lateral parts of the neck
	Supraclavicular nerves (C3–C4): shoulder and clavicular regions

 Cervical plexus

 Superficial nerves of the face and scalp

LYMPHATICS OF THE HEAD AND NECK

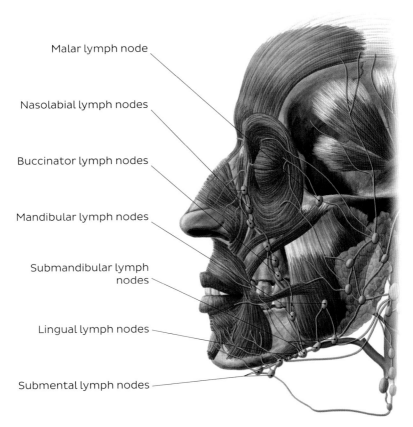

Malar lymph node

Nasolabial lymph nodes

Buccinator lymph nodes

Mandibular lymph nodes

Submandibular lymph nodes

Lingual lymph nodes

Submental lymph nodes

FIGURE 8.106. **Lymph nodes of the head (lateral view).** Lymph nodes of the head are generally divided into three separate groups: The **lingual lymph nodes**, **facial lymph nodes** and a group of five lymph nodes which make up the pericervical lymphatic circle (visible in next image). The lingual lymph nodes are located in the intermuscular spaces of the floor of the mouth and function to drain lymph from the tongue. Its efferent vessels drain to either the superior deep lateral cervical nodes of the neck, submandibular and/or submental lymph nodes. The facial lymph nodes are located along the facial vein and consist of the **buccinator**, **nasolabial**, **malar** and **mandibular lymph nodes**. This group of lymph nodes drain the corresponding regions of the face into the submandibular lymph nodes.

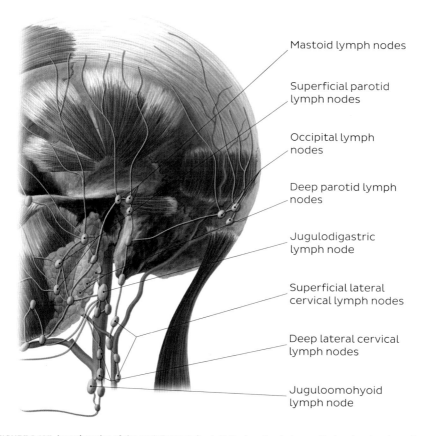

Mastoid lymph nodes

Superficial parotid lymph nodes

Occipital lymph nodes

Deep parotid lymph nodes

Jugulodigastric lymph node

Superficial lateral cervical lymph nodes

Deep lateral cervical lymph nodes

Juguloomohyoid lymph node

FIGURE 8.107. **Lymph nodes of the neck (lateral view).** At the junction between the head and neck are five groups of lymph nodes which form the **pericervical lymphatic circle**. These are the **occipital**, **mastoid**, **superficial** and **deep parotid**, **submandibular** and **submental lymph nodes**. These nodes receive lymph from regions of the nose, cheeks, ear, scalp and chin and drain to either the superficial or deep lymph nodes of the neck.

Lymphatics of the neck can generally be divided into superficial and deep anterior lymph nodes, and superficial and deep lateral lymph nodes. From this lateral perspective, the proximal portions of the superficial and deep lateral cervical lymph nodes can be observed. The **superficial lateral cervical lymph nodes** are situated adjacent to the external jugular vein and receive lymphatic drainage from the pericervical lymphatic circle. This group of lymph nodes extend along the external jugular vein and empty into the supraclavicular lymph nodes at the root of the neck.

The **deep lateral cervical lymph nodes** are located along the course of the internal jugular vein. These are further divided into superior and inferior groups by the superior belly of the omohyoid muscle. The largest node of the superior deep lateral cervical nodes is the **jugulodigastric node**, while the largest node of the inferior group of deep lateral cervical nodes is the **juguloomohyoid node**. This group of lateral nodes receive the majority of lymph from the head and neck region and drain to the jugular trunk at the base of the neck.

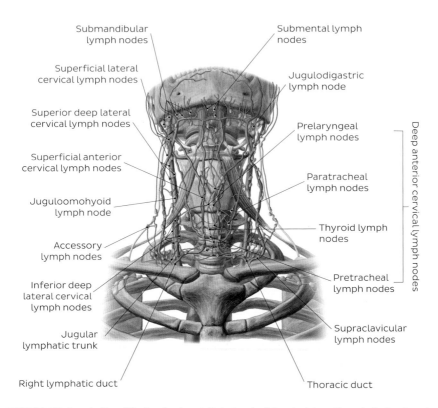

Submandibular
lymph nodes

Submental lymph
nodes

Superficial lateral
cervical lymph nodes

Jugulodigastric
lymph node

Superior deep lateral
cervical lymph nodes

Prelaryngeal
lymph nodes

Superficial anterior
cervical lymph nodes

Paratracheal
lymph nodes

Juguloomohyoid
lymph node

Thyroid lymph
nodes

Accessory
lymph nodes

Inferior deep
lateral cervical
lymph nodes

Pretracheal
lymph nodes

Jugular
lymphatic trunk

Supraclavicular
lymph nodes

Right lymphatic duct

Thoracic duct

Deep anterior cervical lymph nodes

FIGURE 8.108. Lymphatics of the head and neck (Anterior view). Located along the anterior jugular vein are the **superficial anterior cervical lymph nodes**, which drain to the deep lateral cervical lymph nodes or directly to the supraclavicular lymph nodes via efferent vessels. The **deep anterior cervical lymph nodes** are subdivided into the **prelaryngeal**, **thyroid**, **paratracheal** and **pretracheal** lymph nodes depending on their location. These nodes usually drain directly to the deep lateral cervical lymph nodes but in some cases can also drain to the superficial anterior cervical lymph nodes.

The **superficial lateral cervical lymph nodes** are located along the length of the external jugular vein and as a result are also known as the external jugular nodes. These nodes usually drain to the supraclavicular lymph nodes at the root of the neck.

The **deep lateral cervical lymph nodes** are located along the length of the internal jugular vein and are therefore also known as the internal jugular nodes. They are divided into a superior and inferior group. The **superior deep lateral cervical lymph nodes** are located above the superior belly of the omohyoid muscle. One of the largest nodes in this region is known as the **jugulodigastric lymph node**. The **inferior deep lateral cervical node**s are located along the length of the internal jugular vein below the superior belly of the omohyoid muscle. The large **juguloomohyoid lymph** node can be found along the middle portion of the internal jugular vein. Efferent vessels from the deep lateral cervical lymph nodes join to form the jugular trunks which drain into the right lymphatic and thoracic ducts, or directly into the subclavian vein.

Key points about the lymphatics of the head and neck	
Facial lymph nodes	Buccinator, nasolabial, malar and mandibular lymph nodes
Pericervical lymphatic circle	Occipital, mastoid, parotid (superficial and deep), submandibular and submental lymph nodes
Anterior cervical lymph nodes	Superficial anterior cervical lymph nodes, deep anterior cervical lymph nodes (prelaryngeal, thyroid, pretracheal and paratracheal lymph nodes)

Key points about the lymphatics of the head and neck	
Lateral cervical lymph nodes	Superficial lateral cervical lymph nodes, deep lateral cervical lymph nodes (superior and inferior deep lateral cervical lymph nodes), accessory lymph nodes, supraclavicular lymph nodes
Pharyngeal lymphoid ring and nodes	Pharyngeal lymphoid ring (pharyngeal, lingual, palatine and tubal tonsils), retropharyngeal lymph nodes
Lymphatic trunk and ducts	Jugular trunk, right lymphatic duct, thoracic duct

Lymph nodes of the head neck and arm

Lymphatic drainage of the oral and nasal cavities

TRIANGLES OF THE NECK

■ Anterior triangle of neck
■ Carotid triangle
■ Submandibular triangle
■ Submental triangle
■ Muscular triangle

■ Posterior triangle of neck
■ Occipital triangle
■ Omoclavicular triangle

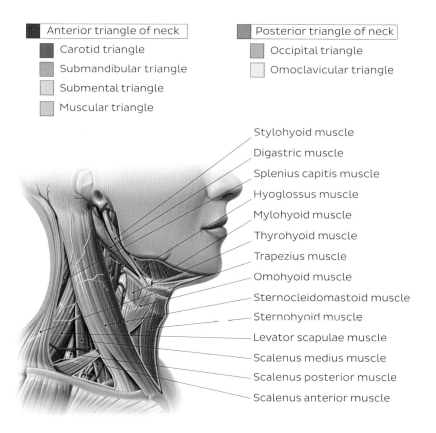

Stylohyoid muscle
Digastric muscle
Splenius capitis muscle
Hyoglossus muscle
Mylohyoid muscle
Thyrohyoid muscle
Trapezius muscle
Omohyoid muscle
Sternocleidomastoid muscle
Sternohyoid muscle
Levator scapulae muscle
Scalenus medius muscle
Scalenus posterior muscle
Scalenus anterior muscle

FIGURE 8.109. **Triangles of the neck (overview).** The midline of the neck divides the anterolateral neck region into two symmetrical halves. On each side there is an anterior and a posterior triangle, separated by the sternocleidomastoid muscle. The **anterior triangle** stretches from the midline of the neck anteriorly

HEAD AND NECK

to the sternocleidomastoid muscle posteriorly and its superior border is the body of the mandible. It is further subdivided into four smaller triangles: The **submandibular**, **submental**, **carotid** and **muscular triangles**. The **posterior triangle** is bordered by the sternocleidomastoid muscle anteriorly, the trapezius muscle posteriorly and the clavicle inferiorly. The inferior belly of the omohyoid muscle passes through and further divides it into a smaller **omoclavicular** (a.k.a. subclavian) and a larger **occipital triangle**.

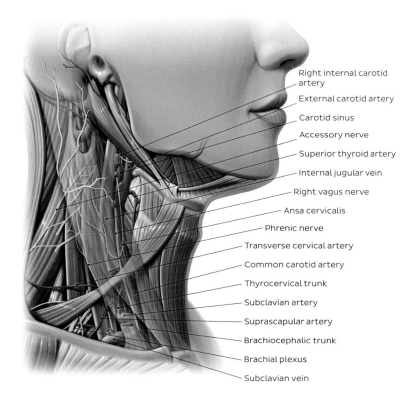

Right internal carotid artery

External carotid artery

Carotid sinus

Accessory nerve

Superior thyroid artery

Internal jugular vein

Right vagus nerve

Ansa cervicalis

Phrenic nerve

Transverse cervical artery

Common carotid artery

Thyrocervical trunk

Subclavian artery

Suprascapular artery

Brachiocephalic trunk

Brachial plexus

Subclavian vein

FIGURE 8.110. **Triangles of the neck: Neurovasculature.** Lateral view of the major arteries, veins and nerves located within the triangles of the neck, with the sternocleidomastoid muscle faded out to reveal the vessels beneath. The **common carotid artery** courses upwards along the sternocleidomastoid muscle into the carotid triangle, where it bifurcates within the carotid sheath into the internal and external carotid arteries. Also located within the sheath are the **internal jugular vein** and **vagus nerve**.

Numerous branches of the **external carotid artery** arise within the carotid triangle, including the superior and inferior thyroid arteries and veins, which travel through the muscular triangle and ultimately supply the thyroid and parathyroid glands; as well as the facial artery, which courses through the submandibular triangle together with the facial vein to supply superficial structures of the face.

Several important nerves are also seen in this image, such as the **vagus nerve** and **ansa cervicalis**, both located anteriorly in the neck, within the carotid triangle. The **accessory nerve** (CN XI) enters the neck in the carotid triangle and courses beneath the sternocleidomastoid muscle to reach the occipital triangle within the posterior neck. Also located posteriorly are the **brachial plexus** and **phrenic nerve**, which pass through the omoclavicular and occipital triangles, as well as branches of the cervical plexus which course through the occipital triangle.

Triangles of the neck: anterior	Borders	Contents
Submandibular triangle	**Superior**: mandible **Anterior**: anterior belly of digastric muscle **Posterior**: posterior belly of the digastric muscle **Floor**: mylohyoid and hyoglossus muscles	Submandibular glands and lymph nodes, facial artery and vein, submental artery and vein, mylohyoid nerve, geniohyoid muscle, hyoglossus muscle, lingual artery, deep lingual vein
Submental triangle	**Lateral**: anterior belly of the digastric muscle **Inferior** (base): hyoid bone **Superior** (apex): mandibular symphysis **Floor**: mylohyoid muscle	Submental veins, submental lymph nodes
Muscular (omotracheal) triangle	**Superior**: hyoid bone **Superolateral**: superior belly of omohyoid muscle **Inferolateral**: sternocleidomastoid muscle **Base**: median line of the neck **Apex**: junction of the sternocleidomastoid and superior belly of the omohyoid muscle	Infrahyoid muscles (thyrohyoid, sternothyroid, sternohyoid), thyroid gland, parathyroid gland, superior thyroid artery and vein, inferior thyroid artery and vein, anterior jugular vein
Carotid triangle	**Anterior**: superior belly of the omohyoid muscle **Superior**: posterior belly of digastric muscle **Posterior**: anterior border of the sternocleidomastoid muscle **Floor**: thyrohyoid, hyoglossus, middle and inferior constrictors of the pharynx muscle	Carotid sheath containing the common carotid artery, internal jugular vein, vagus nerve (CN X), deep cervical lymph nodes; superior thyroid artery, lingual artery, facial artery, ascending pharyngeal artery, occipital artery; hypoglossal nerve (CN XII), accessory nerve (CN XI), ansa cervicalis

Triangles of the neck: posterior	Borders	Contents
Omoclavicular (supraclavicular) triangle	**Superior**: inferior belly of omohyoid muscle **Anterior**: sternocleidomastoid muscle **Inferior**: clavicle **Floor**: anterior and middle scalene muscles	Subclavian artery, transverse cervical artery, dorsal scapular artery, external jugular vein, brachial plexus, phrenic nerve, supraclavicular lymph nodes
Occipital triangle	**Anterior**: posterior border of sternocleidomastoid muscle **Posterior**: trapezius muscle **Inferior**: inferior belly of omohyoid muscle **Floor**: splenius capitis, levator scapulae and middle scalene muscles	Occipital artery, transverse cervical artery, accessory nerve (CN XI), brachial plexus, cervical plexus, phrenic nerve, cervical lymph nodes

COMPARTMENTS OF THE NECK

Fasciae of the neck (cervical fascia) are multilayered sheaths of connective tissue that wrap the structures of the neck and can be divided into two layers: A superficial layer (superficial cervical fascia) and a deep layer (deep cervical fascia). The cervical fasciae provide longitudinal organization by separating the tissues of the neck and therefore largely limit the spread of infection in response to pathology or trauma. The **superficial cervical fascia** (i.e. subcutaneous tissue or tela subcutanea) lies deep to the skin and does not contribute to the formation of the neck compartments. However, the **deep cervical fascia** typically has three separate layers that contribute to the formation of the spaces and compartments of the neck. These layers include:

- The **superficial layer** (investing layer, external layer, parotidomasseteric fascia)
- The **middle layer** (pretracheal layer, buccopharyngeal fascia)
- The **deep layer** (deep investing layer, prevertebral layer)

A compartment is a section of the body bounded by fascia. The internal structures of the neck are divided into **four main compartments**: The visceral compartment, vertebral compartment and two vascular compartments. Each compartment is contained within unique layers of deep cervical fascia.

The fasciae of the neck also contribute to the formation of three **fascial spaces**: The pretracheal space, the retropharyngeal space and the danger space (of Grodinsky). These spaces extend from the base of the skull to the mediastinum and in doing so may provide a conduit for the passage of infection from the neck to the thoracic cavity.

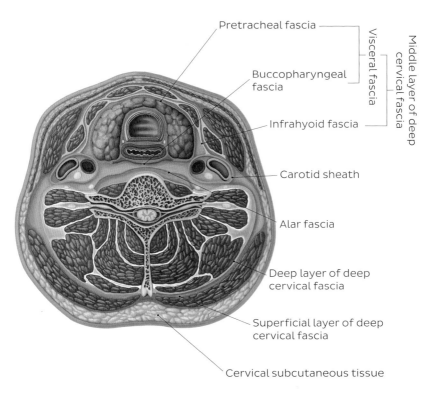

Pretracheal fascia

Buccopharyngeal fascia

Visceral fascia

Middle layer of deep cervical fascia

Infrahyoid fascia

Carotid sheath

Alar fascia

Deep layer of deep cervical fascia

Superficial layer of deep cervical fascia

Cervical subcutaneous tissue

FIGURE 8.111. **Cervical fascia (cross section).** The **superficial layer** of deep cervical fascia is located deep to the superficial cervical fascia and encircles the neck, surrounding the trapezius and sternocleidomastoid muscles. This layer of fascia forms one large compartment which contains the other three smaller compartments of the neck.

The **middle layer** of deep cervical fascia is typically divided into muscular (infrahyoid) and visceral fasciae. The muscular or infrahyoid fascia surrounds the infrahyoid (strap) muscles while the visceral fascia is divided into two parts: A pretracheal layer and a buccopharyngeal layer. The **deep layer** of deep cervical fascia also known as **prevertebral fascia** is a cylindrical layer of fascia which surrounds the cervical verte-bra. Prevertebral fascia passes between the attachment points on the transverse processes of the cervical vertebrae and splits into two layers forming another sheet of fascia known as alar fascia. Alar fascia forms the anterior layer of the prevertebral fascia and delimits the posterior margin of the retropharyngeal space and the anterior margin of the danger space.

Formed by contributions from all three layers of deep cervical fascia is the **carotid sheath**. The carotid sheath extends from the base of the skull caudally to the first rib. It surrounds the major vascular struc-tures of the neck thereby forming the vascular compartment.

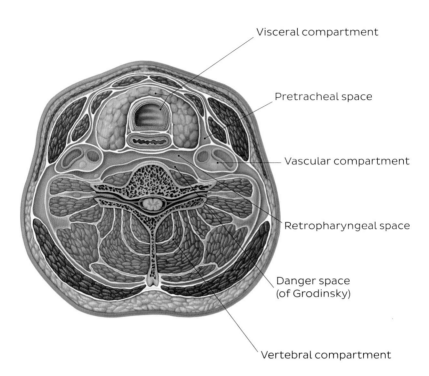

Visceral compartment

Pretracheal space

Vascular compartment

Retropharyngeal space

Danger space
(of Grodinsky)

Vertebral compartment

FIGURE 8.112. **Compartments and spaces of the neck.** The visceral compartment of the neck is surrounded by the visceral cervical fascia, specifically the **pretracheal fascia** anterolaterally and **buccopharyngeal fascia** posteriorly. It extends from the superior part of the hyoid bone superiorly to the superior mediastinum inferiorly. It is the most anteriorly located compartment of the neck.

Posterior to the visceral compartment is the large **vertebral compartment** of the neck. This compartment is surrounded posterolaterally by prevertebral fascia and anteriorly by alar fascia. It is attached superiorly as a continuous circle from the base of the skull and extends to the superior mediastinum inferiorly.

The paired **vascular compartments** (a.k.a. carotid spaces), formed by the carotid sheaths, house the large vascular channels of the neck (common carotid artery, internal jugular vein). Each vascular compartment extends from the base of the skull to the aortic arch within the thoracic cavity.

Between the investing layer of cervical fascia and pretracheal fascia is the most anteriorly located fascial space, the **pretracheal space**. It extends from the thyroid cartilage superiorly to reach the superior mediastinum inferiorly.

The buccopharyngeal fascia together with the carotid sheath and alar fascia of the deep layer of deep cervical fascia form a fat filled space known as the **retropharyngeal space**. The **danger space** which lies between the alar and prevertebral fascia is located just anterior to the cervical vertebral bodies and spans from the base of the skull to the posterior mediastinum where the prevertebral layers of deep cervical fascia fuse. The danger space is so called as its loose areolar tissue provides a route of passage for the rapid down spread of infection from the neck to the thoracic region. The retropharyngeal and danger spaces extend from the base of the skull superiorly to the posterior mediastinum inferiorly.

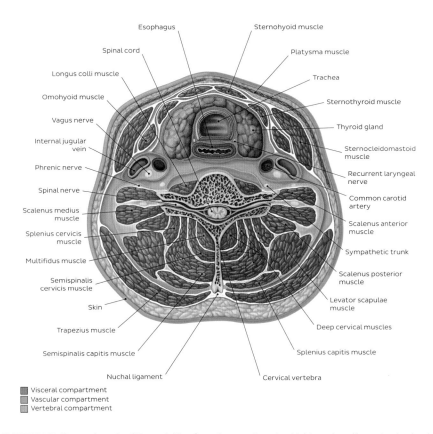

- Esophagus
- Spinal cord
- Longus colli muscle
- Omohyoid muscle
- Vagus nerve
- Internal jugular vein
- Phrenic nerve
- Spinal nerve
- Scalenus medius muscle
- Splenius cervicis muscle
- Multifidus muscle
- Semispinalis cervicis muscle
- Skin
- Trapezius muscle
- Semispinalis capitis muscle
- Nuchal ligament

- Sternohyoid muscle
- Platysma muscle
- Trachea
- Sternothyroid muscle
- Thyroid gland
- Sternocleidomastoid muscle
- Recurrent laryngeal nerve
- Common carotid artery
- Scalenus anterior muscle
- Sympathetic trunk
- Scalenus posterior muscle
- Levator scapulae muscle
- Deep cervical muscles
- Splenius capitis muscle
- Cervical vertebra

- ▨ Visceral compartment
- ▨ Vascular compartment
- ▨ Vertebral compartment

FIGURE 8.113. **Compartments of the neck:** The **visceral compartment**, which is enclosed by pretracheal and buccopharyngeal fascia, contains the thyroid and gland, parathyroid glands, larynx, trachea, hypopharynx, recurrent laryngeal nerve and esophagus.

The **vertebral compartment** contains the cervical vertebrae and deep muscles associated with them, which include the longus colli muscle, the scalenus anterior, medius and posterior muscles, the deep cervical muscles (splenius cervicis, splenius capitis, semispinalis cervicis, semispinalis capitis, multifidus muscle) and the levator scapulae muscle.

The **vascular compartment** of the neck is so called according to its contents. It contains the major vascular structures of the neck which include the common carotid arteries and internal jugular veins. It also contains the vagus nerve, part of the recurrent laryngeal nerve and the deep cervical lymph nodes.

The three spaces of the neck mainly contain a combination of subcutaneous fat, loose connective tissue and lymph nodes.

Cervical fascias

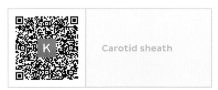

Carotid sheath

NEUROANATOMY 9

The **brain** is an integral part of the central nervous system. It contains three main parts:

- The **cerebrum** is the largest part of the brain. It is responsible for higher-order bodily functions such as vision, hearing, cognition, emotions, learning and fine control of movement.
- The **cerebellum** sits below the cerebrum. It regulates motor functions such as balance, coordination and speech.
- The **brainstem** connects the brain with the spinal cord. It controls the most lower-order bodily functions such as breathing and heart rate.

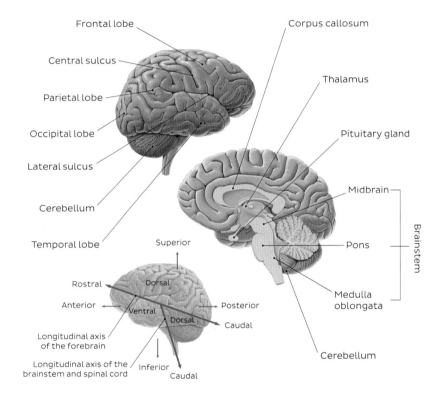

FIGURE 9.1. **Overview of the brain.** The brain consists of three main parts:

- The **cerebrum** is organized into two **hemispheres** that are connected by a large bundle of white matter tissue called the **corpus callosum**. The outer surface of the cerebrum exhibits many elevated ridges of tissue called **gyri**, that are separated by grooves called **sulci**. The gyri and sulci increase the surface area of the cerebrum, providing it with its characteristic convoluted appearance.
  Each hemisphere of the cerebrum contains six lobes: Frontal, temporal, parietal, occipital, insular and limbic. The insular lobe is located internal to the lateral sulcus and is therefore not visible superficially. It is covered by portions of the parietal, temporal and frontal lobes which are collectively referred to as the operculum (lit. 'a covering').

- The **cerebellum** is found inferior to the occipital lobe of the cerebrum. It also has two hemispheres that are connected by the vermis.

- The **brainstem** is the most caudal part of the brain. It is made up of the midbrain, pons, and medulla oblongata, each of which have their own structural and functional organization.

Key points about the brain		
Part	**Structure**	**Functions**
Cerebrum	• Frontal, temporal, parietal, occipital, insular and limbic lobes • Basal nuclei	• Gray matter: process/integrate sensory input, control voluntary/skilled movement, higher mental functions (cognition, emotions, learning) • Modulate voluntary movements
Cerebellum	• Vermis and hemispheres (anterior, posterior, flocculonodular lobes)	• Processes motor/proprioceptive, visual/vestibular input, motor functions (balance/equilibrium, coordination, speech)
Brainstem	• Midbrain • Pons • Medulla oblongata	• Visual/auditory reflexes, nuclei of cranial nerves III/IV • Relays cerebral input to cerebellum, nuclei of cranial nerves V–VII • Relays sensory input to cerebellum, controls heart/breathing rate, nuclei of cranial nerves VIII–XII (all parts of the brainstem carry information between upper and lower parts of the CNS)

Central nervous system

Cerebellum and brainstem

CEREBRAL CORTEX

Each hemisphere of the cerebrum contains **six lobes**: Frontal, temporal, parietal, occipital, insular and limbic. The insular lobe is located internal to the lateral sulcus and is therefore not visible superficially. It is covered by portions of the parietal, temporal and frontal lobes which are collectively referred to as the operculum (*lit. 'a covering'*).

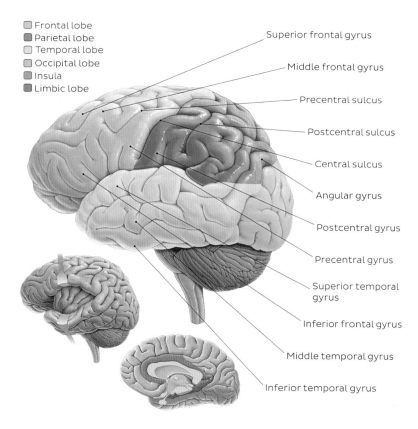

□ Frontal lobe
■ Parietal lobe
□ Temporal lobe
□ Occipital lobe
■ Insula
■ Limbic lobe

Superior frontal gyrus
Middle frontal gyrus
Precentral sulcus
Postcentral sulcus
Central sulcus
Angular gyrus
Postcentral gyrus
Precentral gyrus
Superior temporal gyrus
Inferior frontal gyrus
Middle temporal gyrus
Inferior temporal gyrus

FIGURE 9.2. **Lobes of the cerebrum.** Color-coded representation of the cerebral lobes as well as major gyri and sulci identifiable from a lateral perspective.

Lobes of the cerebrum

	Anatomy	Functions
Frontal lobe	Anterior to central sulcus, superior to lateral sulcus Major gyri: precentral gyrus, superior, middle, inferior frontal gyri	Control of voluntary movement, involved in attention, short term memory tasks, motivation, planning, speech
Parietal lobe	Posterior to the central sulcus Major gyri/areas: postcentral gyrus, superior parietal lobule, inferior parietal lobule (angular gyrus)	Processing of somatosensory input (touch, pain, pressure and temperature), integration of other sensory input (taste, hearing, sight, and smell), visuospatial mapping and attention, processing language and numerical relationships
Temporal lobe	Lateral surface of cerebrum, inferior to lateral sulcus Main gyri: superior, middle, inferior temporal gyri	Decoding sensory input (visual and auditory) into derived meanings for retention of visual memory and language comprehension
Occipital lobe	Posterior to parietal/temporal lobes Main gyri: occipital gyri	Center for visual processing
Insula	Deep to temporal/parietal/frontal lobes Main gyri: long/short gyri of insula	Processing and integration of taste sensation, visceral and pain sensation and vestibular functions
Limbic lobe	Medial surface of each hemisphere, surrounding corpus callosum Main gyri: paraterminal, cingulate, parahippocampal gyri	Modulation of emotions, modulation of visceral and autonomic functions, learning, memory

The cerebral cortex forms the surface of each hemisphere; it is composed of gray matter and is the most complex part of the cerebrum. Functionally, it can be divided into three general areas:

- Primary motor cortex, which is involved in the planning and execution of movement
- Primary sensory cortices, which receive and process sensory input
- Association areas, which serve to integrate information from several structures/areas.

Association areas can be *unimodal*, which integrate information from a single source (typically an adjacent primary motor/sensory area) or *higher-order/multimodal*, which receive information from multiple sources in order to carry out higher cognitive functions. All neurons in the cerebral cortex are interneurons as they synapse with other neurons.

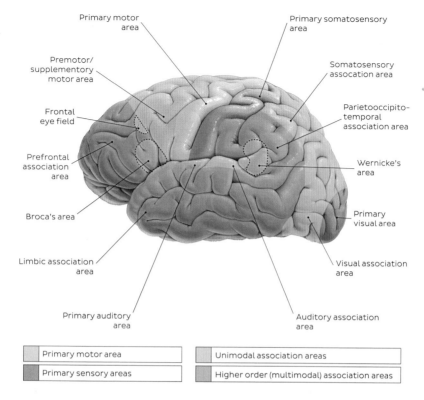

Primary motor area

Primary somatosensory area

Premotor/ supplementory motor area

Somatosensory assocation area

Frontal eye field

Parietooccipito- temporal association area

Prefrontal association area

Wernicke's area

Broca's area

Primary visual area

Limbic association area

Visual association area

Primary auditory area

Auditory association area

	Primary motor area			Unimodal association areas
	Primary sensory areas			Higher order (multimodal) association areas

FIGURE 9.3. **Motor, sensory and association cortices.** Left lateral view of the cerebrum. A map depicting the major functional areas of the cerebrum according to the three main groups.

Motor, sensory and association cortices		
Area	**Location**	**Function**
Motor		
Primary motor area	Precentral gyrus (frontal lobe)	Planning and execution of movement
Sensory		
Primary somatosensory area	Postcentral gyrus (parietal lobe)	Processing of somatic sensory input
Primary visual area	Occipital lobe	Processing of visual input
Primary auditory area	Superior parietal lobule	Processing of auditory input
Olfactory area	Limbic/medial temporal lobes	Processing of olfactory input
Gustatory area	Insular/parietal lobes	Processing of taste stimuli
Vestibular areas	Parietal/temporal lobes	Equilibrium and balance
Association areas		
Premotor area	Anterior to primary motor cortex	Complex movement
Somatosensory association area	Posterior to primary somatosensory cortex	Integration of somatic sensory information
Visual association area	Anterior part of occipital lobe, posterior parts of parietal/temporal lobes	Spatial orientation, perception of depth, location, movement and velocity of objects in space

NEUROANATOMY

Motor, sensory and association cortices		
Area	**Location**	**Function**
Parietalocciptio-temporal association area	Posterior parts of parietal/occipital/temporal lobes	Interpretation of signals from surrounding somatosensory, visual and auditory areas (e.g. visuospatial awareness, visual language (reading), naming of objects), learning of fine motor skills
Wernike's area	Posterolateral part temporal lobe (usually left hemisphere)	Language (comprehension)
Temporal association area	Anterior pole of temporal lobe	Processes of recognition/association, behavior, emotions, and motivation
Prefrontal area	Anterior frontal lobe	Higher mental functions, behavior, personality
Frontal eye fields	Anterior to premotor cortex	Eye movements
Broca's area	Inferolateral frontal lobe (usually left hemisphere)	Language (production/word formation)
Limbic association area	Anterior pole of temporal lobe, ventral part of frontal lobe, cingulate gyrus	Processes of recognition/association, behavior, emotions, and motivation

Cerebral cortex

MOTOR AND SENSORY CORTICAL HOMUNCULUS

The primary motor cortex is somatotopically arranged such that different parts of this gyrus are associated with the motor control of the different parts of the contralateral side of the human body. To reflect this, a spatial map of the body along the primary motor cortex, referred to as the motor homunculus, has been developed. Similar to the primary motor cortex, the neurons in the primary somatosensory cortex are somatotopically arranged; a sensory map of the body along the postcentral gyrus is known as the sensory homunculus.

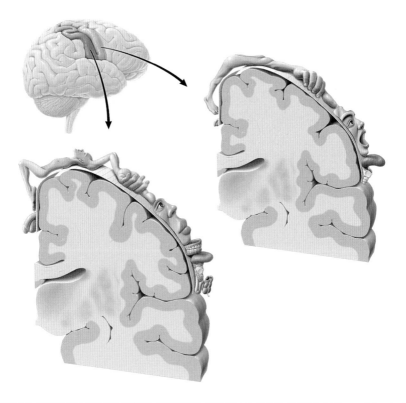

FIGURE 9.4. **Motor and sensory cortical homunculi.** This image shows coronal sections of the brain through the precentral and postcentral gyri. The motor homunculus (upper right image) represents a topographic map of the motor innervation of the body. Note that the body parts of the homunculus are not proportional to the real body parts. This is because the amount of cortex dedicated to each body part is proportional to the intricacy and complexity of the motor function of each body part.

The sensory homunculus (lower left image) is a topographic distribution of the somatosensory innervation of different body parts. Again, the area of the cortex that is responsible for the innervation of the body parts, is not proportional to the dimensions of the body part. The amount of cortex per body part is proportional to the complexity of sensations received from that organ.

WHITE MATTER

Deep to the cerebral cortex (i.e. gray matter containing neuronal cell bodies) is the cerebral white matter which is composed of axons of neurons reaching between different areas of the brain. Most of these nerve fibers are surrounded by a type of fatty sheath/envelope called myelin which gives the white matter its color. While the gray matter facilitates information processing, the white matter serves the important role of function of enabling information transfer.

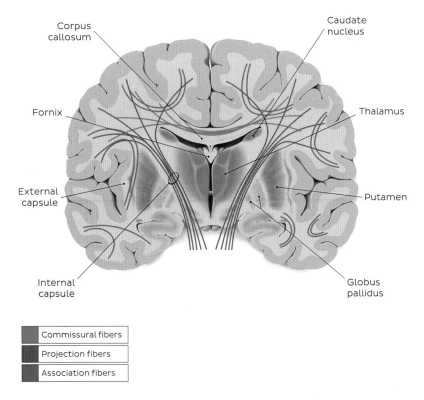

Corpus callosum	Caudate nucleus
Fornix	Thalamus
External capsule	Putamen
Internal capsule	Globus pallidus

- Commissural fibers
- Projection fibers
- Association fibers

FIGURE 9.5. **Cerebral white matter.** Deep to the cerebral cortex (i.e. gray matter) is the cerebral white matter, which is composed of tracts carrying signals to, from or within each cerebral hemisphere. The largest of these is the corpus callosum, a dense plate composed of **commissural fibers** which connect the cerebral hemispheres. Projection fibers, on the other hand, connect different cortical regions within lower regions of the brain or spinal cord, while **association fibers** are those which interconnect different regions of the cerebral cortex within the same hemisphere.

BASAL NUCLEI

The basal nuclei, commonly known as the basal ganglia, are a group of gray matter masses found deep within the white matter of each cerebral hemisphere. The components of basal nuclei are the caudate nucleus, putamen, and globus pallidus. The subthalamic nucleus and substantia nigra are not anatomically part of the basal nuclei but are functionally connected and related to this system.

The basal nuclei play a crucial role in the modulation of voluntary movements. Dysfunction of these structures can lead to several neurologic conditions broadly known as movement disorders.

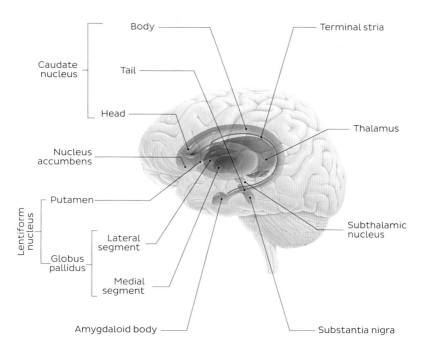

FIGURE 9.6. **Overview of the basal nuclei.** Left lateral perspective of the brain, with the left-sided instances of the different nuclei of the basal nuclei presented. The **caudate nucleus** is an elongated, C-shaped structure that consists of a head, body and tail. The tail extends as far anteriorly/rostrally as far as the amygdaloid body, which is not part of the caudate nucleus. Located close to the head of the caudate nucleus is the nucleus accumbens, a structure involved in the perception of pleasure that is considered to be a part of the limbic system. Continuous with the head of the caudate nucleus is the **putamen**, a rounded nucleus which is the most lateral of the basal nuclei. The globus pallidus is situated medial to the putamen and is divided into lateral (or external) and medial (or internal) segments. Also represented in the image are two important structures functionally related to the basal nuclei: The subthalamic nucleus and the substantia nigra, located in the subthalamus and midbrain, respectively. Central in this image and lying medially to the basal nuclei is the thalamus. The thalamus has important connections with the basal nuclei.

Key points about the basal nuclei	
Definition	Group of subcortical nuclei that fine-tune the voluntary movement
Components	Caudate nucleus
	Putamen
	Globus pallidus
	Functionally related structures:
	Subthalamic nucleus
	Substantia nigra
Function	Planning and modulation of movement, memory, eye movements, reward processing, motivation

Basal ganglia

Direct and indirect pathways of the basal ganglia

DIENCEPHALON

The forebrain can be further divided into two parts: The telencephalon (composed of cerebral cortex, white matter and basal nuclei) and the diencephalon that occupies the central region of the brain (around the third ventricle).

The diencephalon is divided into several distinct parts, most notably the:

- **Thalamus:** Central portion of the diencephalon (many other parts of the diencephalon take their names based on their relevant position compared to the thalamus. It is an ovoid, bilateral gray matter structure, found in the center of the brain, just superior to the brainstem. The thalamus has many important functions, but in general is considered to be the central relay station of the brain, that relays limbic, sensory and motor information between the cerebral cortex and the rest of the nervous system.
- **Epithalamus:** Small dorsal part of the diencephalon that participates in the formation of the roof of the third ventricle. The structures that make up the epithalamus are the pineal gland and habenular nuclei.
- **Subthalamus:** Lies inferior to the posterior part of the thalamus, just posterior and lateral to the hypothalamus. The largest division of the subthalamus is the subthalamic nucleus. This nucleus plays a fundamental role in the circuitry of the basal nuclei (i.e. movement regulation).
- **Hypothalamus:** Inferior most part of the diencephalon, located anteroinferior to the thalamus. It can be divided into several regions each of which is responsible for certain functions. In general, it forms connections with different body systems (endocrine, autonomic and limbic) through which it controls some vital functions of the human body (e.g., homeostasis, energy consumption, hunger, awareness, etc.)

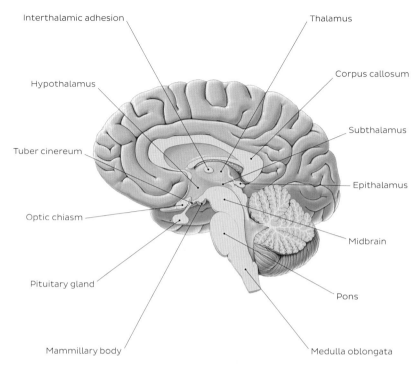

Interthalamic adhesion

Thalamus

Hypothalamus

Corpus callosum

Tuber cinereum

Subthalamus

Epithalamus

Optic chiasm

Midbrain

Pituitary gland

Pons

Mammillary body

Medulla oblongata

FIGURE 9.7. **Overview of the diencephalon.** A sagittal section of the brain showing the diencephalon and surrounding structures. The diencephalon is the central portion of the brain located around the third ventricle, superior to the brainstem (medulla, pons and midbrain), and inferior to the corpus callosum and cerebral cortex.

Four notable parts of the diencephalon include the epithalamus, thalamus, subthalamus, and hypothalamus. The largest and most significant part of the diencephalon is the thalamus, which is an ovoid gray matter structure that relays information from the cortex to the rest of the nervous system and vice versa. The epithalamus is a small portion of the diencephalon located dorsal and caudal to the thalamus. The subthalamus and hypothalamus are both located ventral to the thalamus. The subthalamus is involved in movement regulation, while the hypothalamus controls vital functions such as hunger and thirst.

Key points about the four main parts of the diencephalon		
Part	**Location**	**Function**
Epithalamus	Caudal part of diencephalon	Regulation of circadian rhythms responsible for regular sleep and wake cycles, regulates motivational states and cognition
Thalamus	Superior to brainstem, either side of third ventricle	Relays limbic, sensory and motor information between the cerebral cortex and the rest of the nervous system
Subthalamus	Inferior to posterior part of the thalamus; posterior and lateral to hypothalamus	Regulation of movement
Hypothalamus	Anteroinferior to thalamus	Vital functions of the body (e.g., homeostasis, energy consumption, hunger, awareness, body temperature), regulates hormonal output of the adenohypophysis (anterior pituitary gland), acts as endocrine gland (produces antidiuretic hormone/oxytocin)

Diencephalon

 Hypothalamus

 Thalamus

BRAINSTEM

The brainstem is a stalk-like projection which extends caudally from the base of the diencephalon, connecting it with the spinal cord. It is the oldest part of the brain and is composed of three parts: The midbrain, pons and medulla oblongata.

Vertical division:
☐ Tectum
☐ Tegmentum
☐ Basilar part

Horizontal division:
▦ Midbrain
▨ Pons
▨ Medulla oblongata

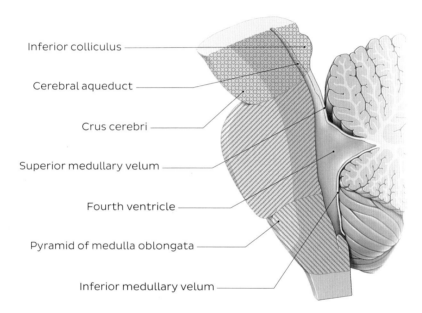

Inferior colliculus

Cerebral aqueduct

Crus cerebri

Superior medullary velum

Fourth ventricle

Pyramid of medulla oblongata

Inferior medullary velum

FIGURE 9.8. **Parts of the brainstem (sagittal view).** The **midbrain** is the shortest segment of the brainstem. It extends caudally from the base of the diencephalon) to the pons. Its functions are associated with motor coordination (in particular eye movements), visual and auditory processing, arousal/consciousness as well as behavioral responses to fear and danger.

The **pons** is located between the midbrain and medulla oblongata and forms the largest component of the brainstem. It houses the nuclei of cranial nerves V–VIII, as well as the pontine nuclei which facilitate corti-copontocerebellar communication. It also participates in the regulation of sleep and breathing.

The **medulla oblongata** is the narrowest and most caudal part of the brainstem. It has a tapered appearance that extends from the pons to the spinal cord. It houses the nuclei of cranial nerves IX–X, and XII and is involved in controlling respiratory function, the cardiovascular system, as well as gastrointestinal and digestive activities.

The brainstem can also be divided vertically into tectum, tegmentum and basilar parts. The tectum (L. roof) and tegmentum (L. covering) are used in relation to the developing central cavity of the neural tube. The **tectum** is the roof of the cavity while the **tegmentum** forms the ventral covering. The central cavity of the neural tube becomes the aqueduct of Sylvius, the fourth ventricle, and the central canal of the spinal cord. Therefore, the tectum is the area dorsal to the cerebral aqueduct, while the tegmentum is ventral to these structures at the respective levels. The **basilar part** is ventral to tegmentum and it spans all three vertical parts of the brainstem.

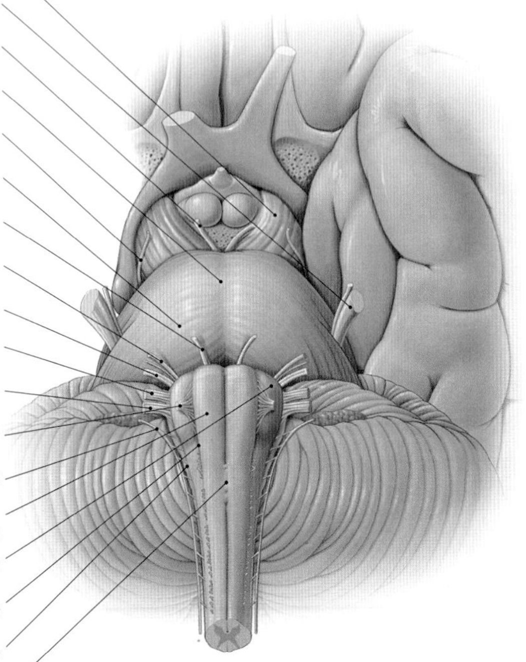

Cerebral peduncle
Trigeminal nerve
Oculomotor nerve
Basilar sulcus
Trochlear nerve
Pons
Abducens nerve
Facial nerve
Vestibulocochlear nerve
Glossopharyngeal nerve
Vagus nerve
Hypoglossal nerve
Accessory nerve
Pyramid of medulla oblongata
Olivary nuclei
Preolivary groove
Retroolivary groove
Decussation of pyramids

FIGURE 9.9. Brainstem (anterior/ventral view). Along its ventral surface, the midbrain is characterized by two prominences known as the cerebral peduncles which connect the cerebral hemispheres to the brainstem. Between each cerebral peduncle is a shallow depression, the interpeduncular fossa; the posterior perforated substance forms the floor of this fossa, while its contents include the oculomotor nerves (CN III) and mammillary bodies.

When viewed from the ventral aspect, the pons resembles a dome-like structure with numerous horizontal striations across its surface. A shallow depression runs along its vertical axis known as the basilar groove, which houses the basilar artery.

An anterior median fissure divides the ventral medulla oblongata into symmetrical halves and is bordered on either side by the medullary pyramids. Lateral to each pyramid is another prominent bulge, the olive, which corresponds to the location of the olivary nuclei. At its caudal/inferior end, the anterior median fissure is interrupted by criss-crossing fibers known as the decussation of pyramids, which mark the termination of the medulla oblongata.

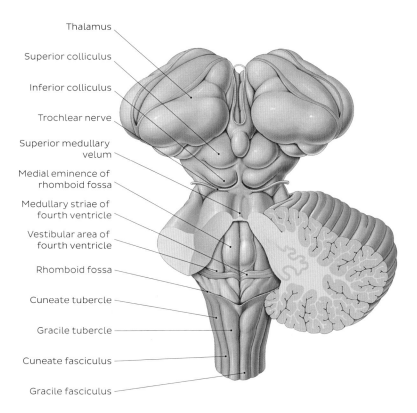

Thalamus

Superior colliculus

Inferior colliculus

Trochlear nerve

Superior medullary velum

Medial eminence of rhomboid fossa

Medullary striae of fourth ventricle

Vestibular area of fourth ventricle

Rhomboid fossa

Cuneate tubercle

Gracile tubercle

Cuneate fasciculus

Gracile fasciculus

FIGURE 9.10. **Brainstem (posterior/dorsal view).** The posterior part (tectum) of the midbrain has two pairs of raised, round protrusions that are collectively known as the quadrigeminal plate. This complex consists of the superior and inferior colliculi.

The dorsal aspect of the pons and upper medulla oblongata forms the floor of the fourth ventricle, forming a large landmark known as the rhomboid fossa. T The cranial/superior limit of the pons is formed by a structure which contributes to the formation of the roof of the fourth ventricle, the superior medullary velum, while the inferior boundary of the pons is formed by the medullary striae of the fourth ventricle.

The dorsal/posterior surface of the medulla oblongata is divided into an open/superior part, which contains the caudal half of the fourth ventricle, and a closed/inferior part, which contains the central canal that continues into the spinal cord. The dorsal aspect of the inferior part of the medulla oblongata is marked by the gracile and cuneate tubercles which are continuations of the gracile and cuneate fasciculi of the spinal cord.

Key points about the brainstem		
	Anatomy	**Functions**
Midbrain	**Major landmarks**: cerebral peduncles, interpeduncular fossa (mamillary body) quadrigeminal plate (inferior colliculus, superior colliculus)	Processes and directs visual/auditory information to thalamus, monitors movement with basal nuclei, contains nuclei of cranial nerves III/IV
Pons	**Major landmarks**: upper rhomboid fossa (median sulcus, sulcus limitans, medial eminence, upper part of vestibular area) intermediate rhomboid fossa (medullary striae of fourth ventricle)	Relays cerebral input to cerebellum, contains nuclei of cranial nerves V–VII Regulates breathing, sleep–wake cycle

NEUROANATOMY

Key points about the brainstem		
	Anatomy	Functions
Medulla oblongata	**Parts:** superior/open (caudal part of fourth ventricle), inferior/closed (contains central canal)	Relays sensory input to cerebellum, regulates several homeostatic functions (e.g. heart/breathing rate), contains nuclei of cranial nerves VIII–XII
	Major landmarks: pyramids, decussation of pyramids, olives, gracile/cuneate tubercles	(all parts of the brainstem carry information (via white matter tracts) between upper and lower parts of the CNS)

The brainstem

CEREBELLUM

The cerebellum is the part of the brain which lies posterior (dorsal) to the pons and medulla. It sits in the posterior cranial fossa beneath the occipital lobe of the cerebrum, from which it is separated by the tentorium cerebelli. It is connected to the brainstem by three sets of large bilateral nerve fiber bundles known as cerebellar peduncles.

At a gross level, the cerebrum is built around a central **vermis** which is flanked on either side by a **cerebellar hemisphere**. It has **three surfaces**: Superior (tentorial), anterior (petrosal) and inferior (suboccipital). All are highly convoluted and bear deep fissures that divide the cerebellum into lobes that are further subdivided into lobules. The surface of the cerebellum is much more tightly folded compared to the cerebral cortex and is marked with fine gyri known as **folia**.

The cerebellum receives input from peripheral receptors and motor centers in the spinal cord, visual and vestibular apparatus as well as cerebrum and brainstem; it is responsible for integrating these inputs to ensure coordination of movement, balance and posture, as well as motor learning.

NEUROANATOMY

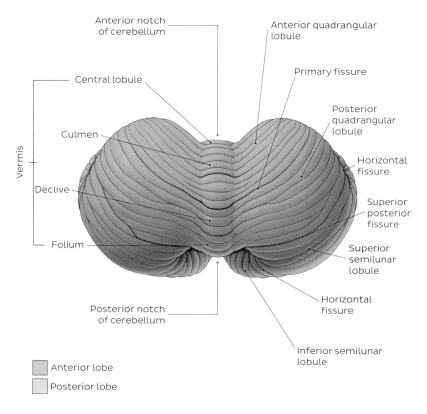

Anterior notch of cerebellum

Anterior quadrangular lobule

Central lobule

Primary fissure

Culmen

Posterior quadrangular lobule

Vermis

Declive

Horizontal fissure

Folium

Superior posterior fissure

Superior semilunar lobule

Posterior notch of cerebellum

Horizontal fissure

Inferior semilunar lobule

Anterior lobe

Posterior lobe

FIGURE 9.11. Cerebellum (superior view). Isolated view of the cerebellum after it has been removed from the posterior cranial fossa and detached from the brainstem.

The superior surface of the cerebellum is generally rounded and broad, except for pronounced anterior and posterior cerebellar notches located between the expanded cerebellar hemispheres. The **anterior cerebellar notch** contains the inferior colliculi of the midbrain in situ, while the **posterior cerebellar notch** contains the falx cerebelli. The **primary fissure** of the cerebellum separates the anterior and posterior lobes. The largest and deepest fissure of the cerebellum, the **horizontal fissure**, extends posterolaterally along each hemisphere separating the superior and inferior semilunar lobules.

NEUROANATOMY

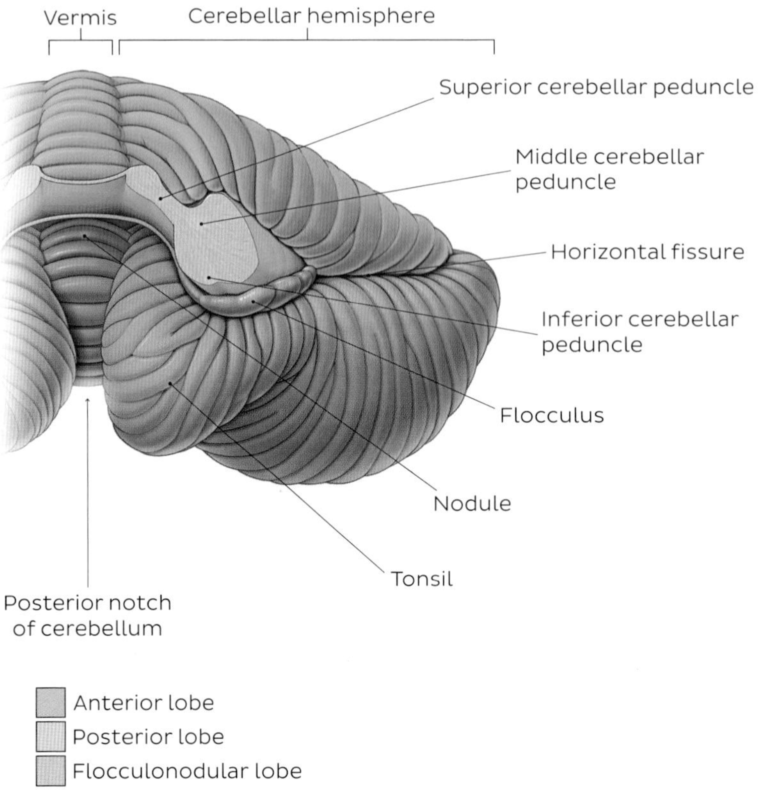

Vermis | Cerebellar hemisphere

Superior cerebellar peduncle

Middle cerebellar peduncle

Horizontal fissure

Inferior cerebellar peduncle

Flocculus

Nodule

Tonsil

Posterior notch of cerebellum

Anterior lobe
Posterior lobe
Flocculonodular lobe

FIGURE 9.12. **Cerebellum (anterior view, left side).** This view of the cerebellum is once again characterized by a central vermis which connects the cerebellar hemispheres. Also visible are three pairs of prominent fiber bundles, the **superior, middle, and inferior cerebellar peduncles** that connect the cerebellum to the midbrain, pons, and medulla oblongata, respectively. The superior and inferior medullary vela are thin sheets of white matter which form the roof of the fourth ventricle. This is the only perspective in which the three lobes of the cerebellum (anterior, posterior and flocculonodular) are collectively visible.

The anterior (petrosal) surface of the cerebellum bears the **tonsils** of the cerebellum which protrude inferomedially between the tuber and uvula of the vermis. The largest and deepest fissure of the cerebellum, the **horizontal fissure**. It extends posterolaterally along each hemisphere dividing the cerebellum into upper and lower parts.

Cerebellum gross anatomy

Afferent and efferent pathways of the cerebellum

NEUROANATOMY

CRANIAL MENINGES

Separating the brain and spinal cord from their surrounding bony enclosures are three membranes known as the meninges. The outermost layer is the dura mater (also known as pachymeninx) which consists of a double layer of thick, dense irregular connective tissue. The middle layer is the arachnoid mater, so-called for its spider web-like appearance, while the innermost layer is the thin and delicate pia mater. The arachnoid and pia mater can also be collectively referred to as the leptomeninges due to their common embryological and cellular structure.

These layers delimitate three clinically important spaces: The epidural (or extradural), subdural, and subarachnoid spaces. The epidural space is located between the bones of the cranium and outer (periosteal) layer of the dura mater, while the subdural space lies between the inner (meningeal) layer of the dura mater and arachnoid mater. Both of these are potential spaces, meaning that under normal circumstances they are closed. The subarachnoid space, located between the arachnoid and pia mater, is a fluid-filled space that contains CSF, as well as cerebral arteries and veins. Finally, separating the pia mater from the surface of the brain is a thin space known as the subpial space.

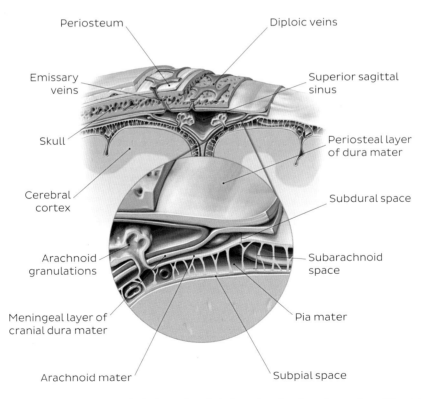

FIGURE 9.13. **Meninges of the brain (coronal section).** Coronal section through a portion of the skull, meninges and cerebral cortex. The cranial dura mater is composed of two layers: The outer periosteal layer

(which adheres tightly to the skull, also known as the endocranium) and inner meningeal layer. The two dural layers are usually directly apposed to one another, except in places where they separate to form the dural venous sinuses, which is represented in this image by the superior sagittal sinus. Deeper to the dura mater is the arachnoid mater with its small protrusions known as arachnoid granulations, that pierce the inner layer of the dura projecting into the lumen of the superior sagittal sinus. The pia mater is a thin membrane composed of a single cell layer which, unlike the dura and arachnoid mater, closely follows all contours (i.e., gyri and sulci) of the brain. Thin projections of connective tissue called arachnoid trabeculae extend from the inner surface of the arachnoid mater, traverse the subarachnoid space and attach to the outer surface of the pia mater.

Key points about the cranial meninges	
Definition	Three membranous layers that envelop the brain
Meninges	Dura mater
	Arachnoid mater
	Pia mater
Meningeal spaces	Epidural space
	Subdural space
	Subarachnoid space
	Subpial space
Function	Mechanical protection of brain
	Support of cerebral blood vessels
	Accommodation and circulation of CSF (subarachnoid space)
Related structures	Dural venous sinuses (venous drainage of the brain)
	Arachnoid granulations (return of CSF to venous circulation)

Meninges of the brain and spinal cord

Meninges ventricles and brain blood supply

VENTRICLES OF THE BRAIN

The ventricles of the brain are an interconnected network of cavities filled with cerebrospinal fluid (CSF) located within the brain parenchyma. The ventricular system consists of the two lateral ventricles, the third ventricle, and the fourth ventricle. The choroid plexuses, located within each ventricle, produce CSF which fills the ventricles and subarachnoid space. This fluid cushions the brain and spinal cord from injury and also serves as a nutrient delivery and waste removal system for the brain.

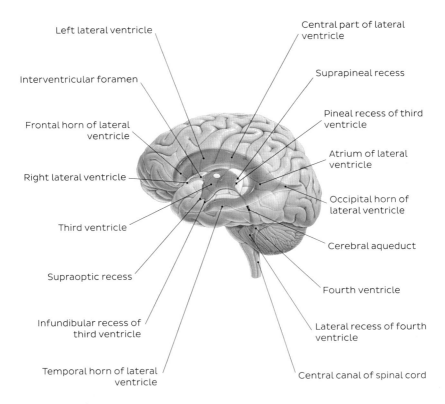

Left lateral ventricle

Central part of lateral ventricle

Interventricular foramen

Suprapineal recess

Frontal horn of lateral ventricle

Pineal recess of third ventricle

Right lateral ventricle

Atrium of lateral ventricle

Third ventricle

Occipital horn of lateral ventricle

Supraoptic recess

Cerebral aqueduct

Infundibular recess of third ventricle

Fourth ventricle

Temporal horn of lateral ventricle

Lateral recess of fourth ventricle

Central canal of spinal cord

FIGURE 9.14. **Ventricles of the brain.** The lateral ventricles are two C-shaped cavities, one in each cerebral hemisphere. Each lateral ventricle has a central part, or body (located in the region of the parietal lobe), an atrium and three horns projecting into the lobes for which they are named: The frontal (or anterior) horn, the occipital (or posterior) horn, and the temporal (or inferior) horn. The interventricular foramen (of Monro) is a Y-shaped channel that connects the paired lateral ventricles with the third ventricle. The third ventricle is a narrow vertical cavity within the diencephalon which bears several outpocketings: The supraoptic, infundibular, suprapineal, and pineal recesses. It is drained by the cerebral aqueduct (of Sylvius) that conveys CSF into the fourth ventricle. The fourth ventricle is a diamond-shaped cavity located in the brainstem. It has two lateral apertures (openings of the lateral recesses) and a single median aperture, both of which empty into the subarachnoid space surrounding the brainstem. This ventricle is the most inferior and is continuous with the central canal of the spinal cord.

Key points about the ventricles of the brain	
Definition	Interconnected cavities within the brain that produce and contain CSF
Function	Protect the brain from injury
	Nutrition of the brain and waste removal
Composition	Lateral ventricles (2)
	Third ventricle
	Fourth ventricle
Related structures	Interventricular foramen (of Monro): lateral ventricles → third ventricle
	Cerebral aqueduct (of Sylvius): third ventricle → fourth ventricle

NEUROANATOMY

Ventricular system of the brain

 Choroid plexus

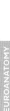

ARTERIES OF THE BRAIN

The arterial supply of the brain is derived from two primary sources: The internal carotid and vertebral arteries. The internal carotid arteries and their branches supply blood to the majority of the forebrain giving them the classification of the anterior cerebral circulation or the internal carotid system. The vertebral arteries and their major branches supply blood to the spinal cord, brainstem and cerebellum, and a significant part of the posterior cerebral hemispheres (usually the occipital and inferior temporal lobes). The vertebral arteries and their branches are commonly referred to as the vertebrobasilar system or the posterior cerebral circulation.

The cerebral arterial circle (of Willis) is an anatomical structure that provides an anastomotic connection between the anterior and posterior circulations, providing collateral flow to affected brain regions in the event of arterial incompetency.

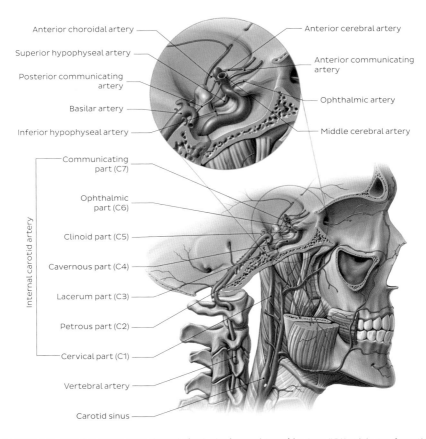

FIGURE 9.15. **Arteries of the head (lateral view).** The **internal carotid artery** (ICA) originates from the common carotid artery. It is usually divided into seven distinct parts based on its course and anatomical relations. Segments C6/C7 provide several branches which supply the anterior circulation of the brain, as well as the orbit: The ophthalmic artery, superior hypophyseal artery, posterior communicating artery, anterior choroidal artery, anterior cerebral artery and middle cerebral artery. The **vertebral artery** provides blood supply for brainstem, cerebellum, and posterior part of the brain.

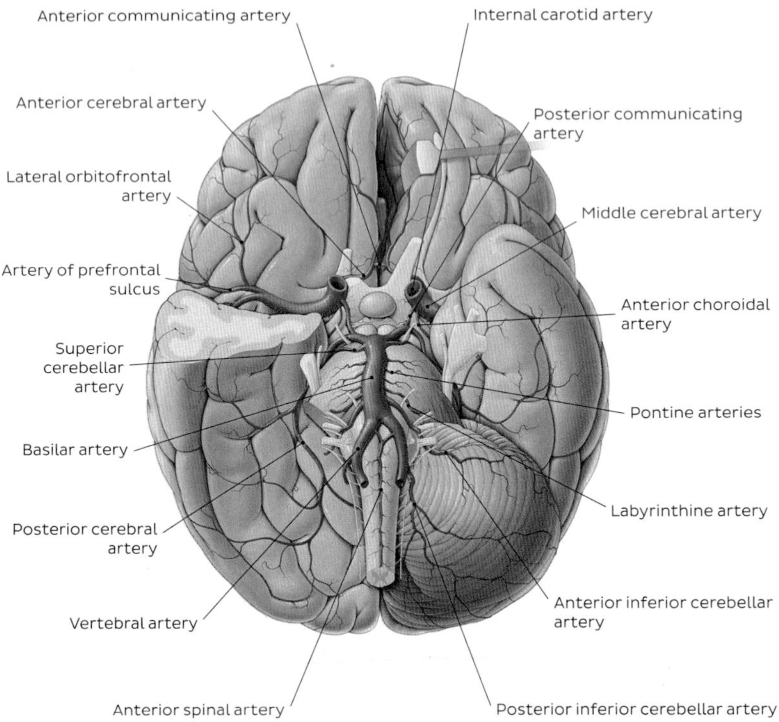

Anterior communicating artery

Internal carotid artery

Anterior cerebral artery

Posterior communicating artery

Lateral orbitofrontal artery

Middle cerebral artery

Artery of prefrontal sulcus

Anterior choroidal artery

Superior cerebellar artery

Pontine arteries

Basilar artery

Posterior cerebral artery

Labyrinthine artery

Vertebral artery

Anterior inferior cerebellar artery

Anterior spinal artery

Posterior inferior cerebellar artery

FIGURE 9.16. **Arteries of the head (inferior view).** The main artery of the anterior circulation of the brain is the **internal carotid artery** (ICA), which terminates as the anterior and middle cerebral arteries.

The main artery of the posterior circulation is the **vertebral artery**. It enters the cranial cavity via the foramen magnum and gives off several branches to the spinal cord, meninges and part of the cerebellum. The two vertebral arteries then converge to form the basilar artery which courses vertically across the pons and posterior cranial fossa where it gives off several branches to the rest of the cerebellum, pons, midbrain and internal ear. The basilar artery terminates as a bifurcation which gives off the paired **posterior cerebral arteries** that contribute to the cerebral arterial circle (of Willis).

The **cerebral arterial circle** (of Willis) is an anastomotic loop/ring formed between four paired arteries and one unpaired artery which facilitates collateral blood between the anterior and posterior cerebral circulations as well as the right and left blood supply. Several small perforating (central) arteries emerge from the cerebral arterial circle (of Willis), many of which pass into the brain directly and supply the cortex and subcortical structures.

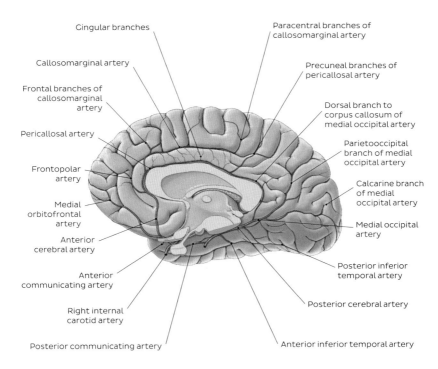

FIGURE 9.17. Arteries of the brain (medial view). Right cerebral hemisphere (without the brainstem and cerebellum) with arteries exposed. The **anterior cerebral artery** (ACA) gives off several branches including the anterior communicating artery and cortical branches to the frontal and medial surfaces of the cerebral cortex (frontal, parietal and limbic lobes) and part of the corpus callosum.

The **posterior cerebral artery** (PCA) gives off several branches to the occipital lobe, the inferolateral surface of the temporal lobe, midbrain, thalamus, choroid plexus (third and lateral ventricle) and cerebral peduncles.

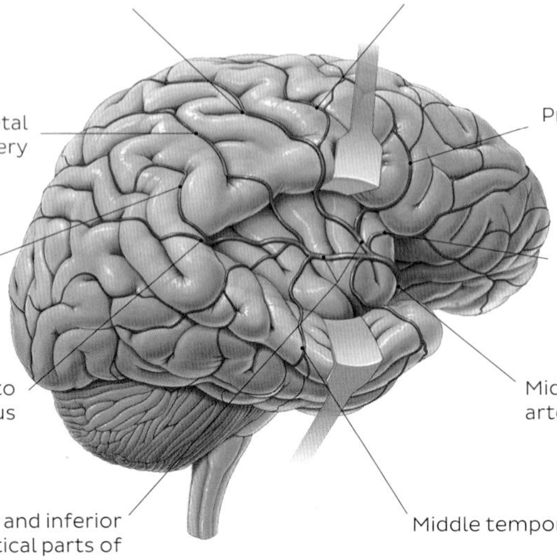

Artery of central sulcus

Artery of precentral sulcus

Anterior parietal artery

Prefrontal artery

Posterior parietal artery

Lateral orbitofrontal artery

Artery to angular gyrus

Middle cerebral artery

Superior and inferior cortical parts of middle cerebral artery

Middle temporal artery

FIGURE 9.18. **Arteries of the brain (lateral view).** Lateral view of the brain with its arterial vessels; the lateral sulcus has been opened to expose the arteries within.

The prominent vessel seen from this view is the **middle cerebral artery** (MCA), a terminal branch of the internal carotid artery. It provides a large number of small central branches (which supply the thalamus, basal nuclei and internal capsule) as well as several larger cortical branches to the frontal, parietal, insular and temporal lobes.

Key points about the arteries of the brain	
Anterior circulation	Main arteries: internal carotid artery, anterior cerebral artery, anterior communicating artery and middle cerebral artery
	Supply: forebrain
Posterior circulation	Main arteries: vertebral artery, basilar artery, posterior cerebral artery and posterior communicating artery
	Supply: posterior cerebral cortex (occipital lobe and partly temporal lobe), midbrain, brainstem
Cerebral arterial circle (of Willis)	**From anterior to posterior**
	Anterior communicating artery (from the anterior cerebral artery)
	Anterior cerebral arteries (from the internal carotid artery)
	Internal carotid arteries (from the common carotid artery)
	Posterior communicating arteries (from the posterior cerebral artery)
	Posterior cerebral arteries (branch of the basilar artery)
Supply	Anterior cerebral artery: frontal, parietal and cingulate cortex; corpus callosum, region of the brain primarily responsible for motor and sensory of the lower limbs
	Middle cerebral artery: most of the lateral surface of the frontal, parietal and temporal lobes (except for the superior border of the former two and inferior border of the latter), basal nuclei and internal capsule
	Posterior cerebral artery: occipital lobe, inferolateral surface of the temporal lobe, midbrain, thalamus, choroid plexus (third and lateral ventricle), cerebral peduncles

Arteries of the brain

 Cerebral arterial circle (of Willis)

 Vertebral artery

 Internal carotid artery

VEINS OF THE BRAIN

The brain is an especially well-vascularised organ, receiving approximately twenty percent of cardiac output. The veins of the brain drain the blood from the entire brain as well as the surrounding structures (meninges, eyeballs etc). The drained blood is then first returned to the dural venous sinuses and then the internal jugular vein. Structurally, the veins of the brain lack a muscular layer (tunica media), which allows them to expand and collapse substantially. There are two types of venous systems that drain the blood from the brain. These are the superficial (external) venous system and the deep (internal) venous system.

- The superficial cerebral veins are found in the subarachnoid space (i.e. between the arachnoid and pia mater) on the external surface of the cerebrum. They are divided into groups in relation to the part of the brain that they drain: The superior, middle and inferior cerebral veins.
- The deep venous system of the cerebrum is composed of a series of venous sinuses and deep cerebral veins. Numerous medullary veins extend throughout the white matter of the cerebrum, and drain into subependymal veins along the inner surface of the lateral ventricles leading to the formation of larger cerebral veins mainly internal cerebral veins, basal vein (of Rosenthal) and great cerebral vein (of Galen). The subependymal veins and subsequent deep medullary veins drain into the dural sinuses before emptying into the internal jugular vein.

Venous drainage of the cerebellum is achieved by the superior and inferior cerebellar veins which drain into the great cerebral vein (of Galen), the straight sinus, the superior petrosal sinus, or the sigmoid sinus.

Veins of the brainstem form an intricate plexus deep to the arteries of the brainstem and drain to the veins of the spinal cord, basal vein, great cerebral vein (of Galen), cerebellar veins and/or the dural venous sinuses.

NEUROANATOMY

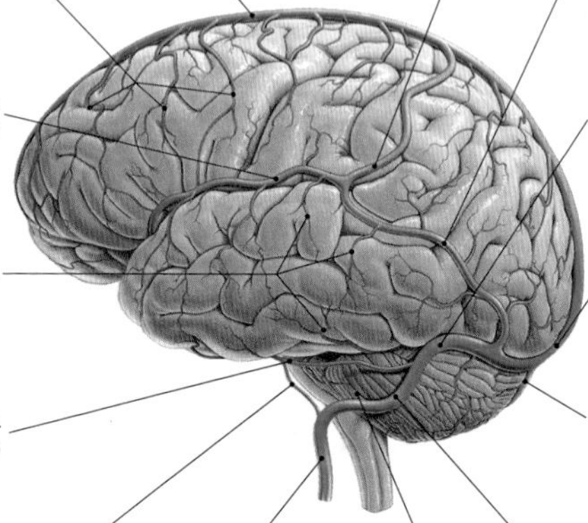

FIGURE 9.19. Superficial veins of the brain (lateral view). There are approximately eight to twelve **superior cerebral veins** that drain the superolateral and upper medial surfaces of each cerebral hemisphere. They are small in caliber, and they usually follow the cerebral sulci towards the superomedial margin of the cerebral hemisphere and drain into the superior sagittal sinus.

The **superficial middle cerebral vein** courses along the lateral cerebral fissure. It drains blood from most of the lateral surface of the cerebral hemisphere and conveys it to the cavernous sinus, following a course along the lateral sulcus.

The **inferior cerebral veins** are variable and numerous; they drain the inferior portion of the cerebral hemisphere.

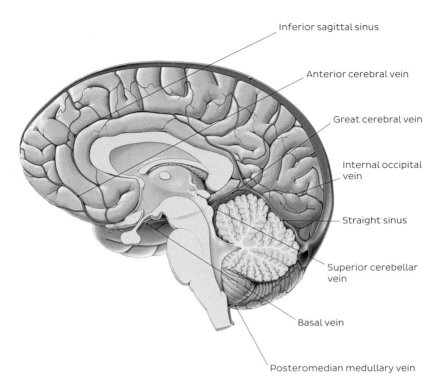

Inferior sagittal sinus

Anterior cerebral vein

Great cerebral vein

Internal occipital vein

Straight sinus

Superior cerebellar vein

Basal vein

Posteromedian medullary vein

FIGURE 9.20. **Deep cerebral veins (medial view).** Located between the periosteal and meningeal layers of dura mater are the dural venous sinuses. Generally venous blood from deeper structures of the cerebrum drain into deep cerebral veins (see previous image) which extend and empty into three dural venous sinuses: The transverse, straight and sigmoid sinuses.

The **straight sinus** receives the inferior sagittal sinus and the great cerebral vein (of Galen). It runs in a posteroinferior direction towards the internal occipital protuberance and contributes to the formation of the confluence of sinuses. Emerging from this confluence are the paired transverse sinuses which travel within the lateral border of the tentorium cerebelli. The **transverse sinuses** terminate as they extend to form the sigmoid sinuses at the point where the tentorium cerebelli ends. The **sigmoid sinuses** course along the floor of the posterior cranial fossa and empty into the internal jugular veins as they leave the cranium via the jugular foramina.

Key points about the veins of the brain	
Superficial cerebral veins	• Superior cerebral veins
	• Superficial middle cerebral vein (of Sylvius)
	• Inferior cerebral veins
Deep cerebral veins	• Great cerebral vein (of Galen):
	Main tributaries: internal cerebral vein, basal vein, inferior sagittal sinus
Veins of cerebellum	• Superior cerebellar veins
	• Inferior cerebellar veins
Veins of brainstem	• Midbrain: veins of midbrain → great cerebral vein (of Galen) or basal vein
	• Pons: pontine veins → basal vein, cerebellar veins, petrosal sinuses or transverse sinus
	• Medulla oblongata: medullary veins → inferior petrosal, occipital sinuses, internal jugular vein or radicular veins of spinal cord

NEUROANATOMY

Veins of the brain

DURAL VENOUS SINUSES

The dural venous sinuses are major vascular channels contained between the meningeal and periosteal layers of the dura mater. Most of the major dural venous sinuses are found adjacent to the falx cerebri and tentorium cerebelli. Major dural venous sinuses include the superior sagittal sinus, inferior sagittal sinus, straight sinus, transverse sinus, sigmoid sinus and superior petrosal sinus (see previous images).

The main function of the dural venous sinuses is to drain all venous blood within the cranial cavity with the ultimate point of drainage being the internal jugular vein. In addition, the dural sinuses also drain cerebrospinal fluid (CSF) via arachnoid granulations.

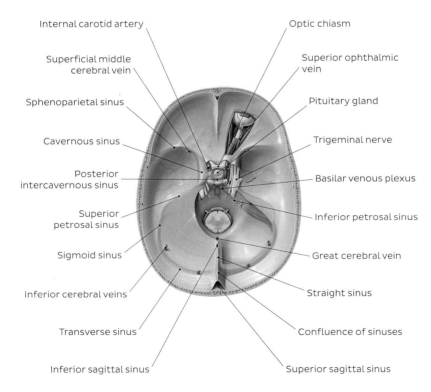

Internal carotid artery
Optic chiasm
Superficial middle cerebral vein
Superior ophthalmic vein
Sphenoparietal sinus
Pituitary gland
Cavernous sinus
Trigeminal nerve
Posterior intercavernous sinus
Basilar venous plexus
Superior petrosal sinus
Inferior petrosal sinus
Sigmoid sinus
Great cerebral vein
Inferior cerebral veins
Straight sinus
Transverse sinus
Confluence of sinuses
Inferior sagittal sinus
Superior sagittal sinus

FIGURE 9.21. **Dural venous sinuses (calvaria removed).** The **cavernous sinus** is a large venous plexus situated on either side of the sella turcica of the sphenoid bone. It drains blood from the superior and

NEUROANATOMY

inferior ophthalmic veins, superficial middle cerebral veins and sphenoparietal sinus. It is then drained by the superior and inferior petrosal sinuses that convey blood to the transverse sinuses and subsequent internal jugular vein.

Key points about the dural venous sinuses	
Definition	A collection of sinuses or blood channels that drains all venous blood from the cranial cavity and returns it towards the heart
Location	Situated between periosteal and meningeal layers of dura mater
Paired venous sinuses	Transverse sinus, cavernous sinus, superior petrosal sinus, inferior petrosal sinus, sphenoparietal sinus, sigmoid sinus, basilar sinus
Unpaired venous sinuses	Superior sagittal sinus, inferior sagittal sinus, straight sinus, occipital sinus, intercavernous sinus

Dural sinuses

TOPOGRAPHY AND MORPHOLOGY
OF THE SPINAL CORD

The spinal cord is a component of the central nervous system (CNS) that arises as a continuation of the medulla oblongata of the brainstem. It is a cylindrical structure enclosed within, and occupying, two-thirds of the length of the vertebral canal.

It extends from the foramen magnum of the skull to vertebra L1/L2, where it terminates as the medullary cone. The spinal cord functions as a conduit for information between the brain and the periphery. It also serves to generate reflexes which ensure the smooth running of daily activities.

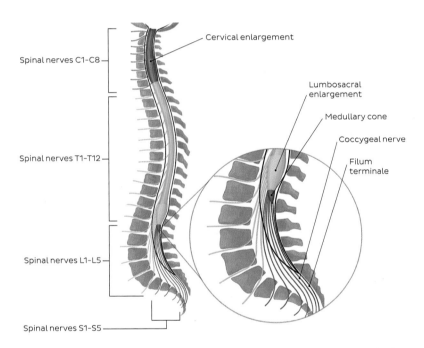

FIGURE 9.22. **Spinal cord (sagittal view).** The spinal cord extends from the brainstem at the foramen magnum and terminates at the level of vertebrae L1/L2. Similar to the vertebral column, the spinal cord is divided into five regions, each providing their sets of spinal nerves: **Cervical** (C1–C8, red), **thoracic** (T1–T12, orange), **lumbar** (L1–L5, green), **sacral** (S1–S5, blue), and **coccygeal** (Co1, purple). The coccygeal nerve originates from the terminal portion of the spinal cord, the medullary cone, and is the last and smallest spinal nerve. Extending from the apex of the medullary cone is the filum terminale, a thin connective tissue structure formed as an extension of pia mater. The filum terminale attaches on the sacrum and functions to anchor and stabilize the distal portion of the spinal cord.

Throughout its length, the spinal cord presents two well defined **enlargements** to accommodate for innervation of the upper and lower limbs: The cervical (C3–T2) and lumbosacral enlargement (L1–S3). As the spinal cord is shorter than the vertebral column, the roots of spinal nerves L2 and onwards descend for varying distances around and beyond the cord resulting in the formation of a nerve root bundle known as the **cauda equina**.

Posterior median sulcus

Posterior intermediate sulcus

Posterolateral sulcus

White matter

Posterior root of spinal nerve

Anterolateral sulcus

Anterior root of spinal nerve

Rootlets of spinal nerve

Anterior median fissure

Gray matter

FIGURE 9.23. **Spinal cord (cross section).** Internally, the spinal cord is made of gray and white matter just like other parts of the central nervous system. Externally, it contains left and right anterolateral and posterolateral surfaces, which feature a number of grooves known as fissures and sulci.

The **anterior median fissure** is a deep groove along the anterior length of the spinal cord that incompletely divides it into symmetrical halves. Lateral to the anterior median fissure is a bilateral shallow groove known as the **anterolateral sulcus** where the anterior rootlets of the spinal nerves emerge.

The **posterior median sulcus** extends along the posterior midline of the spinal cord. On either side of the posterior median sulcus are the **posterolateral sulci**, from which the posterior rootlets of the spinal nerves emerge on either side.

Key points about the topography and morphology of the spinal cord	
Location	Within the vertebral canal of the vertebral column
	Beginning: medulla oblongata of brainstem at foramen magnum
	Termination: medullary cone at vertebral level L1/L2
Parts	Cervical, thoracic, lumbar, sacral, coccygeal
	Cervical enlargement → supplies upper limbs
	Lumbosacral enlargement → supplies lower limbs
Surfaces	Anterolateral → Anterior median fissure, anterolateral sulcus
	Posterolateral → Posterior median sulcus, posterior intermediate sulcus (cervical and upper thoracic levels), posterolateral sulcus
Function	Conducts impulses from the brain to the body and generates reflexes

Ascending tracts of the spinal cord

Descending tracts of the spinal cord

SPINAL MENINGES AND NERVE ROOTS

The spinal cord is enveloped by the three meningeal coverings which, from superficial to deep, are known as the dura mater, arachnoid mater and pia mater. They are continuous with their counterparts surrounding the brain at the foramen magnum and function to suspend and protect the spinal cord within the vertebral canal. They also house blood vessels that supply the spinal cord and form a continuous cerebrospinal fluid (CSF) filled cavity which surrounds the spinal cord.

Also enveloped (partially or fully) by the outer two meningeal layers are the anterior/posterior rootlets of each spinal nerve.

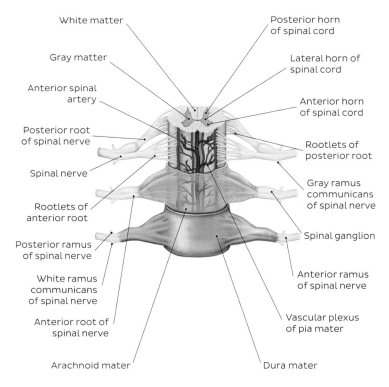

White matter

Gray matter

Anterior spinal artery

Posterior root of spinal nerve

Spinal nerve

Rootlets of anterior root

Posterior ramus of spinal nerve

White ramus communicans of spinal nerve

Anterior root of spinal nerve

Arachnoid mater

Posterior horn of spinal cord

Lateral horn of spinal cord

Anterior horn of spinal cord

Rootlets of posterior root

Gray ramus communicans of spinal nerve

Spinal ganglion

Anterior ramus of spinal nerve

Vascular plexus of pia mater

Dura mater

FIGURE 9.24. **Spinal meninges and nerve roots.** The **pia mater** is the innermost layer of the three meningeal layers which surround the spinal cord. It is highly vascular and closely follows the contours of the spinal cord. The second meninx is the **arachnoid mater**, which is separated from the pia mater by a cerebrospinal fluid filled space known as the subarachnoid space. The thickest and most superficial meninx is the **dura mater**, which lies in close proximity to the arachnoid mater (but is separated from by a potential space known as the subdural space). The space between the vertebral canal and dura mater is known as the epidural space which contains adipose tissue that helps to absorb shock and protect the spinal cord.

The arachnoid and dura mater form a 'sleeve' over the spinal nerve rootlets and roots, whereas the pia mater reflects onto the root complex and blends with their epineurium. The dura, arachnoid and pia mater extend along the spinal cord, beyond the conus medullaris to terminate at the lower border of the second sacral vertebra.

The **anterior rootlets/root of spinal nerve** contain motor/autonomic nerve fibers which carry impulses away from the central nervous system (CNS) towards the periphery. The cell bodies of the anterior root neurons are located in the anterior and lateral horns of the spinal cord.

The **posterior rootlets/root of spinal nerve** contain the central processes of sensory neurons, whose cell bodies are located in the spinal ganglion of the posterior root of each spinal nerve. They carry signals from the periphery to the CNS. Typically, the anterior and posterior roots unite to form a single spinal nerve carrying mixed motor and sensory fibers and exit the vertebral column through the intervertebral foramina.

Key points about the spinal meninges and nerve roots	
Spinal meninges	Dura mater: surrounds filum terminale and terminates at S2 vertebral level
	Arachnoid mater: fuses with dura mater and terminates at S2 vertebral level
	Pia mater: extends as a coating of the filum terminale which reaches S2 vertebra
Spaces	Epidural space, subdural space, subarachnoid space
Nerve rootlets/ roots	Posterior rootlets/roots
	Origin: posterolateral sulcus of spinal cord
	Posterior rootlets → posterior roots (spinal ganglion): sensory fibers
	Anterior rootlets/roots
	Origin: anterolateral sulcus of spinal cord
	Anterior rootlets → anterior roots: motor/autonomic fibers
	Anterior roots + posterior roots → mixed spinal nerve

Meninges of the brain and spinal cord

Spinal nerves

SPINAL NERVES

The spinal nerves are a collection of thirty-one pairs of mixed nerves which arise from the spinal cord. They form the largest component of the peripheral nervous system (PNS), transmitting afferent (sensory) and efferent (motor/autonomic) information between much of the periphery and central nervous system. Neurons within each spinal nerve can be functionally categorized as somatic (related pertaining to skin, skeletal muscle, tendons and joints), or visceral (pertaining to internal organs/smooth muscle, cardiac muscle and glands). Thus, neurons within a typical spinal nerve can be classed as belonging to one of four functional modalities:

- Somatic afferent/efferent, or
- Visceral afferent/efferent

The spinal nerves can be subdivided as follows: Eight pairs of cervical nerves, twelve thoracic, five lumbar, five sacral and one coccygeal.

The spinal nerves exit the vertebral canal through the intervertebral foramen, or via the sacral foramina in the sacral region, and give off two primary branches: A

NEUROANATOMY

small posterior ramus and a larger anterior ramus. These branches supply cutaneous, motor and autonomic innervation to muscles and skin of the neck, trunk and limbs.

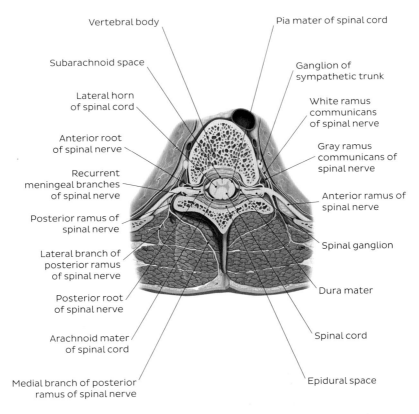

Vertebral body

Pia mater of spinal cord

Subarachnoid space

Ganglion of sympathetic trunk

Lateral horn of spinal cord

White ramus communicans of spinal nerve

Anterior root of spinal nerve

Gray ramus communicans of spinal nerve

Recurrent meningeal branches of spinal nerve

Anterior ramus of spinal nerve

Posterior ramus of spinal nerve

Lateral branch of posterior ramus of spinal nerve

Spinal ganglion

Posterior root of spinal nerve

Dura mater

Arachnoid mater of spinal cord

Spinal cord

Medial branch of posterior ramus of spinal nerve

Epidural space

FIGURE 9.25. **Spinal cord and spinal nerves (superior view).** On exiting the intervertebral foramen, each spinal nerve divides into anterior and posterior rami. The posterior ramus extends in a posterior direction and further divides into medial and lateral branches, which provide innervation to the deep back muscles (epaxial muscles) as well as an associated narrow strip of overlying skin. The anterior ramus provides motor innervation (somatic or visceral) to the rest of the body related to that segmental level, often intermingling with other spinal nerves leading to the formation of the major somatic plexuses (cervical, brachial, lumbar and sacral). Just before the bifurcation into anterior and posterior rami, the spinal nerve also gives rise to one or more recurrent /meningeal branches which re-enter the intervertebral foramen to supply the meninges and other structures of the vertebral canal.

Communicating with the anterior ramus of the spinal nerves are the white and gray rami communicantes which convey sympathetic nerve fibers. The anterior rami of spinal nerves T1-L2 give off the white rami communicantes which carries preganglionic sympathetic fibers from the lateral horn of the spinal cord to an adjacent sympathetic ganglion. Here they can either synapse with a postganglionic sympathetic neuron at the same or a superior/inferior level via the sympathetic trunk, or pass through the sympathetic ganglion (without synapsing) continuing as a preganglionic nerve fiber; in all cases nerve fibers of the sympathetic trunk reenter the spinal nerves via a gray ramus communicans.

Key points about the spinal nerves	
Formation	Anterior root (efferent) + posterior root (afferent) → Spinal nerve (mixed)
Branches	Posterior ramus: lateral and medial branches
	Anterior ramus: recurrent meningeal branch, white ramus communicans (T1–L2 spinal nerves)
	Receives: gray ramus communicans (sympathetic input)
Supply area	Posterior ramus: efferent innervation to the deep back muscles and overlying skin
	Anterior ramus: afferent and autonomic innervation to the rest of the skeletal muscles of the body, including those of the limbs and trunk, and most remaining areas of the skin, except for certain regions of the head

 Spinal nerves

 Spinal cord

BLOOD VESSELS OF THE SPINAL CORD

The spinal cord receives its main arterial supply from the vertebral arteries. The vertebral artery arises from the subclavian artery and gives off three branches for the spinal cord: A single anterior spinal and two posterior spinal arteries. These branches pass longitudinally along the anterior and posterior aspect of the spinal cord, respectively, and are thus deemed as longitudinal vessels.

The spinal cord receives additional arterial supply from segmental spinal arteries that arise in a craniocaudal sequence from the spinal branches of vertebral, deep cervical, posterior intercostal and lumbar arteries. These branches pass through the intervertebral foramina and split into anterior and posterior radicular branches that pass along the anterior and posterior roots, respectively. At some levels of the spinal cord, some radicular arteries give rise to segmental medullary arteries that anastomose with the longitudinal vessels.

Venous blood from the spinal cord is largely drained via a single anterior spinal vein and a single posterior spinal vein, which, in turn, drain into the internal vertebral plexus found in the epidural space. The blood from the internal vertebral plexus continues to drain into the external vertebral plexus, and finally empties into systemic veins of the caval and azygos systems, depending on the location.

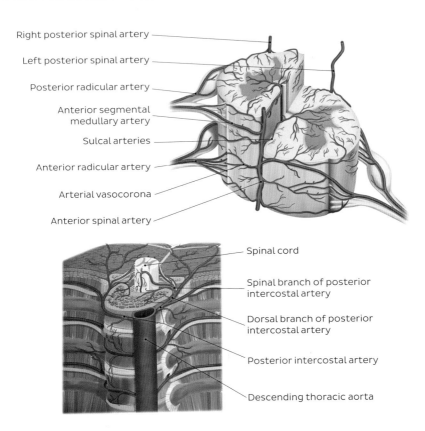

Right posterior spinal artery

Left posterior spinal artery

Posterior radicular artery

Anterior segmental medullary artery

Sulcal arteries

Anterior radicular artery

Arterial vasocorona

Anterior spinal artery

Spinal cord

Spinal branch of posterior intercostal artery

Dorsal branch of posterior intercostal artery

Posterior intercostal artery

Descending thoracic aorta

FIGURE 9.26. **Arteries of the spinal cord.** Top image: The anterior and posterior spinal arteries form pial anastomoses called the 'arterial vasocorona', which encircles the spinal cord and supplies its lateral surface and the spinal meninges.

Lower image: Each segment of the spinal cord receives additional supply from spinal branches of various arteries depending on the region, in this case the posterior intercostal arteries. A spinal branch of the dorsal branch of each posterior intercostal artery passes through the intervertebral foramina into the vertebral canal, where they split into the anterior and posterior radicular branches and pass along the anterior and posterior roots. Most of the radicular branches are small and terminate along the spinal nerve roots. However, some larger radicular branches continue as **segmental medullary arteries** that anastomose the anterior and posterior spinal arteries and provide additional arterial supply to the spinal cord.

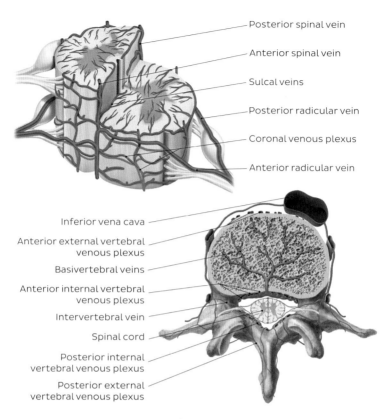

Posterior spinal vein

Anterior spinal vein

Sulcal veins

Posterior radicular vein

Coronal venous plexus

Anterior radicular vein

Inferior vena cava

Anterior external vertebral venous plexus

Basivertebral veins

Anterior internal vertebral venous plexus

Intervertebral vein

Spinal cord

Posterior internal vertebral venous plexus

Posterior external vertebral venous plexus

FIGURE 9.27. **Veins of the spinal cord.** Venous blood from the spinal cord is largely drained via a single anterior spinal vein and a single posterior spinal vein, which, in turn, drain into the internal vertebral plexus found in the epidural space. The blood from the internal vertebral plexus continues to drain into the external vertebral plexus, and finally empties into systemic veins of the caval and azygos systems, depending on the location.

Main blood vessels of the spinal cord	
Arteries	**Longitudinal arteries** (arise from vertebral artery):
	Anterior spinal artery
	Posterior spinal artery (2x)
	Segmental arteries (arise from vertebral, deep cervical, posterior intercostal and lumbar arteries):
	Spinal branches → Anterior and posterior radicular arteries → Segmental medullary arteries
	Arterial vasocorona:
	Anastomosis between the anterior posterior spinal arteries
Veins	Intramedullary venous plexus → coronal plexus (longitudinal veins) anterior and posterior radicular veins (segmental veins) → anterior and posterior internal vertebral plexus → intervertebral veins → anterior and posterior external vertebral plexus → systemic veins

Blood supply of the spinal cord

Veins of the vertebral column

CRANIAL NERVE OVERVIEW

The cranial nerves are a group of 12 nerves that originate directly from the brain and reach the periphery via openings of the skull (i.e. cranium). Each cranial nerve can be denoted by a name (e.g. olfactory nerve) or a number (i.e. Roman numerals: I–XII). The number of each nerve is based on its origin, when the brain and brainstem are observed from rostral to caudal. All 12 nerves are bilateral and collectively function to relay information to/from various parts of the body and brain.

According to the type of nuclei and subsequently the type of nervous fibers that constitute the nerve, we can classify them into seven modalities.

Key points about cranial nerve modalities	
Nerve fiber terminology	**Efferent (motor)**
	Carries information from the brain to the periphery
	Afferent (sensory)
	Carries information from the periphery to the brain
	Mixed
	Carries information both ways
	Special
	Carries information from/to the special senses (vision, smell, taste, hearing and balance)
	General
	Carries information from/to any other part of the body, except the special senses
	Somatic
	Carries information to/from the skin or skeletal muscles
	Visceral
	Carries information to/from internal organs
Nerve fiber types/ modalities	**General somatic afferent (GSA)**
	Conveys general sensation from skin
	(a.k.a. [general] somatic sensory)
	General visceral afferent (GVA)
	Conveys general sensation from viscera
	(a.k.a. [general] visceral sensory)
	Special somatic afferent (SSA)
	Conveys senses derived from ectoderm (e.g. sight, sound, balance)
	(a.k.a. special somatic sensory)
	Special visceral sensory (SVA)
	Conveys senses derived from endoderm (e.g. taste, smell)
	(a.k.a. special visceral sensory)
	General somatic efferent (GSE)
	Conveys motor innervation for skeletal muscles
	(a.k.a. [general] somatic motor)
	General visceral efferent (GVE)
	Conveys motor innervation for smooth muscle, cardiac muscle and glands
	(a.k.a. [general] visceral motor)
	Special visceral efferent (SVE)
	Conveys motor innervation for muscles derived from pharyngeal arches
	(a.k.a. special visceral motor, branchial motor)

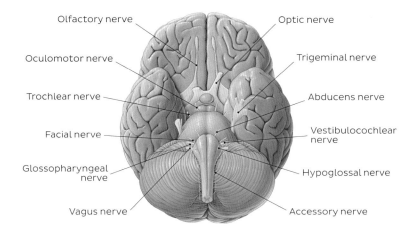

Olfactory nerve

Optic nerve

Oculomotor nerve

Trigeminal nerve

Trochlear nerve

Abducens nerve

Facial nerve

Vestibulocochlear nerve

Glossopharyngeal nerve

Hypoglossal nerve

Vagus nerve

Accessory nerve

FIGURE 9.28. **12 cranial nerves: Anatomy.** Inferior view of the brain and brainstem, summarizing the anatomy of each cranial nerve. The first two cranial nerves, the **olfactory nerve** (CN I) and **optic nerve** (CN II) are the only two cranial nerves that originate from the cerebrum. More specifically, the olfactory nerve (CN I) can be generally used as an umbrella term to describe components extending from the olfactory part of the nasal mucosa to the olfactory cortex (via the cribriform plate of ethmoid bone). The optic nerve (CN II) extends from the retina of the eye to the primary visual cortex (striate area) via the optic canal.

All other cranial nerves originate from the brainstem. The **oculomotor** (CN III) and **trochlear** (CN IV) nerves originate from the midbrain. The **abducens nerve** (CN VI) originates from the pontomedullary region. Since these three nerves act on eye muscles, they extend from the brainstem and exit via the superior orbital fissure. The **trigeminal nerve** (CN V) originates from the pons and gives rise to three nerve divisions: Ophthalmic (V_1), maxillary (V_2), and mandibular (V_3) which exit the cranium via the superior orbital fissure, foramen rotundum and foramen ovale, respectively. The **facial nerve** (CN VII) originates from the pontomedullary junction by two roots: Motor and sensory. The vestibulocochlear nerve (CN VIII) also originates from the pontomedullary junction and consists of the vestibular and cochlear components. Both CN VII and VIII exit via the internal acoustic meatus. The **glossopharyngeal nerve** (CN IX) originates from the superior/rostral portion of the medulla oblongata while the vagus nerve (CN X) also originates from the medulla oblongata, just caudal to CN IX. The **accessory nerve** (CN XI) has traditionally been described as having both spinal and cranial roots. As seen in the illustration, its cranial root emerges from the medulla oblongata, while the spinal root arises from the upper five or six cervical segments of the spinal cord. CN IX-XI all exit the skull via the jugular foramen. Finally, the **hypoglossal nerve** (CN XII) also originates from the medulla oblongata. Its dozen roots pass laterally across the posterior cranial fossa before merging into a single trunk which exits via the hypoglossal canal.

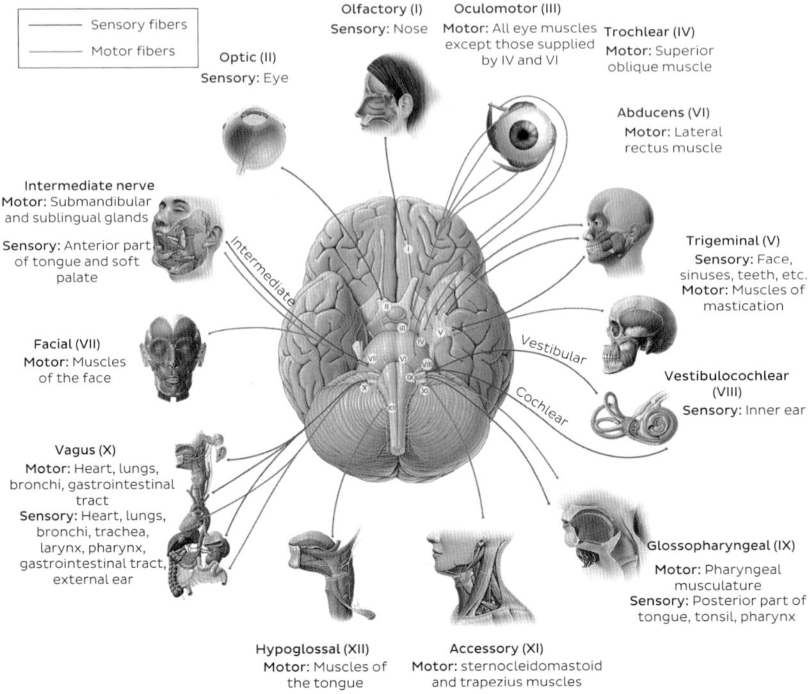

FIGURE 9.29. **12 cranial nerves: Overview of functions.** The olfactory nerve (CN I) is solely sensory and conveys impulses that provide the sense of smell (olfaction). The optic nerve (CN II) is also a sensory nerve, responsible for vision. The oculomotor (CN III), trochlear (CN IV) and abducens (CN VI) nerves can be observed as a group due to their similar functions: All are motor nerves that innervate the eye muscles and thus play a key role in eye movement/accommodation. The trigeminal nerve (CN V) is the first mixed nerve (i.e. has both sensory and motor fibers). This nerve provides the sensation for the face and controls the muscles of mastication. The facial nerve (CN VII) is also a mixed nerve. The function of the sensory portion of this nerve is to provide a taste for the anterior portion of the tongue, while its motor component plays part in the modulation of facial expressions, salivation, and lacrimation. The vestibulocochlear nerve (CN VIII) is a sensory nerve in charge of maintaining balance and hearing. The glossopharyngeal nerve (CN IX) is a mixed nerve that provides sensation to the tongue and pharynx, as well as the control of muscles that facilitate the act of swallowing. The vagus nerve (CN X) is the longest mixed cranial nerve. Its sensory role is to convey sensory information from the external ear, pharynx, larynx, thorax, and abdomen. In contrast, its motor component plays part in acts of swallowing, speech, coughing, and various parasympathetic functions. The accessory nerve (XI) is solely a motor nerve. It controls two muscles involved in head and shoulder movements (sternocleidomastoid and trapezius muscles). The hypoglossal nerve (CN XII) is also a motor nerve that controls muscles that facilitate the movements of the tongue.

Key points about the cranial nerves	
Definition	A set of 12 peripheral nerves emerging from the brain that innervate the structures of the head, neck, thorax and abdomen
12 cranial nerves	Olfactory nerve (CN I): afferent/sensory (SVA)
	Optic nerve (CN II): afferent/sensory (SSA)
	Oculomotor nerve (CN III): efferent/motor (GSE & GVE)
	Trochlear nerve (CN IV): efferent/motor (GSE)
	Trigeminal nerve (CN V): mixed
	Ophthalmic nerve (V_1): afferent/sensory (GSA)
	Maxillary nerve (V_2): afferent/sensory (GSA)
	Mandibular nerve (V_3): afferent/sensory (GSA & SVE)
	Abducens nerve (CN VI): efferent/motor (GSE)
	Facial nerve (CN VII): mixed (GSA, SVA, SVE, GVE)
	Vestibulocochlear nerve (CN VIII): afferent/sensory (SSA)
	Glossopharyngeal nerve (CN IX): mixed (GSA, GVA, SVA, SVE, GVE)
	Vagus nerve (CN X): mixed (GSA, GVA, SVA, SVE, GVE)
	Accessory nerve (CN XI): efferent/Motor (GSE & SVE)
	Hypoglossal nerve (CN XII): efferent/Motor (GSE)

12 cranial nerves

Cranial nerve nuclei

NEUROANATOMY

OLFACTORY NERVE (CN I)

The olfactory nerve (CN I) is a special sensory (special visceral afferent [SVA]) nerve that carries the sensation of smell (olfaction) via a series of nervous structures which make up the olfactory pathway to the brain. This allows us to detect various odors. Each olfactory nerve *proper* is actually one of 15–20 olfactory fiber bundles, which consist of bipolar olfactory sensory neurons located in the olfactory mucosa of the roof of the nasal cavity. These fiber bundles course through small tiny foramina in the cribriform plate of the ethmoid bone to enter the cranial cavity, where they join the olfactory bulb.

In the olfactory bulb, the olfactory nerve fibers synapse with primary dendrites of projection neurons (known as mitral and tufted cells) to form an olfactory glomerulus. Axons from these neurons project posteriorly as the olfactory tract. As it courses posteriorly, each olfactory tract bifurcates at the olfactory trigone into the medial and lateral olfactory striae. The olfactory striae project into areas of the olfactory cortex, allowing perception of smell. The olfactory bulb also receives efferent fibers which synapse on granular cells and subsequently interact with mitral and tufted cells to modulate the sensation of smell.

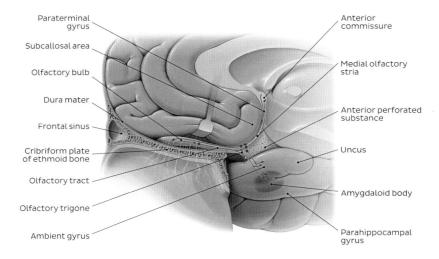

Paraterminal gyrus
Subcallosal area
Olfactory bulb
Dura mater
Frontal sinus
Cribriform plate of ethmoid bone
Olfactory tract
Olfactory trigone
Ambient gyrus

Anterior commissure
Medial olfactory stria
Anterior perforated substance
Uncus
Amygdaloid body
Parahippocampal gyrus

FIGURE 9.30. **Olfactory pathway.** Midsagittal section of the cerebrum and roof of the nasal cavity showing the olfactory structures. The olfactory nerve (CN I) arises from multiple olfactory sensory neurons in the olfactory mucosa whose central processes (axons) combine to form olfactory fiber bundles. These fiber bundles pass through foramina in the cribriform plate (of ethmoid bone), terminating in the olfactory bulb. The olfactory bulb extends caudally/posteriorly as the olfactory tract. This divides at the olfactory trigone into the medial/lateral olfactory striae which form the borders of the anterior perforated substance, and carry sensory information to regions of the olfactory cortex.

NEUROANATOMY

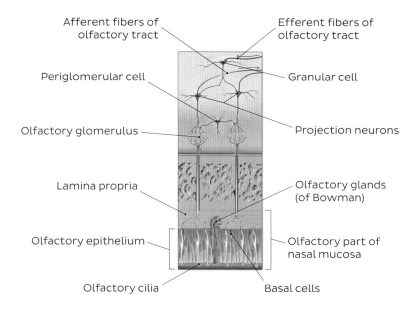

Afferent fibers of olfactory tract

Efferent fibers of olfactory tract

Periglomerular cell

Granular cell

Olfactory glomerulus

Projection neurons

Lamina propria

Olfactory glands (of Bowman)

Olfactory epithelium

Olfactory part of nasal mucosa

Olfactory cilia

Basal cells

FIGURE 9.31. **Olfactory organ and bulb.** Section of nasal mucosa and cribriform plate, with a microscopic view of the olfactory organ (olfactory part of nasal mucosa) and neural pathways of the olfactory bulb. The olfactory epithelium contains olfactory sensory neurons (olfactory receptor cells) that are wedged between supporting and basal epithelial cells. The peripheral processes (dendrites) of each neuron bears dendritic bulbs (sometimes known as olfactory vesicles), with cilia protruding above the epithelial surface which react to odiferous stimuli dissolved with the nasal mucus. The central processes(axons) of each olfactory neuron collect into olfactory fiber bundles (a.k.a. olfactory nerves *proper*) that pass through the cribriform plate and project into the olfactory bulb. Underlying the olfactory epithelium is the lamina propria which contains olfactory glands (of Bowman) that span the olfactory epithelium and secrete mucus. The olfactory bulb contains about 2000 olfactory glomeruli formed by synapses between terminal ends of the olfactory fiber bundles and the primary dendrites of projection neurons (mitral and tufted cells) as well as periglomerular cells, which are involved in odor discrimination. The projection neurons in turn project their axons (afferent fibers) posteriorly/caudally to form the olfactory tract. Additionally, the olfactory bulb contains [amacrine] granular cells which receive efferent fibers from central brain areas (as well as other mitral/tufted cells) and modulates the afferent signals from mitral/tufted cells.

Key points about the olfactory nerve and pathway	
Olfactory organ	(Olfactory part of nasal mucosa)
	Epithelium: olfactory sensory/receptor neurons (contain olfactory cilia), supporting cells, and basal (stem) cells
	Lamina propria: olfactory glands (Bowman's glands)
Olfactory nerve	Cranial nerve I (CN I): collective term for 15–20 olfactory fiber bundles which cross the cribriform plate on each side
Olfactory bulb	Contains olfactory glomeruli, cell bodies of projection neurons (mitral and tufted cells), granule cells, periglomerular cells; serves as a relay station of the olfactory pathway
Olfactory tract	Axons of projection neurons (afferent fibers of olfactory bulb)
	Anterior olfactory nucleus
	Efferent (centrifugal) fibers of olfactory bulb
Olfactory striae	Medial and lateral divisions of olfactory tract
Olfactory cortex	Medial olfactory stria: subcollosal area, paraterminal gyrus, anterior commissure
	Lateral olfactory stria: olfactory tubercle, piriform cortex, anterior cortical amygdaloid nucleus, periamygdaloid cortex, and lateral entorhinal cortex
Function/type of fibers	Smell/olfaction
	Special sensory/special visceral afferent

NEUROANATOMY

The olfactory
pathway

The 12 cranial nerves

OPTIC NERVE (CN II)

The optic nerve (CN II) is a special somatic afferent (SSA) nerve which carries the sensation of sight (vision) from the retina of the eye to the brain. The optic nerve is a part of the visual pathway, which is a route by which light that falls on the retina is transmitted to the occipital lobe of the brain, where it is interpreted as visual information. More specifically, the visual pathway refers to a series of synapses that start in the retina, where light stimuli are converted into action potentials, and transmitted across several nervous structures to reach the primary visual cortex.

The structures of the visual pathway include the retinal neurons (photoreceptors, bipolar cells, ganglion cells) which pass visual stimuli through the optic nerve, optic chiasm, and optic tract to the lateral geniculate nucleus. Axons from the lateral geniculate nucleus then project via the optic radiation to the primary visual cortex of the occipital lobe.

The optic nerve is formed when the axons of retinal ganglion cells pierce the scleral layer of the eyeball. The nerve runs posteromedially within the orbit and through the optic canal to enter the cranial cavity, where together with its contralateral counterpart, forms the optic chiasm.

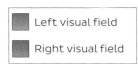

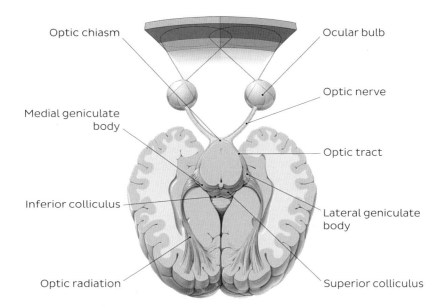

Left visual field

Right visual field

Optic chiasm

Ocular bulb

Optic nerve

Medial geniculate body

Optic tract

Inferior colliculus

Lateral geniculate body

Optic radiation

Superior colliculus

FIGURE 9.32. **The components of the visual pathway.** The visual pathway begins with light entering the ocular bulb from the visual fields and being processed by the retina. Visual information is then passed on from the retina by the optic nerve (CN II) through the optic canal (not shown) to the optic chiasm in the middle cranial fossa. From the optic chiasm, the axons of the optic nerve continue posteriorly as the optic tract, which then synapse at the lateral geniculate nucleus of the thalamus. Axons from the lateral geniculate nucleus travel via the optic radiation to finally reach the primary visual cortex. It is important to note that about 90% of the retinal axons synapse directly at the lateral geniculate nucleus. The remaining 10% project to other subcortical nuclei, mainly the superior colliculus. The superior colliculus is involved in visual reflexes, such as saccadic eye movements or tracking of objects in the visual field. The superior colliculus projects onto the pulvinar of thalamus, which in turn projects onto the secondary visual cortex.

Key points about the visual pathway	
Components	Retina → optic nerve (CN II) → optic chiasm → optic tract → lateral geniculate nucleus (90%) → optic radiation → primary visual cortex
	Retina → optic nerve (CN II) → optic chiasm → optic tract → superior colliculus (10%) → pulvinar of thalamus → secondary visual cortex
Retina	Sensory neural layer of the eyeball
	Neurons: photoreceptors (rod cells and cone cells), bipolar cells, ganglion cells, horizontal cells, and amacrine cells
Optic nerve (CN II)	Formed by axons of ganglion cells coming together at the optic disc
Optic chiasm	Point of decussation of the optic nerves: nasal fibers of retina cross over to the contralateral optic tract, while temporal fibers stay on the same side (ipsilateral)
Optic tracts	Left: carries left temporal and right nasal fibers of retina
	Right: carries right temporal and left nasal fibers of retina

Key points about the visual pathway	
Lateral geniculate nucleus	Receives 90% of the retinal fibers
	Represents a relay center of the thalamus that projects to the primary visual cortex via the optic radiation
Superior colliculus	Receives 10% of the retinal fibers
	Integrates visual, auditory, and somatosensory spatial information and controls reflex movements of the eye
Optic radiation	Large bilateral bundle of fibers each containing two divisions that receive visual input from upper and lower quadrants of the contralateral hemifields
Primary visual cortex	Brodmann area 17: region of the occipital lobe that receives and processes visual information from contralateral visual field

The visual pathway

The optic nerve

OCULOMOTOR, TROCHLEAR AND ABDUCENS NERVES (CN III, IV & VI)

Movements of the eyeball affecting the direction of gaze are controlled by three cranial nerves: The oculomotor (CN III), trochlear (CN IV) and abducens (CN VI) nerves.

To be more specific, these nerves provide motor supply to the extraocular muscles:

- Oculomotor nerve: Superior, medial and inferior recti muscles, as well as the inferior oblique muscle.
- Trochlear nerve: Superior oblique muscle ('trochlear' referring to the pulley-like anatomy of this muscle (Latin: Trochlea = pulley).
- Abducens nerve: Lateral rectus ('abducens' refers to abduction of the eye which is achieved by this muscle).

In addition, the oculomotor nerve also provides motor innervation to the levator palpebrae superioris muscle, as well as parasympathetic innervation to the sphincter pupillae and ciliary muscles. Therefore, it also has a role in elevation of the upper eyelid, pupillary constriction and accommodation of the lens.

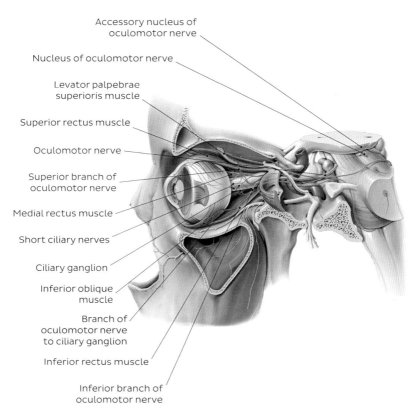

Accessory nucleus of
oculomotor nerve

Nucleus of oculomotor nerve

Levator palpebrae
superioris muscle

Superior rectus muscle

Oculomotor nerve

Superior branch of
oculomotor nerve

Medial rectus muscle

Short ciliary nerves

Ciliary ganglion

Inferior oblique
muscle

Branch of
oculomotor nerve
to ciliary ganglion

Inferior rectus muscle

Inferior branch of
oculomotor nerve

FIGURE 9.33. **Oculomotor nerve (left orbital view).** The oculomotor nerve (CN III) arises from the oculomotor complex located in the midbrain, ventral to the periaqueductal gray substance, at the level of the superior colliculus. It is comprised of two nuclei: The nucleus of oculomotor nerve (contains cell bodies of general somatic efferent (GSE, motor) neurons), and the accessory nucleus of oculomotor nerve (Edinger-Westphal, contains cell bodies of general visceral efferent (GVE, parasympathetic) neurons). Efferent fibers emerge from the midbrain into the interpeduncular fossa/cistern as the oculomotor nerve, which continues through the lateral wall of the cavernous sinus. From here, it enters the orbit the superior orbital fissure (internal to the common tendinous ring) as two branches which innervate the majority of the extraocular muscles:

· Superior branch: Superior rectus and levator palpebrae superioris muscles

· Inferior branch: Medial rectus, inferior rectus and inferior oblique muscles

The inferior branch also carries preganglionic parasympathetic fibers which synapse with postganglionic neurons in the ciliary ganglion; these fibers provide parasympathetic innervation to the ciliary and sphincter pupillae muscles responsible for accommodation and pupillary constriction, via the short ciliary nerves (branch of CN V_1).

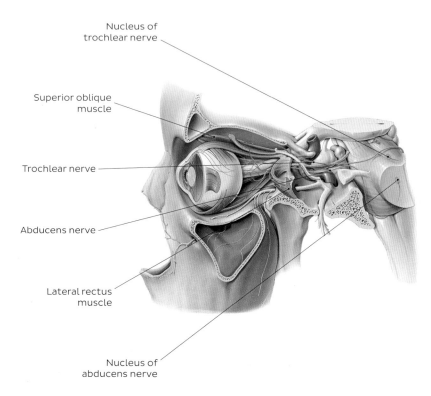

Nucleus of
trochlear nerve

Superior oblique
muscle

Trochlear nerve

Abducens nerve

Lateral rectus
muscle

Nucleus of
abducens nerve

FIGURE 9.34. **Trochlear and abducens nerves.** The trochlear nerve (CN IV) arises from the nucleus of trochlear nerve (containing general somatic efferent (GSE) neurons), which is located in the tegmentum of the caudal midbrain. Fibers from this nucleus decussate posteriorly and emerge from the dorsal midbrain, just below the inferior colliculus. From here, the trochlear nerve curves around the midbrain, passing through the lateral wall of the cavernous sinus, superior and lateral to the oculomotor nerve. It continues into the orbit via the superior orbital fissure, external to the common tendinous ring, before terminating in the superior oblique muscle.

The abducens nerve (CN VI) arises from the nucleus of abducens nerve, which also contains general somatic efferent (GSE) neurons and is located near the rhomboid fossa/floor of the fourth ventricle. Fibers from this nucleus exit the brainstem at the medullopontine sulcus (pontomedullary junction) as the abducens nerve, which courses through the cavernous sinus (along the internal carotid artery). It then enters the orbit via the superior orbital fissure, internal to the common tendinous ring. The abducens nerve then penetrates the medial surface of the lateral rectus muscle, which functions as an abductor of the eyeball.

Key points about the cranial nerves III, IV and VI	
Oculomotor nerve (CN III)	Fiber types: general somatic efferent fibers (GSE), general visceral efferent fibers (GVE)
	Origin: ventral midbrain (interpeduncular fossa)
	Exits skull: superior orbital fissure
	Nuclei: nucleus of oculomotor nerve (GSE); accessory nucleus of oculomotor nerve (Edinger–Westphal) (GVE)
	Branches: superior and inferior branch, branch of oculomotor nerve to ciliary ganglion (parasympathetic root of ciliary ganglion)
	Function: superior branch → Motor innervation to superior rectus, levator palpebrae superioris muscles
	Inferior branch → medial rectus, inferior rectus, inferior oblique muscles (GSE); branch to ciliary ganglion → parasympathetic innervation to ciliary and sphincter pupillae muscles (GVE)

Key points about the cranial nerves III, IV and VI	
Trochlear nerve (CN IV)	Fiber type: general somatic efferent (GSE)
	Origin: dorsal midbrain
	Exits skull: superior orbital fissure
	Nucleus: nucleus of trochlear nerve
	Function: motor innervation to superior oblique muscle
Abducens nerve (CN VI)	Fiber type: general somatic efferent fibers (GSE)
	Origin: medullopontine sulcus (pontomedullary junction)
	Exits skull: superior orbital fissure
	Nucleus: nucleus of abducens nerve
	Function: motor innervation to lateral rectus muscle

Oculomotor nerve

Trochlear nerve and the abducent nerve

TRIGEMINAL NERVE (CN V)

The trigeminal nerve, otherwise known as the 5th cranial nerve (CN V), is a mixed nerve meaning that it is made up of both sensory and motor components. It is formed by three sensory nuclei (mesencephalic/principal sensory/spinal nucleus of trigeminal nerve) and one motor nucleus (motor nucleus of trigeminal nerve). At the level of the pons, efferents of the sensory nuclei merge to form a large sensory root, while those from the motor nucleus continue as a smaller motor root. These roots course anteriorly out of the posterior cranial fossa and travel along the anterior surface of the petrous part of the temporal bone where the sensory root expands to form the trigeminal ganglion, from which arises the three divisions of the trigeminal nerve: The ophthalmic (V_1), maxillary (V_2) and mandibular nerves (V_3).

Ophthalmic nerve (CN V_1)

The ophthalmic nerve is the most superior branch of the trigeminal ganglion, and provides general somatic afferent (GSA) innervation to structures of the upper portion of the face, nasal cavity and mucosa of paranasal sinuses. It extends from the trigeminal ganglion through the lateral wall of the cavernous sinus where it divides into three main branches (the lacrimal, frontal and naso-ciliary nerves) all of which pass through the superior orbital fissure.

NEUROANATOMY

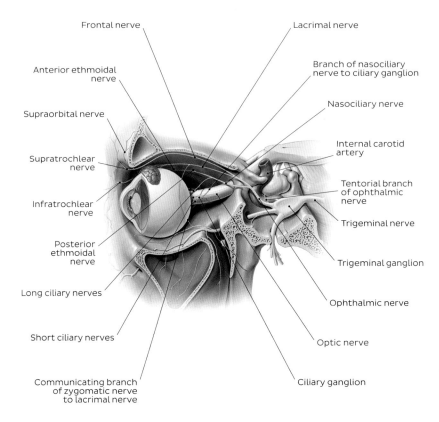

Frontal nerve

Lacrimal nerve

Anterior ethmoidal nerve

Branch of nasociliary nerve to ciliary ganglion

Supraorbital nerve

Nasociliary nerve

Supratrochlear nerve

Internal carotid artery

Infratrochlear nerve

Tentorial branch of ophthalmic nerve

Posterior ethmoidal nerve

Trigeminal nerve

Trigeminal ganglion

Long ciliary nerves

Ophthalmic nerve

Short ciliary nerves

Optic nerve

Communicating branch of zygomatic nerve to lacrimal nerve

Ciliary ganglion

FIGURE 9.35. **Ophthalmic nerve (left lateral view).** The ophthalmic nerve extends in an anterosuperior direction from the trigeminal ganglion and gives rise to a small branch known as the tentorial branch of ophthalmic nerve which provides innervation to the tentorium cerebelli. The **frontal nerve** is the largest branch of the ophthalmic nerve. It enters the orbit via the superior orbital fissure external to the common tendinous ring and divides into two terminal branches: The supraorbital and supratrochlear nerves. The **lacrimal nerve** also enters the orbit external to the common tendinous ring and extends across the roof of the orbit towards the lacrimal gland. Before reaching the gland, it expands into several branches, which either terminate in the lacrimal gland or extend through the gland, terminating in the skin of the upper eyelid. Just behind the lacrimal gland, the lacrimal nerve is joined by the communicating branch of zygomaticotemporal nerve (from V_2) to lacrimal nerve, which provides parasympathetic innervation to the lacrimal gland. The **nasociliary nerve** enters the superior orbital fissure within the common tendinous ring and then crosses over to the medial orbital wall. It gives off several branches which include the long ciliary, posterior ethmoidal, anterior ethmoidal and infratrochlear nerves as well as the branch of nasociliary nerve to ciliary ganglion (sensory root of ciliary ganglion).

Key points about the ophthalmic nerve		
Structure and features	Fibers: general somatic afferent (GSA)
	Origin: trigeminal ganglion
	Exits skull: superior orbital fissure
	Associated nuclei: sensory nuclei (mesencephalic, principal sensory, spinal nuclei of trigeminal nerve) and motor nucleus of trigeminal nerve
	Associated ganglia: trigeminal ganglion, ciliary ganglion
Branches	Frontal nerve (supraorbital and supratrochlear nerves)
	Lacrimal nerve
	Nasociliary nerve (branch of nasociliary nerve to ciliary ganglion, long ciliary nerves, posterior ethmoidal nerve, anterior ethmoidal nerve, infratrochlear nerve)
Function	Provides Innervation to forehead, scalp, eyelids, eye, conjunctiva and nasal cavity

Maxillary nerve (CN V₂)

The maxillary nerve emerges from the anterior portion of the trigeminal ganglion and like its origin, is exclusively composed of general somatic afferent
(sensory) fibers. It passes through the lateral wall of the cavernous sinus and
foramen rotundum to enter the pterygopalatine fossa. Here, it gives rise to the
majority of its branches before extending through the inferior orbital fissure
where it gives rise to its terminal branch, the infraorbital nerve. Through its
intricate pathway the maxillary nerve provides the major sensory innervation to
the skin of the lower eyelid, the prominence of the cheek, part of the temporal
region, alar part of the nose, and upper lip.

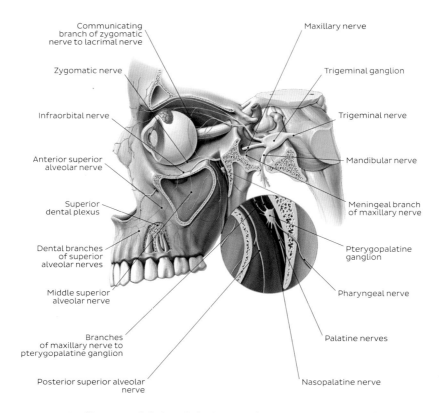

FIGURE 9.36. **Maxillary nerve (left lateral view).** Just before the maxillary nerve exits the middle
cranial fossa, via the foramen rotundum, it gives off a small meningeal branch which carries sensory
impulses from the dura mater of this region. Within the pterygopalatine fossa, the maxillary nerve gives
off a number of branches that can be divided into those which arise directly from the nerve and those

NEUROANATOMY

associated with the pterygopalatine ganglion which is located on the posterior wall of the pterygopalatine fossa (see next image). The maxillary nerve leaves the pterygopalatine fossa by coursing anterior through the pterygomaxillary fissure to enter the infratemporal fossa, where it gives off the **posterior superior alveolar nerve**. It then turns medially to enter the orbit via the inferior orbital fissure, where it continues as the terminal branch of the maxillary nerve, the **infraorbital nerve**. The infraorbital nerve proceeds anteriorly across the floor of the orbit in the infraorbital groove, giving off the middle superior alveolar nerve, before continuing through the infraorbital canal. Here, the anterior superior alveolar nerve arises before the infraorbital nerve continues onto the face via the infraorbital foramen and terminates as groups of palpebral, nasal and superior labial branches.

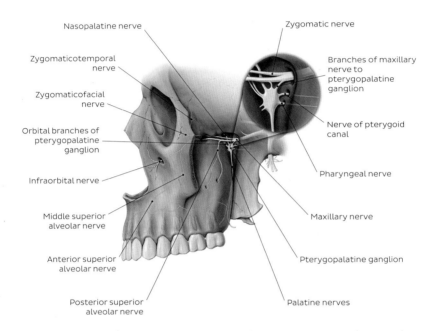

Nasopalatine nerve

Zygomatic nerve

Zygomaticotemporal nerve

Zygomaticofacial nerve

Orbital branches of pterygopalatine ganglion

Infraorbital nerve

Middle superior alveolar nerve

Anterior superior alveolar nerve

Posterior superior alveolar nerve

Branches of maxillary nerve to pterygopalatine ganglion

Nerve of pterygoid canal

Pharyngeal nerve

Maxillary nerve

Pterygopalatine ganglion

Palatine nerves

FIGURE 9.37. **Maxillary nerve (pterygopalatine fossa, left lateral view).** Within the pterygopalatine fossa, branches arise directly from the maxillary nerve including the branches to pterygopalatine ganglion (of which there are usually two) and the zygomatic nerve. Branches associated with the pterygopalatine ganglion include the nasopalatine, posterior superior nasal, greater palatine, lesser palatine and pharyngeal nerves, as well as 2–3 small orbital branches. Parasympathetic and sympathetic fibers are delivered to the pterygopalatine ganglion via the nerve of pterygoid canal (derived from the greater petrosal (facial nerve, CN VII) and deep petrosal nerve (internal carotid plexus), respectively). Postganglionic fibers are then distributed within the aforementioned ganglionic branches of the maxillary nerve to regulate secretomotor and vascular responses in the lacrimal gland as well as mucous membranes of the nasal cavity, naso/oropharynx, and upper oral cavity. While the naso-, greater and lesser palatine nerves mainly convey sensory impulses, they also carry special visceral afferent (taste) fibers from the palate to the pterygopalatine ganglion; these fibers continue to the facial nerve via the nerve of pterygoid canal.

Key points about the maxillary nerve	
Structure and features	Fibers: general somatic afferent (GSA)
	Origin: trigeminal ganglion
	Exits skull: foramen rotundum
	Associated nuclei: sensory nuclei (mesencephalic, principal sensory, spinal nuclei of trigeminal nerve) and motor nucleus of trigeminal nerve
	Associated ganglia: trigeminal ganglion, pterygopalatine ganglion

Key points about the maxillary nerve	
Branches	Directly from maxillary nerve: Meningeal branch, branches of the maxillary nerve to pterygopalatine ganglion, zygomatic nerve, posterior superior alveolar nerve, infraorbital nerve
	Associated with pterygopalatine ganglion: Orbital branches, posterior superior nasal branches, nasopalatine nerve, pharyngeal nerve, greater palatine nerve, lesser palatine nerves
Function	Sensory innervation of skin of lower eyelid, prominence of the cheek, part of the temporal region, alar part of the nose and upper lip

Maxillary branch of
the trigeminal nerve

Mandibular nerve (CN V$_3$)

The mandibular nerve, accompanied by the motor root of the trigeminal nerve, leaves the skull through the foramen ovale, after which both unite within the infratemporal fossa. The mandibular nerve is therefore the only division of the trigeminal nerve to convey both afferent (sensory) and efferent (motor) nerve fibers. It supplies:

- General somatic afferent (GSA, sensory) innervation to the skin over the mandible, cheek and temporal region, mucosa of the oral cavity and tongue, the mandibular teeth, parts of the external ear, as well as the temporomandibular joint
- Special visceral efferent (SVE) innervation is provided to eight muscles: Muscles of mastication (4), mylohyoid, anterior belly of digastric, tensor veli palatini, and tensor tympani muscles
- Other fiber types (special visceral afferent (SVA), general visceral efferent (GVE)) are also carried by the mandibular nerve via anastomoses with branches of other cranial nerves

NEUROANATOMY

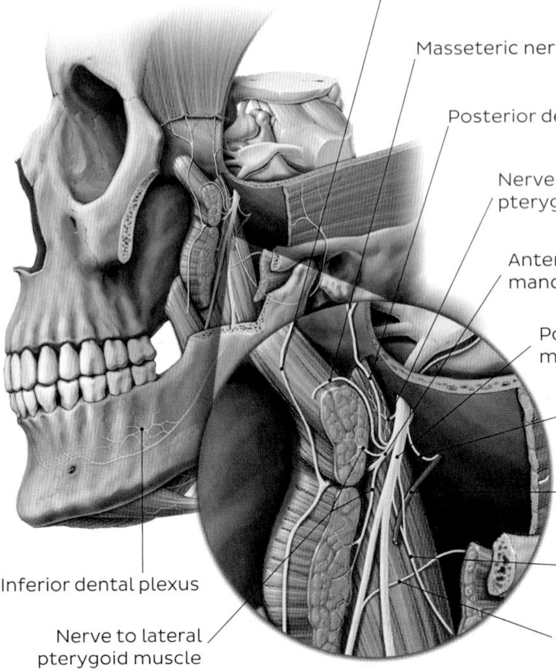

FIGURE 9.38. **Infratemporal branches and anterior division.** The mandibular nerve arises from the anterior portion of the trigeminal ganglion. Accompanied by the motor root of the trigeminal nerve, it exits the skull through the foramen ovale and enters the infratemporal fossa. At this point, the motor root unites with the mandibular nerve, making it a mixed nerve. Within the infratemporal fossa the mandibular trunk immediately gives off two branches: A **meningeal branch** which ascends through the foramen spinosum to supply dura of the middle cranial fossa and a **nerve to medial pterygoid muscle** which passes through the otic ganglion (not shown) to supply the medial pterygoid, tensor veli palatini, and tensor tympani muscles. The mandibular nerve then splits into anterior and posterior divisions. The anterior division passes efferent (motor) fibers to the **masseteric nerve**, **deep temporal nerves** and **nerve to lateral pterygoid** and receives afferent (sensory) fibers from the **buccal nerve** which supplies the skin over the cheek.

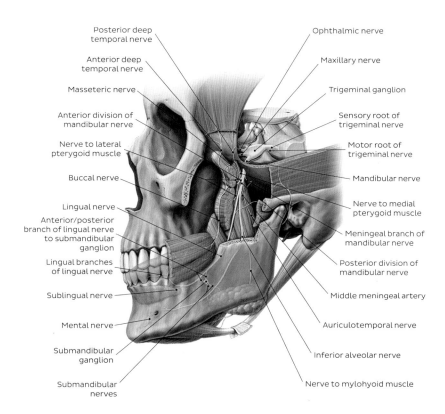

Posterior deep
temporal nerve

Anterior deep
temporal nerve

Masseteric nerve

Anterior division of
mandibular nerve

Nerve to lateral
pterygoid muscle

Buccal nerve

Lingual nerve

Anterior/posterior
branch of lingual nerve
to submandibular
ganglion

Lingual branches
of lingual nerve

Sublingual nerve

Mental nerve

Submandibular
ganglion

Submandibular
nerves

Ophthalmic nerve

Maxillary nerve

Trigeminal ganglion

Sensory root of
trigeminal nerve

Motor root of
trigeminal nerve

Mandibular nerve

Nerve to medial
pterygoid muscle

Meningeal branch of
mandibular nerve

Posterior division of
mandibular nerve

Middle meningeal artery

Auriculotemporal nerve

Inferior alveolar nerve

Nerve to mylohyoid muscle

FIGURE 9.39. **Posterior division.** The posterior division of the mandibular nerve is mainly sensory and is larger than the anterior division. The **auriculotemporal nerve** arises posterior to the temporomandibular joint (usually as two roots which encircle the middle meningeal artery) and supplies parts of the auricle/external acoustic meatus and posterior half of the temporal region. Sympathetic/parasympathetic fibers to the parotid gland (derived from the plexus of the middle meningeal artery and otic ganglion, respectively) are also carried within this nerve. The **lingual nerve** arises from the terminal bifurcation of the posterior division, and carries general somatic afferent/sensory fibers from the anterior two-thirds of the tongue, floor of the oral cavity and lower lingual gingiva. It is joined by the chorda tympani (of facial nerve) which delivers general visceral efferent/parasympathetic fibers to the submandibular and sublingual glands via homonymous/same-named branches of the lingual nerve. Special visceral afferent/taste fibers from the anterior two-thirds of the tongue are carried by the lingual nerve to the chorda tympani. The **inferior alveolar nerve** is a mixed nerve, carrying sensory fibers from the mandibular teeth via the inferior dental plexus (see first image) and lower lip/labial gingiva (via mental nerve), as well as general somatic afferent/motor fibers to the mylohyoid and anterior belly of digastric muscles.

Key points about the mandibular nerve	
Structure and features	Fibers: general somatic afferent (GSA, sensory), special visceral efferent (SVE, branchiomotor) (special visceral afferent/taste (SVA), general visceral efferent/parasympathetic (GVE) fibers also carried to/from other cranial nerves)
	Origin: trigeminal ganglion
	Exits skull: foramen ovale
	Associated nuclei: sensory nuclei (mesencephalic, principal sensory, spinal nuclei of trigeminal nerve) and motor nucleus of trigeminal nerve
	Associated ganglia: trigeminal ganglion, otic ganglion, submandibular/sublingual ganglion

Key points about the mandibular nerve		
Branches		Meningeal branch of mandibular nerve
		Nerve to medial pterygoid
		Anterior division: masseteric nerve, anterior and posterior deep temporal nerves, nerve to lateral pterygoid, buccal nerve
		Posterior division: auriculotemporal nerve, lingual nerve, inferior alveolar nerve
Function		General somatic afferent: skin and mucosa of the lower face, oral cavity, ear and mandibular teeth
		General somatic efferent: muscles of mastication, mylohyoid muscle, anterior belly of digastric, tensor veli palatini muscle, tensor tympani muscle
		(Special visceral afferent: taste from anterior ⅔ of tongue
		General visceral efferent: secretomotor to submandibular/sublingual glands)

Mandibular branch of the trigeminal nerve

FACIAL NERVE (CN VII)

The facial nerve is a mixed nerve carrying several different types of nerve fibers which allow it to participate in a wide range of functions. These include:

- General somatic afferent (sensory) innervation of the skin around the external acoustic meatus, parts of the auricle and retroauricular/mastoid region
- Special visceral afferent (taste) sensation from the anterior two-thirds of the tongue
- General visceral efferent (parasympathetic, or secretomotor) innervation to the lacrimal, submandibular and sublingual glands as well as mucous membranes of the nasal cavity, hard and soft palates
- Special visceral efferent (branchiomotor) innervation of the muscles of facial expression and scalp, as well as the stapedius, stylohyoid and posterior belly of the digastric muscles

The facial nerve arises at the cerebellopontine angle as two separate roots. Its motor root is associated with neurons originating in the large motor nucleus of facial nerve, located in the pons. The sensory root contains somatic sensory and visceral sensory (taste) fibers, the cell bodies of which are located in the geniculate ganglion. The central processes of these fibers terminate at the sensory nucleus of trigeminal nerve and nucleus of solitary tract, respectively. Efferent parasympathetic roots (from the superior salivatory nucleus) are also carried within the sensory root, therefore it is not actually completely sensory in composition; hence the term 'intermediate nerve' is often used instead.

NEUROANATOMY

Along its pathway, the facial nerve can be divided into three different segments: An intracranial (cisternal) part, intratemporal part (enclosed within the temporal bone) and an extracranial part that describes the facial nerve after it emerges from the temporal bone.

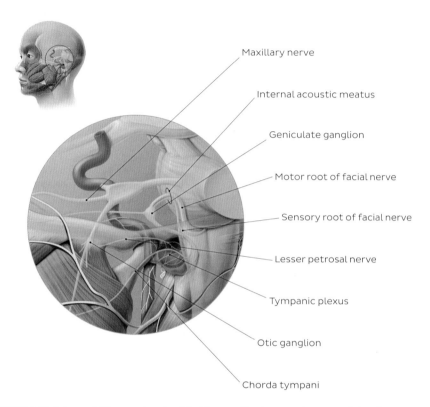

Maxillary nerve

Internal acoustic meatus

Geniculate ganglion

Motor root of facial nerve

Sensory root of facial nerve

Lesser petrosal nerve

Tympanic plexus

Otic ganglion

Chorda tympani

FIGURE 9.40. **Intracranial/temporal parts of facial nerve.** The larger and more medial motor root as well as the smaller, more lateral, sensory root (intermediate nerve) arise at the cerebellopontine angle and traverse the posterior cranial fossa, forming the branchless, intracranial part of the facial nerve. The roots then enter the temporal bone via the internal acoustic meatus together with the vestibulocochlear nerve, as well as the labyrinthine artery and vein. The sensory and motor components usually merge at, or within the internal acoustic meatus, and then continue into the facial canal located along the medial wall of the tympanic cavity. Here, the facial nerve expands into the geniculate ganglion, which contains the cell bodies of the sensory neurons related to the nerve. The greater petrosal nerve arises directly from the **geniculate ganglion** and carries general visceral efferent (parasympathetic) fibers destined for the lacrimal, nasal and palatine glands, as well as special visceral afferent (taste) fibers from the palate (both via the pterygopalatine ganglion). The facial nerve then gives off two further intratemporal branches (**nerve to stapedius muscle** and the **chorda tympani**) which arise before the facial nerve exits the temporal bone via the stylomastoid foramen. The chorda tympani carries both parasympathetic fibers destined for the submandibular/sublingual glands as well as special visceral afferent (taste) fibers from the anterior two-thirds of the tongue via the lingual nerve (see next image).

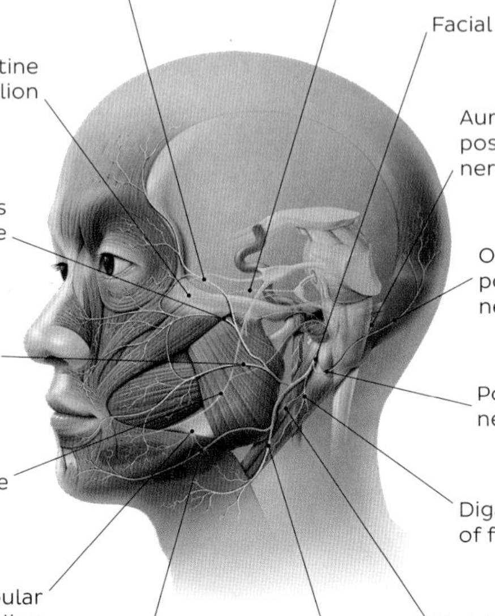

FIGURE 9.41. **Extracranial part of facial nerve.** After it emerges from the stylomastoid foramen, the facial nerve gives off the **posterior auricular nerve** (which provides motor innervation to the occipital part of occipitofrontalis muscle and auricular muscles, as well as sensory innervation to the variable amounts of the auricle and retroauricular region), as well as other motor branches to the digastric (posterior belly) and stylohyoid muscles. It then enters the parotid gland and bifurcates into two trunks, which give off five terminal branches collectively known as the **parotid plexus**. These are the temporal, zygomatic, buccal, marginal mandibular, and cervical branches, all of which innervate the muscles of facial expression but do not innervate the parotid gland itself.

Key points about the facial nerve	
Structure and features	Fibers: general somatic afferent (GSA), special visceral afferent (SVA), general visceral efferent (GVE), special visceral efferent (SVE, branchiomotor)
	Origin: cerebellopontine angle (Motor and sensory (intermediate nerve) roots)
	Exits skull: stylomastoid foramen
	Associated nuclei: motor nucleus of facial nerve, superior salivatory nucleus, nucleus of solitary tract
	Associated ganglia: geniculate ganglion (pterygopalatine ganglion, otic ganglion, submandibular ganglion)

Key points about the facial nerve	
Parts & branches	Intracranial: origin → internal acoustic meatus
	(no branches)
	Intratemporal: internal acoustic meatus → stylomastoid foramen
	Greater petrosal nerve, nerve to stapedius, chorda tympani
	Extracranial: after stylomastoid foramen
	Posterior auricular nerve, digastric branch, stylohyoid branch
	Parotid plexus: temporal branch, zygomatic branch, buccal branch, marginal mandibular branch, cervical branch
Functions	Main: motor innervation to muscles of facial expression (SVE)
	Others: taste innervation of anterior two-thirds of tongue and palate (SVA), parasympathetic innervation of lacrimal, nasal, palatine and salivary glands (except parotid) (GVE), sensation to parts of auricle and retroauricular region (GSA)

Facial nerve

Superficial nerves of the face and scalp

VESTIBULOCOCHLEAR NERVE (CN VIII)

The vestibulocochlear nerve, also known as the 8th cranial nerve (CN VIII) is a sensory nerve that consists of two divisions: The vestibular and cochlear nerves. The function of the vestibulocochlear nerve is to provide special somatic afferent (SSA) innervation of the internal ear, with each division serving a specific role:

- The vestibular nerve conveys information from the vestibular apparatus of the internal ear to the vestibular nuclei in the pons and brainstem in order to maintain balance, spatial orientation and coordination
- The cochlear nerve is part of the auditory pathway, conveying auditory information from the cochlea of the internal ear to the cochlear nuclei in the brainstem in order to enable the sense of hearing

NEUROANATOMY

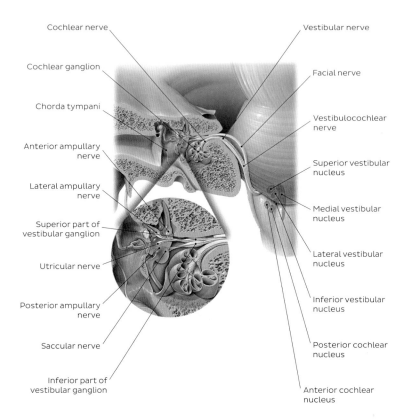

Cochlear nerve

Cochlear ganglion

Chorda tympani

Anterior ampullary nerve

Lateral ampullary nerve

Superior part of vestibular ganglion

Utricular nerve

Posterior ampullary nerve

Saccular nerve

Inferior part of vestibular ganglion

Vestibular nerve

Facial nerve

Vestibulocochlear nerve

Superior vestibular nucleus

Medial vestibular nucleus

Lateral vestibular nucleus

Inferior vestibular nucleus

Posterior cochlear nucleus

Anterior cochlear nucleus

FIGURE 9.42. **Vestibulocochlear nerve.** The vestibulocochlear nerve (CN VIII) arises from the brainstem at the pontomedullary junction/cerebellopontine angle. It exits the cranium via the internal acoustic meatus of the temporal bone, where it divides into the vestibular and cochlear nerves.

The **vestibular nerve** contains the axons of neurons whose cell bodies are found in the vestibular ganglion, found at the lateral end/fundus of the internal acoustic meatus. The vestibular ganglion consists of superior and inferior parts, from which the superior and inferior branches of vestibular nerve arise and proceed to innervate the vestibular apparatus (utricle, saccule and semicircular ducts). The anterior ampullary, lateral ampullary and utricular nerves arise from the superior branch, while the posterior ampullary and saccular nerves are given off from the inferior component. These nerves collect information related to motion and position of the head and transmit it to the vestibular nuclei (the superior, inferior, medial and lateral vestibular nuclei) in the lower pons/upper medulla oblongata in order to maintain balance and equilibrium.

The **cochlear nerve** contains the axons of neurons whose cell bodies are located in the cochlear/spiral ganglion that lies in the spiral canal of the modiolus of the cochlea. Peripheral processes of these neurons send terminal endings to receptors in the spiral organ (of Corti), that collect auditory information and transmit it via the cochlear nerve to the cochlear nuclei (anterior and posterior cochlear nuclei) in the brainstem, and ultimately to the primary auditory cortex of the temporal lobe.

Key points about the vestibulocochlear nerve (CN VIII)	
Structure and features	Fibers: special sensory afferent nerve (SSA)
	Origin: pontomedullary junction/cerebellopontine angle
	Enters skull: internal acoustic meatus
	Associated nuclei: Vestibular nerve: superior vestibular nucleus (of Bechterew), lateral vestibular nucleus (of Deiters), inferior vestibular nucleus (of Roller), medial vestibular nucleus (of Schwalbe)
	Cochlear nerve: anterior and posterior cochlear nuclei
	Associated ganglia: Vestibular nerve: vestibular ganglion (receives the inputs from the utricular, saccular, lateral, anterior and posterior ampullary nerves)
	Cochlear nerve: spiral ganglion (receives the inputs from the spiral organ (of Corti))
Function	Vestibular nerve: transmits information about motion and position of the head to maintain balance and equilibrium
	Cochlear nerve: transmits auditory information/enables the sense of hearing

Auditory pathway

Vestibular system

GLOSSOPHARYNGEAL NERVE (CN IX)

The glossopharyngeal nerve (CN IX) is a mixed cranial nerve that carries both motor and sensory fibers. Its functions include:

- general somatic afferent (GSA) innervation of the tongue and throat
- special visceral afferent (SVA) sensation of taste to the posterior third of the tongue
- general visceral afferent (GVA) sensation from specific structures of the common carotid artery (carotid sinus and carotid body)
- general somatic efferent (GSE) innervation is also provided to the stylopharyngeus muscle
- general visceral efferent (GVE) secretomotor (parasympathetic) innervation to the parotid gland

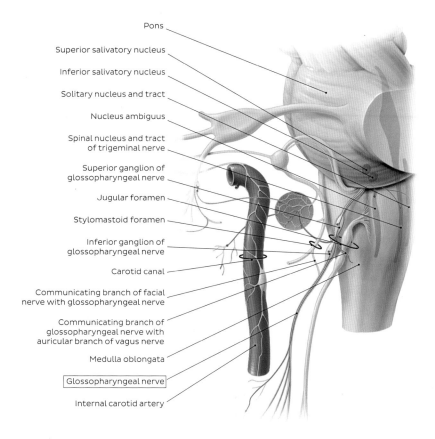

Pons

Superior salivatory nucleus

Inferior salivatory nucleus

Solitary nucleus and tract

Nucleus ambiguus

Spinal nucleus and tract of trigeminal nerve

Superior ganglion of glossopharyngeal nerve

Jugular foramen

Stylomastoid foramen

Inferior ganglion of glossopharyngeal nerve

Carotid canal

Communicating branch of facial nerve with glossopharyngeal nerve

Communicating branch of glossopharyngeal nerve with auricular branch of vagus nerve

Medulla oblongata

Glossopharyngeal nerve

Internal carotid artery

FIGURE 9.43. **Glossopharyngeal nerve (origin and proximal branches).** The glossopharyngeal nerve (CN IX) carries motor fibers from the inferior salivatory nucleus (general visceral efferent) and nucleus ambiguus (general somatic efferent fibers), and sensory fibers from the spinal trigeminal nucleus (general somatic afferent) and solitary nucleus (general visceral sensory).

The glossopharyngeal nerve emerges from the lateral aspect of the rostral medulla and leaves the skull via the anterior part of the jugular foramen. Here, it bears its associated sensory ganglia: The superior and inferior ganglia.

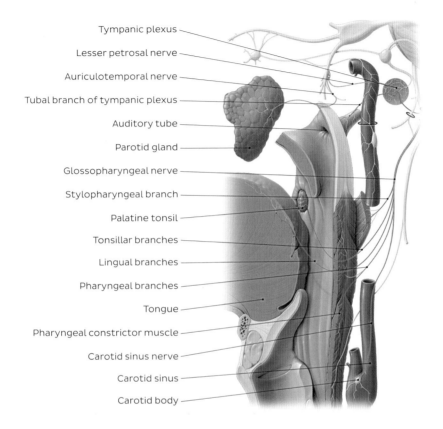

Tympanic plexus

Lesser petrosal nerve

Auriculotemporal nerve

Tubal branch of tympanic plexus

Auditory tube

Parotid gland

Glossopharyngeal nerve

Stylopharyngeal branch

Palatine tonsil

Tonsillar branches

Lingual branches

Pharyngeal branches

Tongue

Pharyngeal constrictor muscle

Carotid sinus nerve

Carotid sinus

Carotid body

FIGURE 9.44. **Glossopharyngeal nerve (distal branches).** After exiting the jugular foramen, the glossopharyngeal nerve gives off the **tympanic nerve**, which joins the tympanic plexus in providing general sensory innervation to the mucosa of the middle ear, auditory tube, and mastoid air cells. The tympanic plexus gives rise to the lesser petrosal nerve, which carries the parasympathetic component of the glossopharyngeal nerve and supplies it to the otic ganglion to innervate the parotid gland via the auriculotemporal nerve (CN V_3). CN IX then descends into the anterior triangle of the neck, where it gives rise to several branches.

The **stylopharyngeal branch** provides somatic motor innervation to the stylopharyngeus muscle. The **carotid branch** carries general visceral afferent fibers from the carotid sinus and carotid body. **Pharyngeal and tonsillar branches** provide general sensory supply to the mucosa of the pharynx and the palatine tonsil region, respectively. The **lingual branch** provides general sensory supply to the base of the tongue and special visceral afferent (taste) innervation to the posterior one-third of the tongue. Finally, the glossopharyngeal nerve gives off communicating branches that form connections with the sympathetic trunk, vagus (CN X) and facial nerves (CN VII).

Key points about the glossopharyngeal nerve (CN IX)	
Structure	Fiber types: general somatic efferent (GSE), special visceral afferent (SVA), general somatic afferent (GSA), general visceral afferent (GVA), general visceral efferent (GVE)
	Origin: medulla oblongata
	Exists skull: jugular foramen
	Associated nuclei: Motor: nucleus ambiguus (SVE) and inferior salivatory nucleus (GVE)
	Sensory: nucleus of trigeminal nerve (GSA) and nuclei of solitary tract (SVA)
	Associated ganglia: Sensory: superior and inferior ganglia of glossopharyngeal nerve
	Parasympathetic: otic ganglion
Branches	Tympanic nerve
	Carotid branch
	Pharyngeal branches
	Stylopharyngeal branch
	Tonsillar branches
	Lingual branch
Function	Motor innervation: stylopharyngeus muscle
	Taste innervation: posterior third of tongue
	General sensation: tympanic cavity, eustachian tube, fauces, tonsils, nasopharynx, uvula and posterior third of tongue
	Visceral sensation: carotid body and sinus
	Parasympathetic innervation: parotid gland

Glossopharyngeal nerve

Anatomy of taste

VAGUS NERVE (CN X)

The vagus nerve is the longest cranial nerve, and as its name suggests (Latin = wandering nerve). It has an extensive course and wide distribution in the body, traversing the neck, thorax and abdomen. It is a mixed nerve, whose functions include:

- general somatic afferent (GSA, sensory) innervation of the laryngopharynx, larynx and root of the tongue
- special visceral afferent (SVA, taste) innervation of the root of the tongue and epiglottal taste buds
- general visceral afferent (GVA, sensory) innervation of thoracic and abdominal organs
- general visceral efferent (GVE, parasympathetic) innervation to thoracoab-dominal organs and mucosa of the palate, pharynx, larynx and trachea
- special visceral efferent (SVE, branchiomotor) innervation to the palatoglos-sus muscle of the tongue and several muscles of the soft palate, pharynx and larynx

The vagus nerve arises from the lateral aspect of the medulla oblongata and exits the cranial cavity through the jugular foramen. From here, each vagus nerve descends through the neck, providing innervation to the palate, pharynx, and larynx along the way, before continuing into the thorax to innervate the heart, bronchi, and lungs. The right and left vagus nerves intermingle around the esophagus before going on to form the posterior and anterior vagal trunks which subsequently pass into the abdomen to supply abdominal viscera of the foregut and midgut (i.e. stomach as far as the left colic flexure of large intestine) and other abdominal organs (liver, spleen, pancreas etc.).

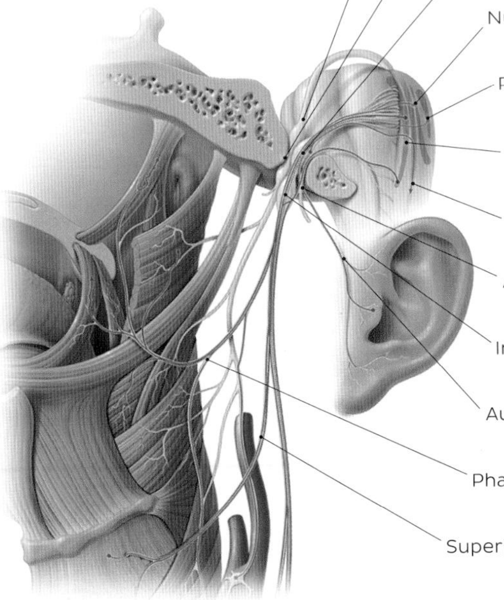

Glossopharyngeal nerve

Jugular foramen

Superior ganglion

Nucleus of solitary tract

Posterior nucleus

Nucleus ambiguus

Spinal nucleus of trigeminal nerve

Accessory nerve

Inferior ganglion

Auricular branch

Pharyngeal branch

Superior laryngeal nerve

FIGURE 9.45. **Vagus nerve: Intracranial and upper cervical parts.** The vagus nerve carries special visceral efferent/branchiomotor fibers from the nucleus ambiguus and general visceral efferent/parasympathetic fibers from the posterior (dorsal) nucleus of vagus nerve. General somatic afferent/sensory fibers are carried to the spinal nucleus of trigeminal nerve, while both general and special visceral afferent fibers arrive at the nucleus of solitary tract.

The vagus nerve emerges from the lateral surface of the medulla as a group of rootlets that merge before exiting the skull via the jugular foramen between the glossopharyngeal (CN IX) and accessory (CN XI) nerves. In this region, the vagus nerve bears the **superior (jugular) ganglion** that contains the cell bodies of GSA fibers and has connections to the glossopharyngeal nerve, cervical sympathetic trunk and cranial root of accessory nerve (which is nowadays considered as a functional component of the vagus nerve). The superior ganglion gives off a meningeal branch (not shown) as well as an auricular branch, which supplies parts of the auricle and tympanic membrane. Below the superior ganglion is the **inferior (nodose) ganglion** which contains cell bodies of visceral and special sensory fibers of the vagus nerve and has connections with the hypoglossal nerve (CN XII).

After exiting the jugular foramen, the vagus nerve gives off a **pharyngeal branch** which supplies motor function to pharyngeal constrictor and palatine muscles, as well as receiving some GVA/sensory fibers from the pharyngeal plexus also. It also communicates with the carotid branch (of CN IX). The final upper cervical branch seen here is the **superior laryngeal nerve**.

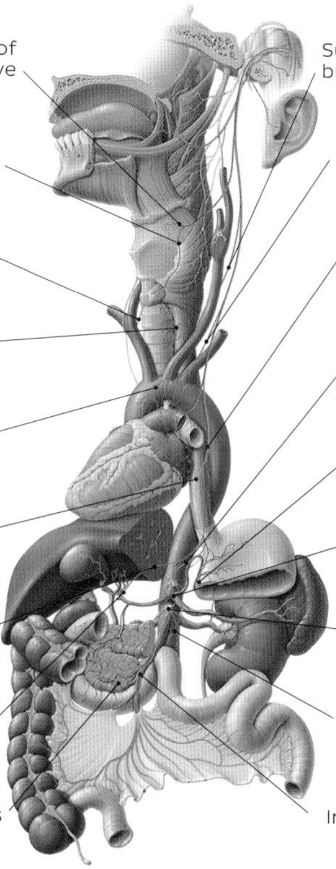

Internal branch of
superior laryngeal nerve

External branch of
superior laryngeal nerve

Right recurrent
aryngeal nerve

Left recurrent
laryngeal nerve

Cardiac plexus

Esophageal plexus

Hepatic branch of
anterior vagal trunk

Hepatic plexus

Pancreatic plexus

Superior cervical cardiac
branch

Inferior cervical cardiac
branch

Anterior vagal trunk

Celiac branches of
posterior vagal trunk

Anterior gastric branches of
anterior vagal trunk

Splenic plexus

Superior mesenteric
ganglion

Intermesenteric plexus

Intestinal branch

FIGURE 9.46. **Vagus nerve: Cervical and thoracoabdominal branches.** The **superior laryngeal nerve** terminates via an internal branch (which carries sensory information from the supraglottic part of the larynx and epiglottis), and an external branch (which innervates the cricothyroid muscle). The vagus nerve then descends through the anterior triangle of the neck in the carotid sheath, traveling posterior to the internal jugular vein and common carotid artery, where superior and inferior cervical cardiac branches are given off carrying GVE (parasympathetic) to and GVA (reflex) fibers from the cardiac plexus.

At the root of the neck, the vagus nerve passes anterior to each subclavian artery to enter the thorax, after which the right and left vagus nerves follow asymmetric courses. On the right side, the **recurrent laryngeal nerve** loops under the subclavian artery, while its counterpart on the left courses under the aortic arch before ascending through the neck. Both nerves innervate the intrinsic muscles of the larynx (except cricothyroid) as well as the mucosa of the infraglottic part of the larynx and trachea. In the thorax, the vagus nerve also gives rise to thoracic cardiac branches, bronchial and esophageal branches which together with branches of the sympathetic trunk, form the cardiac, pulmonary (not shown) and esophageal plexuses, respectively.

The right and left vagus nerves, after contributing to the esophageal plexus, re-form and continue into the abdomen as the posterior and anterior vagal trunks, respectively. The **posterior vagal trunk** gives rise to the posterior gastric branch, most of the fibers of the celiac, pancreatic, splenic, renal, suprarenal (not shown) and intermesenteric plexuses, as well as the intestinal branches of the vagus nerve. The **anterior vagal trunk** gives off the anterior gastric branch and the hepatic branch which contributes to the hepatic plexus, but not the superior mesenteric ganglion which contains sympathetic fibers.

Key points about the vagus nerve (CN X)	
Structure	Fiber types: general somatic afferent (GSA), special visceral afferent (SVA), general visceral afferent (GVA), general somatic efferent (GSE), general visceral efferent (GVE)
	Origin: medulla oblongata
	Motor nuclei: nucleus ambiguus (SVE), dorsal vagal nucleus (GVE)
	Sensory nuclei: spinal nucleus of trigeminal nerve (GSA), nucleus of solitary tract (GVA/SVA)
	Associated ganglia: superior and inferior ganglia of CN X
Branches	Jugular fossa: meningeal, auricular branches
	Neck: pharyngeal, superior laryngeal, recurrent laryngeal nerve (right only); superior/inferior cervical cardiac branches
	Thorax: recurrent laryngeal nerve (left only), thoracic cardiac branches, bronchial branches, esophageal branches
	Abdomen: posterior vagal trunk (posterior gastric, celiac, renal branches), anterior vagal trunk (anterior gastric branches, hepatic, pyloric branches), intestinal branches (up to left colic flexure)
Function	General somatic afferent (GSA): larynx, laryngopharynx, part of the external acoustic meatus, and dura mater of posterior cranial fossa
	General visceral afferent (GVA): aortic body chemoreceptors/aortic arch baroreceptors, esophagus, bronchi, lungs, heart, and abdominal viscera of foregut and midgut
	Special visceral afferent (SVA): taste from root of tongue and epiglottis
	General somatic efferent (GSE): palatoglossus muscle, muscles of soft palate (except tensor veli palatini), muscles of pharynx (except stylopharyngeus) and muscles of larynx
	General visceral efferent (GVE): parasympathetic/secretomotor fibers to smooth muscle and glands of the pharynx and larynx, parasympathetic innervation of thoracic viscera, and abdominal viscera of the foregut and midgut

Vagus nerve

NEUROANATOMY

ACCESSORY NERVE (CN XI)

The accessory nerve is primarily a motor nerve meaning that it supplies efferent motor function to muscles. Traditionally, it has been considered to have
two parts, a cranial root and a spinal root. The classification of the cranial root
is somewhat controversial however, with many anatomists nowadays considering these fibers to be part of the vagus nerve. Therefore, when clinicians and
textbooks refer to the accessory nerve, they usually are specifically referring to
the spinal part only (making the accessory nerve the only cranial nerve *not to*
originate within the cranium). Consequently, many no longer technically con-
sider the accessory nerve to be a cranial nerve but continue to include it as one,
so as not to defy traditional convention.

When considering the spinal part only, the function of the accessory nerve is to
supply motor innervation to two muscles, the sternocleidomastoid and trapezius. The type of innervation carried by the accessory nerve to these muscles
is disputed however. Some references describe it as carrying special visceral
efferent (SVE, branchiomotor) fibers (due to a close relationship between the
nucleus of accessory nerve with the nucleus ambiguous), while others describe
it as carrying general somatic efferent (GVE) fibers (due to the unknown/dis-
puted embryological origins of the sternocleidomastoid and trapezius muscles).

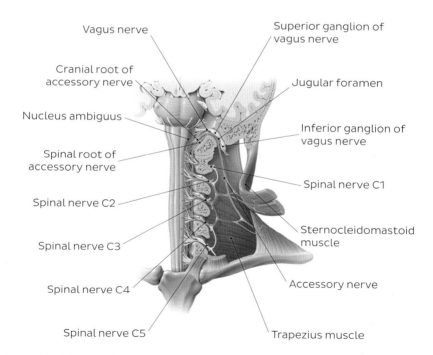

Vagus nerve

Superior ganglion of
vagus nerve

Cranial root of
accessory nerve

Jugular foramen

Nucleus ambiguus

Inferior ganglion of
vagus nerve

Spinal root of
accessory nerve

Spinal nerve C1

Spinal nerve C2

Spinal nerve C3

Sternocleidomastoid
muscle

Spinal nerve C4

Accessory nerve

Spinal nerve C5

Trapezius muscle

FIGURE 9.47. **Pathway of the accessory nerve.** The spinal root of the accessory nerve originates from the
cell bodies of motor neurons located in the upper five or six cervical segments of the spinal cord which
collectively form the nucleus of accessory nerve. Multiple rootlets exit the spinal cord between the
anterior and posterior spinal nerve roots and combine to form the nerve trunk, which ascends the spinal
cord and passes through the foramen magnum to enter the cranium. The cranial root arises from motor

neurons originating in the nucleus ambiguus of the medulla oblongata. Rootlets from this nucleus exit from the dorsolateral medulla oblongata and temporarily join with the fibers of the spinal root. Together, they then exit the skull via the jugular foramen.

The nerve then divides into two again: The internal branch (cranial root) joins with the vagus nerve to innervate the muscles of soft palate/larynx while the external branch (spinal root) descends into the lateral cervical region of the neck, passing superficially through its posterior triangle. Here the accessory nerve passes deep to the sternocleidomastoid muscle, which it innervates via a muscular branch. It continues to descend in a posterolateral direction, before terminating as a trapezius branch which spans out across the trapezius muscle, supplying it with motor function.

Supplementary innervation of the sternocleidomastoid and trapezius muscles is also delivered via homonymous branches of the cervical plexus. These branches contain afferent/sensory neurons, whose cells bodies are located in the spinal ganglia of spinal nerves C2–C4. Some motor fibers are also believed to be delivered to the muscles via this pathway.

Key points about the accessory nerve	
Structure and features	Fibers: special visceral efferent (SVE) (or general somatic efferent (GSE))
	Origin: rootlets along upper cervical spinal cord (spinal root), dorsolateral medulla oblongata (cranial root)
	Exits skull: jugular foramen
	Associated nuclei: nucleus ambiguus (cranial root); Nucleus of accessory nerve (spinal root)
Branches	Internal branch → joins vagus nerve
	External branch → sternocleidomastoid and trapezius branches
Function	Spinal root: motor innervation to sternocleidomastoid and trapezius muscles
	Cranial root: motor innervation to muscles of soft palate and larynx

Accessory nerve

Motor cranial nerves

HYPOGLOSSAL NERVE (CN XII)

The hypoglossal nerve is primarily a motor nerve which arises as a series of rootlets from the lateral surface of the medulla oblongata, between the pyramid and olive.

It supplies motor innervation (GSE) to the extrinsic muscles of the tongue with the exception of palatoglossus (i.e. genioglossus, hyoglossus and styloglossus muscles) as well as all of the intrinsic muscles of the tongue (superior longitudinal muscle of tongue, inferior longitudinal muscle of tongue, transverse muscle of tongue and vertical muscle of tongue).

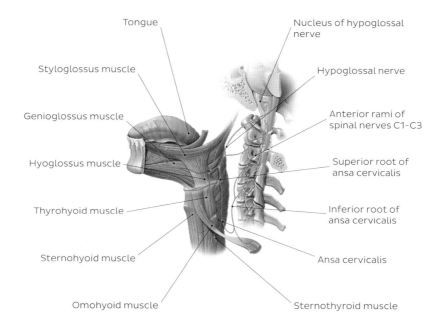

Tongue

Nucleus of hypoglossal nerve

Styloglossus muscle

Hypoglossal nerve

Genioglossus muscle

Anterior rami of spinal nerves C1-C3

Hyoglossus muscle

Superior root of ansa cervicalis

Thyrohyoid muscle

Inferior root of ansa cervicalis

Sternohyoid muscle

Ansa cervicalis

Omohyoid muscle

Sternothyroid muscle

FIGURE 9.48. **Hypoglossal nerve: Overview.** The hypoglossal nerve (CN XII) arises as a series of rootlets from the hypoglossal nucleus of the medulla oblongata. The rootlets combine to form the nerve *proper*, which then exits the cranium via the hypoglossal canal.

During its course, the hypoglossal nerve receives the fibers from spinal nerve C1 (and/or C2) which 'piggy-back' the nerve, but do not mix with it. They leave the hypoglossal nerve as a series of branches: Meningeal branch, superior root of ansa cervicalis, thyrohyoid branch and geniohyoid branch.

The only 'true' branches of the hypoglossal nerve are the terminal lingual branches that innervate the muscles of the tongue. These branches supply all extrinsic and intrinsic muscles of the tongue, with the exception of the palatoglossus muscle, which is supplied by the vagus nerve.

Key points about the hypoglossal nerve (CN XII)	
Structure and features	Fibers: general somatic efferent (GSE)
	Origin: medulla oblongata (between pyramid and olive)
	Exits skull: hypoglossal canal
	Associated nuclei: nucleus of hypoglossal nerve
Branches	Lingual branches of hypoglossal nerve
	Note that whilst the following branches are given off by the hypoglossal nerve, their fibers originate from the cervical plexus (C1–2):
	Meningeal branch Superior root of ansa cervicalis
	Thyrohyoid branch
	Geniohyoid branch
Function	Motor innervation: Extrinsic muscles of the tongue: genioglossus, hyoglossus and styloglossus
	Intrinsic muscles of the tongue: superior longitudinal lingual, inferior longitudinal lingual, transversus linguae and verticalis linguae muscle

The hypoglossal nerve

TASTE PATHWAY

After reviewing the anatomy of the facial, glossopharyngeal and vagus nerves, the various pathways of taste sensation will now be summarized.

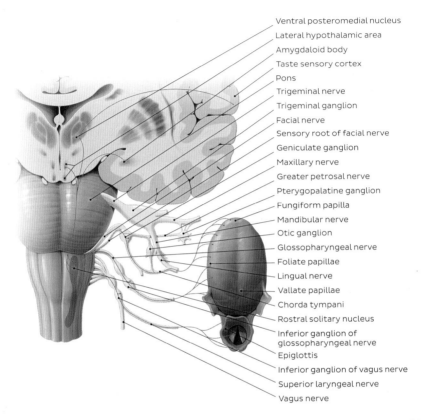

Ventral posteromedial nucleus
Lateral hypothalamic area
Amygdaloid body
Taste sensory cortex
Pons
Trigeminal nerve
Trigeminal ganglion
Facial nerve
Sensory root of facial nerve
Geniculate ganglion
Maxillary nerve
Greater petrosal nerve
Pterygopalatine ganglion
Fungiform papilla
Mandibular nerve
Otic ganglion
Glossopharyngeal nerve
Foliate papillae
Lingual nerve
Vallate papillae
Chorda tympani
Rostral solitary nucleus
Inferior ganglion of glossopharyngeal nerve
Epiglottis
Inferior ganglion of vagus nerve
Superior laryngeal nerve
Vagus nerve

FIGURE 9.49. **Taste pathway: Overview.** Taste sensation from taste buds of the anterior two-thirds of the tongue (fungiform and foliate papillae), travels via the chorda tympani of the **facial nerve**. Additionally, the greater petrosal branch of the facial nerve supplies the taste buds of the soft palate. Cell bodies of these neurons are located in the geniculate ganglion; their central processes continue towards the brainstem as the sensory root of facial nerve, also known as the intermediate nerve.

Taste sensation from the posterior third of the tongue is carried by the lingual branch of the **glossopharyngeal nerve**; the cell bodies of these neurons are located in the inferior ganglion of glossopharyngeal nerve. Taste sensation from the laryngeal surface of the epiglottis is carried by the superior laryngeal branch of the **vagus nerve**; cell bodies of these neurons are located in the inferior ganglion of vagus nerve.

Upon entering the brainstem, central processes of the gustatory elements: Afferents of the facial, glossopharyngeal and vagus nerve fibers form the solitary tract and synapse in the rostral third of the **nucleus of solitary tract** of the medulla oblongata. Second-order fibers then ascend via three pathways. The majority of the fibers go on to synapse in the ventral posteromedial nucleus of the thalamus, which synapse with third-order fibers destined for the insular cortex for interpretation of taste. Other fibers travel to the lateral hypothalamic area, involved in appetite and satiety mechanisms. The rest of the fibers pass to the amygdala, which is involved in emotions and memory formation in relation to food.

INDEX

Amnion, 319–320, *fig 7.13–7.14*
Amniotic sac, 319, *fig 7.13*
Ampulla
   of urethra, 329, *fig 7.20*
   of uterine tube, 313, *fig 7.10*
Ampulla of Vater *see* Hepatopancreatic ampulla
   (ampulla of Vater)
Ampullary nerve
   anterior, 436, *fig 8.71*, 554, *fig 9.42*
   lateral, 436, *fig 8.71*, 554, *fig 9.42*
   posterior, 436, *fig 8.71*, 554, *fig 9.42*
Amygdaloid body, 501, *fig 9.6*, 536, *fig 9.30*, 566,
   fig 9.49
Anal aperture, 338
Anal canal, 235, 268, **269–270**, **fig 6.34**
   blood vessels of, 275–276, *fig 6.37–6.38*
   function of, 270
   innervation of, 276, *fig 6.38*
   landmarks of, 270
Anal nerve
   inferior
     of female, 341, *fig 7.28*
     of male, 344–345, *fig 7.30*
Anal pecten, 269, *fig 6.34*
Anal region, 114, *fig 4.1*
Anal sphincter
   external, 269, *fig 6.34*, 307, *fig 7.6*
     of female, 310, *fig 7.7*
     of male, 334, *fig 7.22*
   internal, 269, *fig 6.34*
Anal triangle, 336, *fig 7.24*
Anastomotic network elbow joint, 51, *fig 2.32*
Anastomotic vein
   inferior, 520, *fig 9.19*
   superior, 520, *fig 9.19*
Anatomical neck of humerus, 13–14, *fig 2.3*
Anatomical position, 2
Anatomical relations of heart, 198, *fig 5.38*
Anatomical snuffbox *see* radial roveola
Anconeus muscle, 19–21, *fig 2.9*
Angle of mandible, 380, *fig 8.22*
Angular artery, 388, *fig 8.27*, 396, *fig 8.35*
Angular gyrus(i), 495–496, *fig 9.2*
   artery to, 518, *fig 9.18*
Angular vein, 391, *fig 8.30*
Ankle joint, 89, *fig 3.21*, **92–93**, **fig 3.24–3.25**
   articulating surfaces of, 93
   ligaments of, 93
   movements of, 93
   synovial hinge joint, 92–93
Ankle joint *see also* talocrural joint
Anococcygeal ligament, 338
Anococcygeal nerve, 341, *fig 7.28*
Anocutaneous line, 269, *fig 6.34*
Anorectal artery
   inferior, 275, *fig 6.37*, 339, *fig 7.26*
     female, 349, *fig 7.33*
     male, 347–348, *fig 7.32*
   superior of male, 347, *fig 7.32*
Anorectal junction, 269
Anorectal vein(s), 275
   inferior, 276, *fig 6.38*
     female, 349–350, *fig 7.33*
   middle, 276, *fig 6.38*
     female, 349–350, *fig 7.33*
     male, 347–348, *fig 7.32*
   superior, 276, *fig 6.38*
     female, 349–350, *fig 7.33*
     male, 347–348, *fig 7.32*

Anorectal venous plexus
   inferior of male, 344–345, *fig 7.30*
   middle
     of female, 346, *fig 7.31*
     of male, 344–345, *fig 7.30*
Ansa cervicalis, 462, **477–478**, **fig 8.103–8.104**,
   479, *fig 8.105*, 484–485, *fig 8.110*, 565,
   fig 9.48
   omohyoid branch of
     inferior, 479, *fig 8.105*
     superior, 479, *fig 8.105*
   sternocleidomastoid branch of, 479, *fig 8.105*
   sternothyroid branch of, 479, *fig 8.105*
Ansa pectoralis, 43, *fig 2.24*, 48, *fig 2.29*
Anserine bursa of the knee, 77, *fig 3.12*
Antebrachial cutaneous nerve(s)
   lateral, 54, *fig 2.35*
     anterior branch of, 54, *fig 2.35*
     posterior branch of, 54–55, *fig 2.35–2.36*
   medial, 43, *fig 2.24*, 48–50, *fig 2.29–2.30*
     anterior branch of, 54, *fig 2.35*
     posterior branch of, 54–55, *fig 2.35–2.36*
   posterior, 49, *fig 2.30*, 55, *fig 2.36*
Antebrachial region
   anterior, 10–11, *fig 2.1*
   posterior, 10–11, *fig 2.1*
Antebrachial vein, 52, *fig 2.33*
Anterior arch of atlas (C1), 120–121, *fig 4.6–4.8*
Anterior atlantooccipital ligament, 122–123,
   fig 4.8
Anterior branch of renal arteries, 279–280,
   fig 6.41
Anterior cardiac vein, 212–213, *fig 5.47*
Anterior cerebral vein, 521, *fig 9.20*
Anterior cervical lymph nodes
   superficial, 482, *fig 8.108*
Anterior chamber of eyeball, 420, *fig 8.55*
Anterior ciliary arteries, 422, *fig 8.57*
Anterior clinoid process, 369, *fig 8.11*
   of sphenoid bone, 369, *fig 8.11*, 376, *fig 8.18*
Anterior crus of ear, 431, *fig 8.66*
Anterior extremity of spleen, 246, *fig 6.18*
Anterior interventricular artery, 197, *fig 5.37*, 212,
   213, *fig 5.47*
Anterior lateral malleolar artery, 108, *fig 3.37*
Anterior longitudinal ligament, 117–118, *fig 4.4*,
   122, *fig 4.8*, 304, 306, *fig 7.4–7.5*
Anterior medial malleolar artery, 108, *fig 3.37*
Anterior median fissure of spinal cord, 525,
   fig 9.23
Anterior nasal spine of maxilla, 360, *fig 8.2*, 370,
   fig 8.12
Anterior rami of spinal nerves C1–C3, 565, *fig 9.48*
Anterior rami of spinal nerves C1–C4, **479**,
   fig 8.105, 528
Anterior semicircular duct of membranous
   labyrinth, 436, *fig 8.71*
Anterior talofibular ligament, 93, *fig 3.25*
Anterior tibial artery, 108, 110, *fig 3.37–3.38*
Anterior tibiotalar ligament, 93, *fig 3.25*
Anterior tubercle of atlas, 120, *fig 4.6*
Anterior vagal trunk, 264, *fig 6.31*, 561–562,
   fig 9.46
   celiac branches of, 264, *fig 6.31*
   gastric branches of, 561–562, *fig 9.46*
   hepatic branch of, 264, *fig 6.31*, 561, *fig 9.46*
   pyloric branch, 264, *fig 6.31*, 561, *fig 9.46*
Antihelix of ear, 430–431, *fig 8.65–8.66*
   crura of, 430–431, *fig 8.65–8.66*

Bronchial arteries and veins, 190–191, *fig 5.32–5.33*
Bronchomediastinal lymph trunk, 194–195, *fig 5.35*
Bronchopulmonary lymph nodes, 190–191, *fig 5.32–5.33*, 194, *fig 5.35*, 217, *fig 5.50*
Buccal artery, 388–389, *fig 8.27–8.28*, 396, *fig 8.35*
Buccal nerve, 394–395, *fig 8.33–8.34*, 548–550, *fig 9.39*
Buccal region, 359, *fig 8.1*
Buccal vein, 392, *fig 8.31*
Buccinator lymph nodes, 480, *fig 8.106*
Buccinator muscle, 359, 383–384, *fig 8.25*, 388–389, 395, 446, *fig 8.80*
Buccopharyngeal fascia, 486–489, *fig 8.111*
Buck's fascia *see* Deep fascia of penis (Buck's fascia)
Bulbar conjunctiva, 420, *fig 8.55*, 424, *fig 8.58*
Bulb of penis, 329–330, *fig 7.20*, 334–335, *fig 7.22–7.23*
Bulb of vestibule, 317–318, *fig 7.12*, 331, *fig 7.21*, 338
    artery of, 339, *fig 7.26*
    vein of, 340, *fig 7.27*
Bulb of vorticose vein, 422, *fig 8.57*
Bulbospongiosus muscle, 307–308, *fig 7.6*, 317–318, *fig 7.12*, 330–331, *fig 7.21*, 333–334, 338
Bulbourethral gland, 329–330, *fig 7.20*, 335–335, *fig 7.23*, 352–353
Bundle branch
    left, 215, *fig 5.49*
    right, 215, *fig 5.49*
Bursa(e) of the knee, 77, *fig 3.12*
    anserine, 77, *fig 3.12*
    deep infrapatellar, 81, *fig 3.16*
    prepatellar, 81, *fig 3.16*
    subcutaneous infrapatellar, 81, *fig 3.16*
    subtendinous
        of biceps femoris
            inferior, 77, *fig 3.12*
    subtendinous
        of gastrocnemius muscle
            lateral, 81, *fig 3.16*
    subtendinous
        of iliotibial tract, 77, *fig 3.12*
    suprapatellar, 81, *fig 3.16*

C

Caecal recesses, 235
Calcaneal sulcus, 90, *fig 3.22*
Calcaneal tuberosity, 90–91, *fig 3.22–3.23*
    lateral process, 90–91, *fig 3.22–3.23*
    medial process, 90–91, *fig 3.22–3.23*
Calcaneocuboid joint, 91
Calcaneofibular ligament, 93, *fig 3.25*, 95
Calcaneus, 83, 85–89, *fig 3.19–3.20*, **90–91**, **fig 3.22–3.23**, 92–94, *fig 3.24–3.25*, 97–99, 101
    articular surface for cuboid, 90–91, *fig 3.22–3.23*
    body of calcaneus, 90, *fig 3.22*
    calcaneal sulcus, 90, *fig 3.22*
    calcaneal tuberosity, 90–91, *fig 3.22–3.23*
        lateral process, 90–91, *fig 3.22–3.23*
        medial process, 90–91, *fig 3.22–3.23*
    calcaneocuboid joint, 91
    fibular trochlea, 90–91, *fig 3.22–3.23*
    groove for flexor hallucis longus tendon, 90–91, *fig 3.22–3.23*

Calcaneus
(*continued*)
    subtalar joint, 91
    sustentaculum tali, 90–91, *fig 3.22–3.23*
    talar articular surface, 90, *fig 3.22*
        anterior, 90–91, *fig 3.22–3.23*
        middle, 90–91, *fig 3.22–3.23*
        posterior, 90–91, *fig 3.22–3.23*
Callosomarginal artery, 517, *fig 9.17*
    frontal branches of, 517, *fig 9.17*
    paracentral branches of, 517, *fig 9.17*
Calvaria, 363, *fig 8.5*
Canine teeth, 448–449, *fig 8.81–8.82*
Capitate bone, 31–32, *fig 2.16*, 34, 40–41
Capitohamate interosseous ligament, 35, *fig 2.3*, 37
    palmar, 37
Capitulum, 13–14, *fig 2.3*, 22, 24–25
Capsular ligaments, 68, *fig 3.7*
Capsule of cricoarytenoid joint, 465, *fig 8.92*
Capsule(s) of cerebral cortex
    external, 500, *fig 9.5*
    internal, 500, *fig 9.5*
Cardiac impression of left lung, 190–191, *fig 5.32–5.33*
Cardiac notch of lung, 190–191, *fig 5.32–5.33*
Cardiac plexus, 214, *fig 5.48*, 561, *fig 9.46*
Cardiac veins, 212–213, *fig 5.47*
    anterior, 212–213, *fig 5.47*
    atrial, 212
    coronary sinus, 201–206, *fig 5.40–5.41*, *fig 5.43*, 210, *fig 5.46*, 212–213, *fig 5.47*
        orifice of, 203, *fig 5.41*
        valve of, 203, *fig 5.41*
    great, 201, *fig 5.40*, 212–213, *fig 5.47*
    inferior of left ventricle, 213
    marginal of heart
        left, 212, *fig 5.47*
        right, 212, *fig 5.47*
    middle, 212–213, *fig 5.47*
    oblique of left atrium, 212, *fig 5.47*
    small, 212–213, *fig 5.47*
    smallest
        atrial, 212–213
        ventricular smallest (thebesian veins) 212–213
Cardia of stomach, 243–244, *fig 6.16–6.17*
Cardinal ligament, 312, *fig 7.9*, 316–318, *fig 7.12*
Caroticotympanic nerves, 434
Carotid artery
    branches of, 389
    common, 144, *fig 4.18*, 396, *fig 8.35*, 456, *fig 8.87*, 472, *fig 8.99*, 474–475, *fig 8.101*, 478, *fig 8.104*, 484–485, *fig 8.110*, 488, 489, *fig 8.113*, 561
        left, 175–177, *fig 5.21–5.22*, 196, *fig 5.36*, 200–201, *fig 5.39–5.40*
        right, 175–177, *fig 5.21–5.22*, 196, *fig 5.36*, 200–201, *fig 5.39–5.40*
    external, 386–389, *fig 8.27–8.28*, 396, *fig 8.35*, 398, 422, *fig 8.57*, 427, *fig 8.62*, 445–447, *fig 8.79–8.80*, 456, *fig 8.87*, 472–473, *fig 8.99*, 474–475, *fig 8.101*, 478, *fig 8.104*, 484, *fig 8.110*
    internal, 366, 386, 389, *fig 8.28*, 396–398, *fig 8.35–8.36*, 412, *fig 8.47*, 456, *fig 8.87*, 472, *fig 8.99*, 474–476, *fig 8.101*, 478, *fig 8.104*, 515–516, *fig 9.15–9.16*, 518, 522, *fig 9.21*, 544, *fig 9.35*, 556, *fig 9.43*

Digital vein(s) of hand
dorsal, 58, *fig 2.40*
palmar, 58, *fig 2.40*
Dilator pupillae muscle, 420, *fig 8.55*
Diploë, 363, *fig 8.5*
Diploic veins, 511, *fig 9.13*
Directional terms of the brain, 493, *fig 9.1*
Distal as term of relationship, 2, *fig 1.1*
Distal end of femur, 67, *fig 3.6*
intercondylar fossa, 67, *fig 3.6*
intercondylar line, 67
patellar surface, 66, *fig 3.5*
Distal end of ulna, 22–24, *fig 2.10–2.11*
Distal part of duodenum, 235
Distal phalanx of hand, 31, *fig 2.16*
Dorsal artery of penis, 347, *fig 7.32*
Dorsal as term of relationship, 2, *fig 1.1*
Dorsal cutaneous nerve of foot, 112
intermediate, 112
lateral, 107, *fig 3.36*, 111, *fig 3.40*
medial, 112
Dorsal digital branches, 112
Dorsal digital nerves of foot, 111, *fig 3.40*
Dorsalis pedis artery, 109, 111–112, *fig 3.39*
Dorsal metatarsal arteries, 111, *fig 3.39*
Dorsal nerve of clitoris, 341, *fig 7.28*
Dorsal nerve of penis, 344–345, *fig 7.30*
Dorsal radial tubercle of radius, 23–24, *fig 2.11*
Dorsal scapular artery, 45, *fig 2.26*
Dorsal vein
deep
of clitoris, 311, *fig 7.8*
of penis, 347, *fig 7.32*
Dorsum sellae, 369, *fig 8.11*, 376, *fig 8.18*
Duct of Santorini *see* **Accessory pancreatic duct (of Santorini)**
Duct of Wirsung *see* **Pancreatic duct (of Wirsung)**
Ductus deferens, 228–229, *fig 6.4*, 321–325, *fig 7.15–7.17*
artery of, 325, *fig 7.17*
right, 321, *fig 7.15*
Ductus reuniens (of Hensen), 436, *fig 8.71*
Duodenal flexure
inferior, 256–258, *fig 6.26–6.27*
superior, 256–258, *fig 6.26–6.27*
Duodenal papilla
major, 253, *fig 6.24*, 256–258, *fig 6.26–6.27*
minor, 256–258, *fig 6.26–6.27*
Duodenal recesses, 235
Duodenojejunal flexure, 248, *fig 6.20*, 256–260, *fig 6.26–6.28*
related liver, 248, *fig 6.20*
Duodenum, 222, 243, *fig 6.16*, 248, *fig 6.20*, **257–258**, **fig 6.27**, 259, *fig 6.28*, 261–262
arterial supply of, 262, 287–288, *fig 6.45*
ascending part of, 241, *fig 6.15*, 254–258, *fig 6.25–6.27*
descending part of, 240–241, *fig 6.14–6.15*, 254–258, *fig 6.25–6.27*
distal part of, 235
horizontal part of, 235, *fig 6.10*, 241, *fig 6.15*, 248, *fig 6.20*, 254–258, *fig 6.25–6.27*
related liver, 248, *fig 6.20*
lymphatics of, 266, *fig 6.32*, 290–291, *fig 6.47*, 297
muscular coat of
circular layer of, 257, *fig 6.27*
longitudinal layer of, 244, *fig 6.17*

Duodenum
(*continued*)
recesses of, 235
related gallbladder, 253, *fig 6.24*
related liver, 248–249, *fig 6.20*
related pancreas, 254–255, *fig 6.25*
superior part of, 235, 244, *fig 6.17*, 248, *fig 6.20*, 254–256, *fig 6.26*, 257–258, *fig 6.27*
venous drainage of, 262
wall of, 257
Dural venous sinuses, 512, 519, 521, **522–523**, **fig 9.21**
paired venous sinuses, 523
unpaired venous sinuses, 523
Dura mater of cranial meninges, 511–512, *fig 9.13*
Dura mater of spinal meninges, 526, *fig 9.24*, 528, *fig 9.25*, 536, *fig 9.30*

E
Ear
anterior crus of, 431, *fig 8.66*
antihelix of, 430–431, *fig 8.65–8.66*
crura of, 431, *fig 8.66*
external ear, 430–431, *fig 8.65–8.66*
internal ear, 435–438, *fig 8.70–8.73*
middle ear, 432–434, *fig 8.67–8.69*
Efferent ductules of testis, 323, *fig 7.16*
Ejaculatory duct opening, 329, *fig 7.20*, 335, *fig 7.23*
Elbow and forearm, 3, 10, *fig 2.1*, 20, 22–30, *fig 2.10–2.15*
bones of, 22–24, *fig 2.10–2.11*
elbow joint, 25–26, *fig 2.12–2.13*
muscles of, 27–30, *fig 2.14–2.15*
neurovasculature of, 44–49, *fig 2.25–2.30*
Elbow as region, 10, *fig 2.1*
Elbow joint, 25–26, *fig 2.12–2.13*
articular capsule of, 25, *fig 2.12*
bones of, 25–26, *fig 2.12–2.13*
joint of, 25–26, *fig 2.12–2.13*
ligaments of, 25–26, *fig 2.12*
movements of, 26, *fig 2.13*
Emissary veins, 366, 379, 511, *fig 9.13*
Enamel of teeth, 451, *fig 8.83*
Endocrine system
pancreas, 254–255, *fig 6.25*
Endolymph, 435–437
Endometrium, 313–315, *fig 7.11*
Enteric nervous system, 263–264, *fig 6.31*, 272
of anal canal, 276
of rectum, 276
Enteric plexus (of Auerbach)
of anal canal, 276
of rectum, *276*
Epicondyle(s)
of femur
lateral, 66–67, *fig 3.5–3.6*
medial, 66–67, *fig 3.5–3.6*
of humerus
lateral, 13–14, *fig 2.3*, 20, 25, *fig 2.12*, 28–30
medial, 13–14, *fig 2.3*, 25, *fig 2.12*, 28–30
Epicranial aponeurosis, 383, *fig 8.25*, 385–386
Epididymis, 323–324, *fig 7.16*
body of, 323–324, *fig 7.16*
function of, 324
head of, 323–324, *fig 7.16*
tail of, 323–324, *fig 7.16*
Epidural space, 511–512, 526–529, *fig 9.25*, 531

Infraglenoid tubercle of scapula, 15, *fig 2.5–2.6*, 20
Infrahyoid fascia, 487, *fig 8.111*
Infraorbital artery, 388–389, *fig 8.27*, 396,
    fig 8.35, 406, *fig 8.43*, 412, *fig 8.47*,
    417–418, *fig 8.52–8.53*
Infraorbital foramen of maxilla, 360, *fig 8.2*, 408,
    fig 8.45
Infraorbital groove, 408, *fig 8.45*
Infraorbital nerve, 394–395, *fig 8.33–8.34*,
    405, *fig 8.42*, 414, *fig 8.49*, 417–418,
    fig 8.52–8.53, 545–546, *fig 9.36–9.37*
Infraorbital region, 359, *fig 8.1*
Infraorbital vein, 407, *fig 8.44*, 412–413, *fig 8.47*,
    417–418, *fig 8.52–8.53*
Infrascapular branches of brachial plexus, 43,
    fig 2.24
Infrascapular region, **114**, *fig 4.1*
Infraspinatus muscle, 17–18, *fig 2.7–2.8*
Infraspinous fossa of scapula, 15, *fig 2.5*
Infratemporal crest of sphenoid bone, 365, *fig 8.7*,
    375–376, *fig 8.17–8.18*
Infratemporal region, 399–400, *fig 8.38*
Infratemporal surface of greater wing of
    sphenoid bone, 365, *fig 8.7*
Infratrochlear nerve, 394–394, *fig 8.33–8.34*,
    414–415, *fig 8.49–8.50*, 544, *fig 9.35*
Infundibulum
    gallbladder, 253, *fig 6.24*
    uterine tube, 313–315, *fig 7.10–7.11*
Inguinal canal, 228–229, *fig 6.4*
Inguinal ligament, 223–225, *fig 6.2*, 228–229,
    fig 6.4, 304–306, *fig 7.4–7.5*
Inguinal lymph nodes
    deep, 296, *fig 6.50*
        female, 354, *fig 7.36*
        male, 353, *fig 7.35*
    inferior superficial
        male, 353, *fig 7.34–7.35*
    superficial, 296, *fig 6.50*
        female, 354, *fig 7.36*
    superolateral
        male, 353, *fig 7.35*
    superomedial
        male, 353, *fig 7.35*
Inguinal region, 221–222, *fig 6.1*
Inguinal ring
    deep, 228, *fig 6.4*, 311, *fig 7.8*
    superficial, 228, *fig 6.4*
Inner border cell of cochlear duct, 438, *fig 8.73*
Inner hair cell of cochlear duct, 438, *fig 8.73*
Inner layer (internal tunic) of eyeball, 420, *fig 8.55*
Inner phalangeal epithelial cell of cochlear duct,
    438, *fig 8.73*
Internal pillar epithelial cell of cochlear duct, 438,
    fig 8.73
Inner spiral sulcus of cochlear duct, 438, *fig 8.73*
Inner sulcus cells of cochlear duct, 438, *fig 8.73*
Inner tunnel of cochlear duct, 438, *fig 8.73*
Innervation of diaphragm, 160, 479
Innervation of ear, 431, *fig 8.66*
Innervation of heart
    conduction service of, 215–216
        atrioventricular (AV) node, 215–216
        atrioventricular bundles, 215–216
        AV bundle, 215–216
        sinuatrial (SA) node, 215–216
        subendocardial (Purkinje) fibers, 215–216
    efferent parasympathetic, 215–216
        vagal cardiac nerves, 215–216

Innervation of heart
(*continued*)
    efferent sympathetic fibers, 215–216
        lower cervical ganglia, 215–216
        thoracic ganglia, 215–216
    parasympathetic fibers, 215–216
        vagus nerve, 215–216
    sympathetic fibers, 215–216
        cardiac nerves, 215–216
Innervation of larynx, 470
Innervation of parathyroid gland, 473, *fig 8.100*
Innervation of thyroid gland, 473, *fig 8.100*
Innervation of tongue, 445, *fig 8.79*
Insula of cerebrum, 496
Insular lobe of brain, 493, 495, *fig 9.1*
Interalveolar septa of mandible, 381, *fig 8.23*
Interarytenoid notch, 453, *fig 8.85*, 465, *fig 8.92*
Interatrial septum, 203, *fig 5.41*
Intercapitular veins of hand, 58, *fig 2.39*
Intercarpal interosseous ligaments, 37
Intercarpal joints, 32, 37
Intercarpal ligament
    dorsal, 35, *fig 2.19*, 37
    palmar, 37
Intercavernous septum
    of deep fascia of penis, 334, *fig 7.22*
Intercavernous sinus
    posterior, 522, *fig 9.21*
Intercondylar areas of tibia
    anterior, 75
    posterior, 75
Intercondylar eminence of tibia, 74, *fig 3.10*
Intercondylar fossa of femur, 67, *fig 3.6*
Intercondylar line, 67
Intercostal artery
    anterior, 230, *fig 6.5*, 233, *fig 6.8*
    lateral cutaneous branches of
        anterior branches of, 230, *fig 6.5*
    posterior, 131, 145, *fig 4.19*, 231, *fig 6.6*, 530,
        fig 9.26
        dorsal branch, 530, *fig 9.26*
        spinal branch of, 530, *fig 9.26*
    supreme, 398, *fig 8.37*
Intercostal nerves, 43, *fig 2.24*, 145, *fig 4.19*, 214,
    fig 5.48, 232, *fig 6.7*
    cutaneous branch
        anterior, 231–232, *fig 6.7*
        lateral, 145, *fig 4.19*, 232, *fig 6.7*
Intercostal veins
    anterior, 233, *fig 6.8*
    posterior, 132, *fig 4.14*, 145, *fig 4.19*, 231, *fig 6.6*
Intercrural joints
    tibiofibular joint
Interdental cells, 437, *fig 8.72*
Intergluteal cleft, 62, *fig 3.10*
Interlobar arteries of kidney, 279, *fig 6.41*
Intermaxillary suture of skull, 360, *fig 8.2*
Intermediate dorsal cutaneous nerve of foot, 112
Intermediate tunnel of cochlear duct, 438, *fig 8.73*
Intermesenteric plexus, 273, *fig 6.36*, 561, *fig 9.46*
Intermetacarpal joint, 32, 37
Internal acoustic meatus, 369, *fig 8.11*
Internal capsule of cerebral cortex, 500, *fig 9.5*
Internal carotid artery, 389, *fig 8.28*, 397–398,
    fig 8.36, 412, *fig 8.47*, 422, 456, *fig 8.87*,
    472, *fig 8.99*, 474–475, *fig 8.101*,
    477–478, *fig 8.104*, **515**, ***fig 9.15***,
    515–516, *fig 9.15–9.16*, 518, 544, *fig 9.35*
    right, 478, *fig 8.104*, 484, *fig 8.110*, 517, *fig 9.17*

Q

Quadrangular membrane, 465, *fig 8.92*
Quadrate lobe, 248, *fig 6.20, 251, fig 6.22*
Quadratus lumborum muscle, 223–225, *fig 6.2*
Quadriceps femoris muscle, 5, **69**, **fig 3.8**, 74
  nerve to, 342–343, *fig 7.29*
  rectus femoris muscle, **69**, **fig 3.8**, 72
  vastus lateralis muscle, **69**, **fig 3.8**, 72
  vastus intermedius muscle, **69**, **fig 3.8**
  vastus medialis muscle, **69**, **fig 3.8**, 72

R

Radial artery, 50–51, *fig 2.31–2.32*
  carpal branch of
    dorsal, 57, *fig 2.38*
    palmar, 56, *fig 2.37*
  muscular branches, 50, *fig 2.31*
  radial digital artery of thumb
    dorsal, 57, *fig 2.38*
    palmar, 56, *fig 2.37*
  recurrent, 50, *fig 2.31*
  superficial branch of
    palmar, 56, *fig 2.37*
Radial as term of relationship, 2, *fig 1.1*
Radial collateral artery, 44, *fig 2.25*
Radial collateral ligament
  of elbow joint, 24–26, *fig 2.12*
  of wrist joint, 37
Radial digital artery of thumb
  palmar, perforating branches, 56, *fig 2.37*
Radial fossa, 13–14, *fig 2.3*
Radial foveola, 10–11, *fig 2.1*
Radial groove, 14, *fig 2.4*
Radialis indicis artery, 56, *fig 2.37*
Radial nerve, 29–30, 43, *fig 2.24, 45, 48–49,*
      fig 2.29–2.30, 54–55, fig 2.35–2.36
  deep branch of, 54–55, *fig 2.35–2.36*
  dorsal digital branches of, 59, *fig 2.40*
  muscular branches of, 54, *fig 2.35*
  superficial branch of, 54–55, *fig 2.35–2.36, 59,*
      fig 2.40
Radial notch of ulna, 24
Radial tuberosity of radius, 22, 24, *fig 2.10*
Radial veins, 52, *fig 2.33*
Radiate carpal ligament, 37
Radicular artery(ies)
  anterior, 131, 530, *fig 9.26*
  posterior, 131, 530, *fig 9.26*
Radicular vein, 132, *fig 4.14*
  anterior, 531, *fig 9.27*
  posterior, 531, *fig 9.27*
Radiocarpal anastomosis
  dorsal, 57, *fig 2.38*
Radiocarpal joint, 32, 37
Radiocarpal ligament, 37
  dorsal, 35, *fig 2.19*
  palmar, 37, *fig 2.17*
Radiolunate ligaments, 37
Radioscaphocapitate ligament, 2, 33, *fig 2.17*, 37
Radioscapholunate ligament, 33, *fig 2.17*, 37
Radioulnar joint, distal, 37
Radioulnar ligament, 24, 33, *fig 2.17*
  palmar, 24, 33, *fig 2.17*, 37
  dorsal, 24, 35, *fig 2.19*, 37
Radioulnate ligament
  long, 33, *fig 2.17*, 37
  short, 33, *fig 2.17*, 37
Radius, 22–25, *fig 2.10–2.12*
  anterior border of, 22, *fig 2.10*
  anular ligament of, 24–26, *fig 2.12*

Radius
(continued)
  body of, 22–24, *fig 2.10–2.11*
  carpal articular surface, 24
  distal end of, 22–24, *fig 2.10*
  dorsal radial tubercle, 23–24, *fig 2.11*
  elbow joint, 25–26, *fig 2.12*
  head of, 22–24, *fig 2.10–2.11*
  ligaments of (radius and ulna), 24
  neck of, 22, *fig 2.10*
  pronator tuberosity of, 22–24, *fig 2.10*
  proximal end of, 22–24, *fig 2.10*
  radial styloid process of, 22–24, *fig 2.10–2.11*
  radial tuberosity of, 22, 24, *fig 2.10*
  shaft of, 22
  styloid process of, 22–23, *fig 2.10*
  suprastyloid crest of, 24
  ulnar notch of, 23
Radius and ulna ligaments, **24**
  anular ligament of radius, 24
  dorsal radioulnar ligament, 24
  interosseous membrane of forearm, 24
  oblique cord, 24
  palmar radioulnar ligament, 24
  radial collateral ligament of elbow joint, 24
  ulnar collateral ligament of the elbow joint, 24
Rami communicantes
  of spinal nerve
    gray, 283, *fig 6.43, 344, fig 7.30*
      of female pelvis, 346, *fig 7.31*
    white, 283, *fig 6.43*
Ramus(i)
  iliac tuberosity, 64, *fig 3.3*
  ischiopubic, 303, *fig 7.3*
  of lumbar nerves
    anterior
      of female pelvis, 346, *fig 7.31*
  of spinal nerves C5–C8
    anterior, 477
  pubis
    inferior, 64, *fig 3.3*, 310, *fig 7.7*
    superior, 64, *fig 3.3*, 309–312, *fig 7.7–7.8*
Ramus of mandible, 360, *fig 8.2, 380, fig 8.22*
Ramus(i) communicans of spinal nerve
  gray, 526, *fig 9.24, 528, fig 9.25*
  white, 526, *fig 9.24, 528, fig 9.25*
Ramus(i) of spinal nerve
  anterior, 526, *fig 9.24*
  posterior, 526, *fig 9.24, 528, fig 9.25*
Recesses of duodenum, 235
Rectal ampulla, 269, *fig 6.34*
Rectal fascia, 312, *fig 7.9*
Rectal venous plexus
  external, 269, *fig 6.34*
  internal, 269, *fig 6.34*
Rectosigmoid junction, 269, *fig 6.34*
Rectouterine pouch, 310, *fig 7.9, 312, fig 7.7*
Rectovesical pouch, 321–322, *fig 7.15*
Rectum, 235–236, *fig 6.10–6.11, 241, fig 6.15,*
      *267–268, fig 6.33, **269–270**, **fig 6.34**,*
      309–312, fig 7.7–7.8, 316–318, fig 7.12,
      319–322, fig 7.13–7.15, 322
  blood vessels of, 275
  function of, 270
  landmarks of, 270
  transverse folds of, 269, *fig 6.34*
Rectus abdominis muscle, 5, 164, *fig 5.13, 223,*
      fig 6.2, 228, fig 6.4, 311, fig 7.8, 319,
      fig 7.13, 321, fig 7.15
Rectus femoris muscle, 69, *fig 3.8*

Rectus sheath, 312, *fig 7.9*
Recurrent branches of deep palmar arch, 56, *fig 2.37*
Recurrent laryngeal nerve, 489, *fig 8.113*
Recurrent meningeal branches of spinal nerve,
      528, *fig 9.25*
Refractive media of eyeball, 420, *fig 8.55*
Renal arteries
      anterior branch of, 279–280, *fig 6.41*
      branches of, 279–281, *fig 6.41–6.42*
      functions of, 279–280, *fig 6.41*
      pelvic branches of, 279–280, *fig 6.41*
      right, 277–280, *fig 6.39–6.41*
      ureteric arteries, 281, *fig 6.42*
      ureteric branches of renal artery, 281, *fig 6.42*
      ureteric branches of superior, 281, *fig 6.42*
Renal calyx
      major, 278, *fig 6.40*
      minor, 278, *fig 6.40*
Renal capsule, 277–278, *fig 6.39–6.40*
Renal column, 277–278, *fig 6.39–6.40*
Renal cortex, 277–278, *fig 6.39–6.40*
Renal impression on spleen, 246, *fig 6.18*
Renal medulla, 278, *fig 6.40*
Renal papilla, 277, *fig 6.39–6.40*
Renal pelvis, 277, *fig 6.39–6.40*
Renal plexus, 278, *fig 6.40*
Renal pyramid
      base of, 278, *fig 6.40*
Renal vein
      right, 277, *fig 6.39*
Reproductive system
      female, 309–320, *fig 7.7–7.14*
      male, 321–326, *fig 7.15–7.17*
Respiratory system
      lungs, 184–195, *fig 5.27–5.35*
Rete testis, 323–324, *fig 7.16*
Retina
      optic part of, 418, *fig 8.53*, 421, *fig 8.56*
Retinal artery
      central, 413, *fig 8.48*, 418, *fig 8.53*, 422, *fig 8.57*
Retinal vein
      central, 413
Retroaortic lymph nodes, 296, *fig 6.50*
      female, 354, *fig 7.36*
Retrocaval lymph nodes, 296, *fig 6.50*, 351, *fig 7.34*
      female, 354, *fig 7.36*
Retroduodenal arteries, 288
Retromalleolar region
      lateral, 62, *fig 3.10*
      medial, 62, *fig 3.10*
Retromandibular vein, 392, *fig 8.31*, 407, *fig 8.44*,
      445, *fig 8.79*
      anterior division, 392, *fig 8.31*, 446, *fig 8.80*
      posterior division of, 392, *fig 8.31*, 446, *fig 8.80*
Retroolivary groove, 506, *fig 9.9*
Retroperitoneal organs, 235, *fig 6.10*
      primary, 242
      secondary, 242
Retroperitoneum, 241–242, *fig 6.15*
      anterior pararenal space, 241, *fig 6.15*
      definition, 242
      perirenal space, 241, *fig 6.15*
      posterior pararenal space, 241, *fig 6.15*
Retropharyngeal space, 488, *fig 8.112*
Retropubic space, 312, *fig 7.9*
Rhomboid fossa, 507, *fig 9.10*
      medial eminence of, 507, *fig 9.10*
Rhomboid muscle
      major, 135–136, *fig 4.15*
      minor, 135–136, *fig 4.15*

Rhythm of heart, 202
Rib(s), 150–153, *fig 5.2–5.5*
      11th, 226, *fig 6.3*
      12th, 226, *fig 6.3*
      joints of, 154–155, *fig 5.6–5.7*
Right atrioventricular valve
      fibrous ring, 208, *fig 5.44*
      inferior leaflet, *fig 5.44*
      septal leaflet, *fig 5.44*
      superior leaflet, *fig 5.44*
Right colic artery, 271, *fig 6.35*
      descending branch, 271, *fig 6.35*
Right hepatic artery, 251–252, *fig 6.22–6.23*, 285,
      fig 6.44
Right inferolateral branch of right coronary
      artery, 213
Right lobe of liver, 238, *fig 6.12*, 243, *fig 6.16*, 248,
      fig 6.20
Right lower quadrant of abdomen, 222, *fig 6.1*
Right marginal branch of right coronary artery,
      213, *fig 5.47*
Right (pulmonary) surface of heart, 201, *fig 5.40*
Right upper quadrant of abdomen, 222, *fig 6.1*
Rima glottidis, 465, 467, *fig 8.94*, 469, *fig 8.97*
Risorius muscle, 383–384, *fig 8.25*
Root canal, 451, *fig 8.83*
Root of ansa cervicalis
      inferior, 565, *fig 9.48*
      superior, 565, *fig 9.48*
Root of spinal nerve
      posterior, 528, *fig 9.25*
Root of tongue, 440, *fig 8.75*, 453, *fig 8.85*
Root of tooth, 451, *fig 8.83*
Rostral as term of relationship, 2, *fig 1.1*
Rostral solitary nucleus, 566, *fig 9.49*
Rotator cuff muscles
      infraspinatus muscle, 17–18, 21, *fig 2.7–2.8*
      subscapularis muscle, 17–18, 21, *fig 2.7–2.8*
      supraspinatus muscle, 17–18, 21, *fig 2.7–2.8*
      teres minor muscle, 17–18, 21, *fig 2.7–2.8*
Rotatores muscles
      breves, 139, *fig 4.17*, 142
      longi, 139, *fig 4.17*, 142
Round ligament
      of liver, 238, *fig 6.12*, 243, *fig 6.16*, 248–251,
      fig 6.20–6.22
      of uterus, 310, *fig 7.7*, 317, *fig 7.12*, 331, *fig 7.21*

S

Saccular nerve, 436, *fig 8.71*, 554, *fig 9.42*
Sacral arteries
      lateral, 131, *fig 4.13*
      median, 131, *fig 4.13*, 232, *fig 6.7*, 275, *fig 6.37*,
            311, *fig 7.8*, 322
            female, 349, *fig 7.33*
            male, 347, *fig 7.32*
Sacral crest
      median, 128, 302, *fig 7.2*
Sacral foramina
      anterior, 128
Sacral horns, 129
Sacral kyphosis, 115, *fig 4.2*
Sacral lymph nodes, 296, *fig 6.50*
      female, 354, *fig 7.36*
      lateral
            male, 353, *fig 7.35*
      median
            male, 353, *fig 7.35*
Sacral plexus, 104–105, 283, **342–343**, ***fig 7.29***, 345
      branches of, 343